Muscle Disorders of Horses

Editors

STEPHANIE J. VALBERG
ERICA C. MCKENZIE

VETERINARY CLINICS OF NORTH AMERICA: EQUINE PRACTICE

www.vetequine.theclinics.com

Consulting Editor
RAMIRO E. TORIBIO

April 2025 • Volume 41 • Number 1

ELSEVIER

1600 John F. Kennedy Boulevard • Suite 1800 • Philadelphia, Pennsylvania, 19103-2899

http://www.vetequine.theclinics.com

VETERINARY CLINICS OF NORTH AMERICA: EQUINE PRACTICE Volume 41, Number 1
April 2025 ISSN 0749-0739, ISBN-13: 978-0-443-29316-0

Editor: Taylor Hayes
Developmental Editor: Akshay Samson

Publication information: *Veterinary Clinics of North America: Equine Practice* (ISSN 0749-0739) is published in April, August, and December by Elsevier, 230 Park Avenue, Suite 800, New York, NY 10169. Periodicals postage paid at New York, NY and additional mailing offices. USA POSTMASTER: Send address changes to *Veterinary Clinics of North America: Equine Practice,* Elsevier Customer Service Department, 3251 Riverport Lane, Maryland Heights, MO 63043, USA. Subscription prices are $317.00 per year (domestic individuals), $100.00 per year (domestic students/residents), $361.00 per year (Canadian individuals), $395.00 per year (international individuals), $100.00 per year (Canadian students/residents), and $180.00 per year (international students/residents). For institutional access pricing please contact Customer Service via the contact information below. To receive student/resident rate, orders must be accompanied by name of affiliated institution, date of term, and the signature of program/residency coordinator on institution letterhead. Orders will be billed at individual rate until proof of status is received. Foreign air speed delivery is included in all *Clinics* subscription prices. All prices are subject to change without notice. Orders, claims, and journal inquiries: Please visit our Support Hub page https://service.elsevier.com for assistance.

Reprints. For copies of 100 or more of articles in this publication, please contact the Commercial Reprints Department, Elsevier Inc., 360 Park Avenue South, New York, NY 10010-1710. Tel.: 212-633-3874; Fax: 212-633-3820; E-mail: reprints@elsevier.com.

Veterinary Clinics of North America: Equine Practice is covered in *MEDLINE/PubMed (Index Medicus), Excerpta Medica, Current Contents/Agriculture, Biology and Environmental Sciences, and ISI.*

Printed in the United States of America.

Contributors

CONSULTING EDITOR

RAMIRO E. TORIBIO, DVM, MS, PhD
Diplomate, American College of Veterinary Internal Medicine; Professor and Trueman Endowed Chair of Equine Medicine and Surgery, College of Veterinary Medicine, The Ohio State University, Columbus, Ohio, USA

EDITORS

STEPHANIE J. VALBERG, DVM, PhD
Diplomate, American College of Veterinary Internal Medicine; Diplomate American College of Veterinary Sports Medicine and Rehabilitation; Emeritus Professor, Mary Anne McPhail Dressage Chair in Equine Sports Medicine, Department of Large Animal Clinical Sciences, College of Veterinary Medicine, Michigan State University, East Lansing, Michigan, USA

ERICA C. McKENZIE, BSc, BVMS, PhD
Diplomate, American College of Veterinary Internal Medicine; Diplomate American College of Veterinary Sports Medicine and Rehabilitation; Professor, Large Animal Internal Medicine, Department of Clinical Sciences, Carlson College of Veterinary Medicine, Oregon State University, Corvallis, Oregon, USA

AUTHORS

MONICA ALEMAN, MVZ Cert, PhD
Diplomate, American College of Veterinary Internal Medicine (Large Animal Internal Medicine, Neurology); Professor, Terry Holliday Equine and Comparative Neurology Endowed Presidential Chair, SVM: Department of Medicine and Epidemiology, University of California, Davis, California, USA

DOUGLAS CASTRO, DVM, MSc, DSc
Diplomate, American College of Veterinary Anesthesia and Analgesia; Assistant Clinical Professor of Anesthesiology, Department of Clinical Sciences, Auburn University College of Veterinary Medicine, Auburn, Alabama, USA

STUART CLARK-PRICE, DVM, MS, EMBA
Diplomate, American College of Veterinary Internal Medicine (Large Animal Internal Medicine); Diplomate American College of Veterinary Anesthesia and Analgesia; Professor of Anesthesiology, Department of Clinical Sciences, College of Veterinary Medicine, Auburn University, Auburn, Alabama, USA

SANDRO COLLA, DVM, MSc
Post-Doctoral Fellow, Department of Clinical Sciences, College of Veterinary Medicine and Biomedical Sciences, Colorado State University, Colorado State University Veterinary Teaching Hospital, Equine Orthopaedic Research Center, Fort Collins, Colorado, USA

SIAN A. DURWARD-AKHURST, BVMS, MS, PhD, MRCVS
Diplomate, American College of Veterinary Internal Medicine - Large Animal Medicine; Assistant Professor of Genetics, Genomics, and Large Animal Internal Medicine, Department of Veterinary Clinical Sciences, University of Minnesota, St Paul, Minnesota, USA

CARRIE J. FINNO, DVM, PhD
Diplomate, American College of Veterinary Internal Medicine (Large Animal); Professor, Department of Veterinary Population Health and Reproduction, School of Veterinary Medicine, University of California Davis, Davis, California, USA

ANNA M. FIRSHMAN, BVSc, PhD
Diplomate, American College of Veterinary Internal Medicine; Clinical Professor, Department of Veterinary Population Medicine, University of Minnesota, Saint Paul, Minnesota, USA

MELISSA R. KING, DVM, PhD
Diplomate, American College of Veterinary Sports Medicine and Rehabilitation; Associate Professor, Department of Clinical Sciences, College of Veterinary Medicine and Biomedical Sciences, Colorado State University, Colorado State University Veterinary Teaching Hospital, Equine Orthopaedic Research Center, Fort Collins, Colorado, USA

CATHERINE McGOWAN, BVSc, MANZCVSC, DEIM, PhD, PgCertVBM, FHEA, FRCVS
Diplomate, European College of Equine Internal Medicine; Emeritus Professor, Department of Equine Clinical Science, The University of Liverpool, Leahurst Campus, Neston, United Kingdom

ERICA C. McKENZIE, BSc, BVMS, PhD
Diplomate, American College of Veterinary Internal Medicine; Diplomate American College of Veterinary Sports Medicine and Rehabilitation; Professor, Large Animal Internal Medicine, Department of Clinical Sciences, Carlson College of Veterinary Medicine, Oregon State University, Corvallis, Oregon, USA

JOE D. PAGAN, MS, PhD
President, Kentucky Equine Research, Versailles, Kentucky, USA

AMY PORTER, HT (ASCP) QIHC
Supervisor, Investigative HistoPathology Laboratory, Division of Pathology, Department of Physiology, Michigan State University, East Lansing, Michigan, USA

STEPHANIE J. VALBERG, DVM, PhD
Diplomate, American College of Veterinary Internal Medicine; Diplomate American College of Veterinary Sports Medicine and Rehabilitation; Emeritus Professor, Mary Anne McPhail Dressage Chair in Equine Sports Medicine, Department of Large Animal Clinical Sciences, College of Veterinary Medicine, Michigan State University, East Lansing, Michigan, USA

ZOË J. WILLIAMS, DVM, PhD
Postdoctoral Research Fellow, Department of Clinical Sciences, College of Veterinary Medicine and Biomedical Sciences, Colorado State University, Fort Collins, Colorado, USA

Contents

The equine muscle system is complex and prone to a large range of hereditary and acquired diseases that often have overlapping clinical signs with orthopedic, neurologic, and other disorders. Obtaining a clinical history that fully outlines the client concerns and any known information about the disorder and following with a comprehensive physical examination and screening clinical pathology tests are fundamental to achieve definitive diagnosis. A methodical and comprehensive approach aids accurate diagnosis and development of an optimal treatment and management plan. This article describes the clinical examination approach and clinical pathology relevant to evaluating muscle disease in horses.

In the field of equine muscle disorders, many conditions have a genetic basis. Therefore, genetic testing is an important part of the diagnostic evaluation. Validated genetic tests are currently available for 5 equine muscle disorders: hyperkalemic periodic paralysis, malignant hyperthermia, glycogen branching enzyme disease, type 1 polysaccharide storage myopathy, and myosin heavy chain myopathy. These diseases should be tested for in the appropriate breeds with clinical signs of disease or as part of breeding management. Genetic testing in veterinary medicine is not regulated, and therefore, any new genetic test offered in horses should be carefully evaluated and confirmed to be a valid test before use.

Muscle biopsy is often required to provide a definitive diagnosis for neuromuscular disorders and can be performed using open surgical or percutaneous needle biopsy techniques. Fresh samples that are subsequently frozen in the laboratory are preferred by laboratories engaged in research, whereas formalin-fixed muscle is processed by diagnostic laboratories with specialized tinctorial and immunohistochemical techniques. Interpretation by an experienced histopathologist, combined with the signalment, history, and clinical input, is essential for establishing a diagnosis. This article outlines best practices to select, obtain, and ship a muscle sample to a laboratory and a summary of laboratory techniques.

Muscle disease has various clinical manifestations that range from exertional and non-exertional rhabdomyolysis, fasciculations, weakness, rigidity, stiffness, gait abnormalities, poor performance, and alterations in muscle mass and tone. Neurogenic disorders and non-neurogenic disorders such as primary muscle disease can cause muscle atrophy and changes in muscle tone. Myotonic disorders can have a genetic (eg, inherited channelopathies) or acquired (eg, electrolyte derangements) origin. Normal muscle enzyme activities do not rule out a myopathic disorder as the underlying cause of muscle atrophy and changes in muscle tone. Genetic testing to facilitate responsible breeding practices is recommended.

Several inflammatory myopathies have an infectious or immune-mediated basis in the horse. Myosin heavy chain myopathy is caused by a codominant missense variant in *MYH1* and has 3 clinical presentations: immune-mediated myositis, calciphylaxis, and nonexertional rhabdomyolysis in Quarter Horse-related breeds. An infarctive form of purpura hemorrhagica affects numerous breeds, presenting with focal firm, painful muscle swelling, and subsequent infarction of multiple tissues. While *Streptococcus equi equi* is often the inciting cause, anaplasmosis, sarcocystis, piroplasmosis, viruses, and vaccines can also be inciting agents. This article describes the diagnosis, pathophysiology, and treatment of these inflammatory myopathies.

Nutritional deficiencies of vitamin E and selenium can occur alone or concurrently. Prolonged and sustained deficiency of either or both nutrients can lead to profound clinical disease. Selenium deficiency can also result in signs of cardiac disease, upper gastrointestinal dysfunction, and abortion or the birth of weak foals. Deficiencies can usually be readily established by evaluating the dietary intake of individuals and by measurement of blood concentrations of these nutrients. Treatment of clinical disease is not always successful and prolonged morbidity and mortality can be encountered; hence, prevention is of the utmost importance.

Although horses most commonly develop exertional rhabdomyolysis, there are numerous causes for nonexertional rhabdomyolysis (nonER) that pose a serious health threat to horses. Their etiologies can be broadly categorized as toxic, genetic, inflammatory/infectious, nutritional, and traumatic and a variety of diagnostic tests are available to discern among them. This study discusses causes of nonER as well as diagnostics and treatments that are specific to each etiology. General treatment of acute rhabdomyolysis is covered in detail in the study in this issue on sporadic and recurrent exertional rhabdomyolysis.

Stephanie J. Valberg

Horses are particularly susceptible to developing exertional rhabdomyolysis (ER) characterized by muscle stiffness, pain, and reluctance to move. Diagnosis requires establishing abnormal increases in serum creatine kinase activity when horses exhibit clinical signs. The 2 main categories of ER include sporadic ER arising from extrinsic causes and chronic ER that arises from intrinsic continuous or episodic abnormalities in muscle function. This article focuses on treatment of acute ER and causes and management of sporadic ER. Differential diagnoses for chronic ER as well as the pathophysiology, diagnosis, and management of recurrent ER, and malignant hyperthermia are also discussed in this article.

Anna M. Firshman and Stephanie J. Valberg

Type 1 Polysaccharide Storage Myopathy (PSSM1) is an autosomal dominant glycogen storage disorder affecting more than 20 breeds of horses that can present with a variety of signs, including exertional rhabdomyolysis (ER). It is diagnosed by genetic testing or muscle biopsies containing muscle fibers with abnormal amylase-resistant polysaccharide. Type 2 PSSM has recently been subdivided. PSSM2-ER is a glycogen storage disorder identified in Quarter Horses that causes ER and is diagnosed by muscle biopsy as its genetic basis is unknown. Both PSSM1 and PSSM2-ER respond well to a low nonstructural carbohydrate, high fat diet combined with regular exercise. These forms of PSSM are discussed in this article.

Stephanie J. Valberg and Zoë J. Williams

Myofibrillar myopathy (MFM) is characterized by segmental disarray of myofibrils and ectopic accumulation of a protein called desmin. Previously thought to be a glycogen storage disease, MFM is now recognized as a stand-alone myopathy. Endurance Arabians with MFM usually present with exertional rhabdomyolysis (MFM-ER) at the end of races, elevated serum muscle enzymes, and myoglobinuria. Warmblood horses with MFM (MFM-WB) usually present with pain-associated behaviors such as exercise intolerance, reluctance to engage hind quarter muscles, shifting lameness and normal serum muscle enzymes. Both forms have evidence of decreased cysteine-based antioxidants and, additionally, MFM-WB has molecular signatures of a maladaptive training response.

Joe D. Pagan and Stephanie J. Valberg

Many myopathies in horses can be managed by exercise regimes and dietary modifications. This includes modifying the amount of nonstructural carbohydrate, fat, amino acids, vitamin E, and selenium based on the horse's specific myopathy, metabolic status, exercise program, and optimal body weight. Because dietary recommendations differ substantially between myopathies, it is imperative to establish a specific diagnosis. A nutritionist will help practitioners select from the myriad of offered products to ensure a balanced diet. This article provides detailed recommendations for a variety of myopathies affecting performance horses.

Pre-existing muscle disorders in horses can often be subtle and may only become evident during or after anesthesia. Advancements in veterinary medicine, along with increased knowledge and research in this field, help minimize anesthesia-related problems. Adequate preanesthesia assessment, early disease diagnosis, and proper management are crucial in minimizing risks to the neuromuscular system during general anesthesia.

Traumatic muscle injuries are likely to be frequent in athletic horses yet are often overlooked. These injuries usually involve internal (intrinsic) trauma, and particularly occur in athletic horses exercising at higher intensities, at unaccustomed workloads, or performing work requiring sudden acceleration, deceleration, and/or direction changes. These injuries can present with signs ranging from acute pain and lameness in a localized region to unexplained elevations of muscle enzymes on routine blood tests with or without poor performance. They include exercise-induced muscle damage such as delayed-onset muscle soreness and muscle injury such as muscle tears.

Rehabilitation following muscle injury is critical in restoring the equine athlete to full function. Rehabilitation protocols should be tailored to each patient's global functional assessment, taking into account sports-specific demands, goals for return-to-performance, and overall prognosis. Rehabilitation protocols are often designed to modulate pain, enhance repair, improve proprioception, increase flexibility, restore muscle strength, joint range-of-motion, and neuromotor control. This article will review mechanisms of muscle injury, various physical modalities commonly employed in the rehabilitation period following muscle injury, and injury prevention.

Successful rehabilitation of muscle injury requires a comprehensive understanding of the injury process, healing phases, and resources to be employed. The initial phase is characterized by acute inflammatory signs, followed by the regenerative and remodeling phases. Therapeutic exercises can be utilized in all 3 phases, progressing from isometric exercises to aquatic therapies. The classification and phase of injury and the individual response to the applied therapies will guide the progression of the therapeutic exercises through the rehabilitation program.

VETERINARY CLINICS OF NORTH AMERICA: EQUINE PRACTICE

SERIES OF RELATED INTEREST

Veterinary Clinics of North America: Food Animal Practice
https://www.vetfood.theclinics.com/

THE CLINICS ARE NOW AVAILABLE ONLINE!
Access your subscription at:
www.theclinics.com

Preface

Untying the Knots in Muscle Diseases

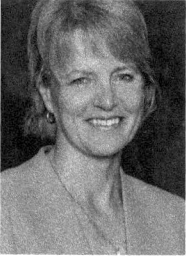

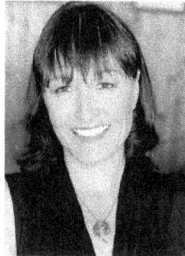

Stephanie J. Valberg, DVM, PhD   Erica C. McKenzie, BSc, BVMS, PhD
Editors

Horses are supreme athletes, whose beauty and performance depend upon their powerful musculature. Through careful genetic selection, equine breeders have shaped muscle form and function to produce breeds with muscles fine-tuned for extreme endurance, an elegant piaffe, or a bold stretch across the finish line. Even minor or intermittent perturbations in muscle function can have a major impact in athletic horses because they are constantly being exercised and asked for maximal performance. The past 30 years have produced exciting discoveries with regard to equine exercise physiology, muscle biopsy, muscle histopathology, and genomics that led the way for an explosion of knowledge with regard to muscle diseases. Many clinician scientists, past and present, have provided the building blocks that have led to the discovery of specific muscle disorders in horses. In the early twentieth century, elegant scientific studies by Birger Carlström were precursors to the discovery of polysaccharide storage myopathy. Although initially only one muscle disease "azoturia" was recognized in horses, a gradual recognition of the complexity of exertional rhabdomyolysis (ER) disorders in this species arose in the twentieth century through work by Drs Gary Carlson and Jill Beech and others. The advent of the percutaneous needle biopsy technique by Drs Arne Lindholm and David Snow in the 1970s, the application of frozen-section staining techniques by Dr George Cardinet III in the 1980s, and the sequencing of the equine genome in 2009 have led to an exponential growth of information on equine muscle diseases. The development of equine neuromuscular diagnostic laboratories and the routine submission of muscle biopsies by practitioners provided an opportunity to assimilate thousands of muscle biopsies from horses, categorize their causes, and develop strategies to manage these disorders.

This issue of *Veterinary Clinics of North America: Equine Practice* features the latest information on the pathophysiology, diagnosis, treatment, and management of a broad

Vet Clin Equine 41 (2025) xi–xii
https://doi.org/10.1016/j.cveq.2025.01.001
0749-0739/25/© 2025 Published by Elsevier Inc.

vetequine.theclinics.com

spectrum of inherited and acquired muscle disorders in horses written by a spectrum of renowned clinicians. Clinical examination of the equine muscle system, the genetics of equine myopathies, and equine muscle biopsy techniques are thoroughly described. Muscle disorders impacting muscle tone and mass, immune-mediated muscle diseases, and nutritional myopathies are also featured. Differentiating causes of nonexertional rhabdomyolysis and causes and management of various forms of ER as well as the role of nutrition in their management are also thoroughly reviewed in this issue. Finally, anesthesia-related myopathies, traumatic muscle injuries, and the role of rehabilitation in restoring horses to full function are presented. Armed with the knowledge acquired from this issue, veterinarians will be able to recognize and manage equine myopathies well into the future. To the horse! And to the brightest of futures!

DISCLOSURES

S.J. Valberg directs the Valberg Neuromuscular Disease Laboratory (ValbergNMDL. com) and receives remuneration for analyzing muscle biopsies. S.J. Valberg's professional web site is sponsored by Kentucky Equine Research, and she receives royalties from the PSSM1 genetic test and the feed products Re-Leve and MFM Pellet developed in association with Kentucky Equine Research.

Stephanie J. Valberg, DVM, PhD
College of Veterinary Medicine
Michigan State University
East Lansing, MI, USA

Erica C. McKenzie, BSc, BVMS, PhD
Large Animal Internal Medicine
Carlson College of Veterinary Medicine
Oregon State University
Corvallis, OR 97331, USA

E-mail addresses:
Valbergs@msu.edu (S.J. Valberg)
erica.mckenzie@oregonstate.edu (E.C. McKenzie)

Clinical Examination of the Muscle System

Erica C. McKenzie, BSc, BVMS, PhD

KEYWORDS

- Rhabdomyolysis • Atrophy • Neuropathy • Clinical pathology • Muscle enzymes

KEY POINTS

- A standardized approach to evaluating the muscle system optimizes the potential to correctly identify disorders.
- Evaluation should commence with thorough history, methodical examination, and assessment of any pre-existing results.
- Differentiating muscle, neurologic, and orthopedic disorders that can have overlapping signs helps establish the most appropriate diagnostic pathway.
- Physical examination is aided by screening clinical pathology, including muscle enzyme activities to detect acquired and hereditary causes of rhabdomyolysis or other disorders.

INTRODUCTION

Examination of the equine muscle system is an important skill for equine clinicians, particularly those who work with performance horses. Muscle disorders are a common cause of disease and reduced athletic performance.[1–3] They can be challenging to characterize, as clinical signs can be subtle, nebulous, and fluctuating, and commonly overlap with other clinical disorders, particularly orthopedic and neurologic disorders. As a result, definitive diagnosis can require an array of diagnostic techniques.[1–3] Thorough anamnesis (history taking) and a comprehensive physical examination are critical first steps in establishing an appropriate differential list and facilitating the accurate selection of additional diagnostics. Because the diagnostic pathway can differ for muscle versus neurologic or orthopedic issues, and because diagnostic procedures can be expensive and invasive and may incur enforced rest from performance, it is important to select them effectively and collaboratively with the client. Specific objectives of the history assessment and physical examination as they relate to the muscle system are outlined:

1. To determine the primary clinical concerns of the client and any triggering events that might have been associated with their onset, including exercise.

Department of Clinical Sciences, Carlson College of Veterinary Medicine, Oregon State University, 227 Magruder Hall, Corvallis, OR 97331, USA
E-mail address: erica.mckenzie@oregonstate.edu

Vet Clin Equine 41 (2025) 1–15
https://doi.org/10.1016/j.cveq.2024.10.001
0749-0739/25/© 2024 Elsevier Inc. All rights are reserved, including those for text and data mining, AI training, and similar technologies.

2. To determine if there is a true medical issue, rather than a behavior, management, or equipment (tack) issue.
3. To determine if disease is primarily based in the muscle system, in another body system, or from a combination of disrupted systems.
4. To determine which diagnostic procedures will be most useful in distinguishing and defining causes, commencing with less invasive and less expensive techniques and escalating in a stepwise fashion, as needed and in collaboration with the client.

OBTAINING AN EFFECTIVE CLINICAL HISTORY

A thorough and helpful clinical history is often obtained in stages, commencing before the appointment, continuing during the appointment, and following up with additional questions after the appointment if new information or results become available. A conversation with the client in advance of the appointment can allow time for thorough historical investigation, effective note taking, and procurement of any existing records and results. It also aids development of understanding what events or procedures might occur during the evaluation, which is helpful in preparing clinician and client. Pre-evaluation conversations might lead to discontinuation of any analgesic agents or other drugs ahead of clinical evaluation. It can also be determined if exercise testing might be indicated and safe, so that the owner can bring and supply any specific equipment that might be needed to achieve this.[1] An idea of how readily the horse can be handled and moved through necessary evaluations including lunge line work can be obtained. Owners may be able to provide photos and footage of their concerns, which are often revealing. Excellent reviews of equine muscle function and structure, and the current knowledge regarding equine muscle diseases, can be valuable in preparing for upcoming investigations, particularly when specific details regarding the case are already known.[1–4]

Information sought in an individual case history will vary with the signalment, clinical concerns, and if the horse is presenting on an emergent basis or as an elective appointment. Separating information questing into categories and pursuing questions relevant to the case help achieve the most useful facts. Suggested categories are

1. Signalment (sex, breed, age). Many prevalent muscle disorders of the horse are breed specific and may have characteristics influenced by sex and age.[1,3] Confirm the signalment with the owner to ensure it is accurately recorded, which can aid development of an appropriate differential diagnosis list.
2. Management factors. Many muscle disorders of the horse are evoked or influenced by dietary composition.[5,6] Establishing the complete ration details, including vitamin E and selenium supplementation, is important as this is a common point of modification in treatment steps.[7] Other details to collect include vaccination history, housing features (eg, stall or pasture), and any potential toxins horses have access to (eg, plants or ionophores).
3. Exercise routine. Type of exercise, when the horse was last exercised, and any changes in exercise routine or rider can be relevant. In rhabdomyolysis cases, it is critical to determine if exercise was a triggering feature or not, to establish an accurate differential diagnosis list and to direct diagnostic testing.
4. Clinical signs of concern. Establish what the client has noticed most prominently. Is it loss of muscle mass (and where)? Reluctance to work or change in performance? Tremors or gait abnormalities? Difficulty prehending or swallowing? Stiffness or stretching out with exercise? Are there photos or other footage?
5. Onset and duration. Attempting to determine if clinical signs developed chronically or acutely, and if any known event preceded their development such as a fall or

injury, competition event, signs of respiratory infection, change in housing location, or other factor is helpful in delineating differential diagnoses.[8–10]

6. Previous results. Evaluating past records such as routine blood work from annual health assessments can be revealing, as even mild persistent increases in muscle enzyme values can signify disease. Prior results from genetic testing can also be informative, and duplication of testing can be avoided.[4]

7. Medication history. Establish if the horse is or has received any medications (type, route, dose, frequency) and if there is evidence of response to any treatment. Improvement with a course of analgesia is usually suggestive of an orthopedic disorder rather than a primary muscle disorder. Also establish if any intramuscular injections recently occurred, or if there has been increased recumbency or rolling, which can aid interpretation of muscle enzyme elevations.[11]

Not infrequently, horses with muscle disorders present for clinical complaints that do not typify muscle disease, such as colic, weight loss, misbehavior during exercise, or even signs of cardiac disease. Physical examination findings are not always leading, and it is not uncommon to recognize muscle disease only after screening serum chemistry returns elevated muscle enzyme values, or spontaneous myoglobinuria is observed. Collecting additional relevant history retrospectively has strong value in these cases.

Fig. 1A, B demonstrates the importance of collecting a thorough history, evaluating all available information, and determining what information needs repeating or collecting to ensure accurate diagnosis and resolution of all client concerns and disease processes. The algorithm displays the case flow of a 2-year-old Quarter Horse gelding

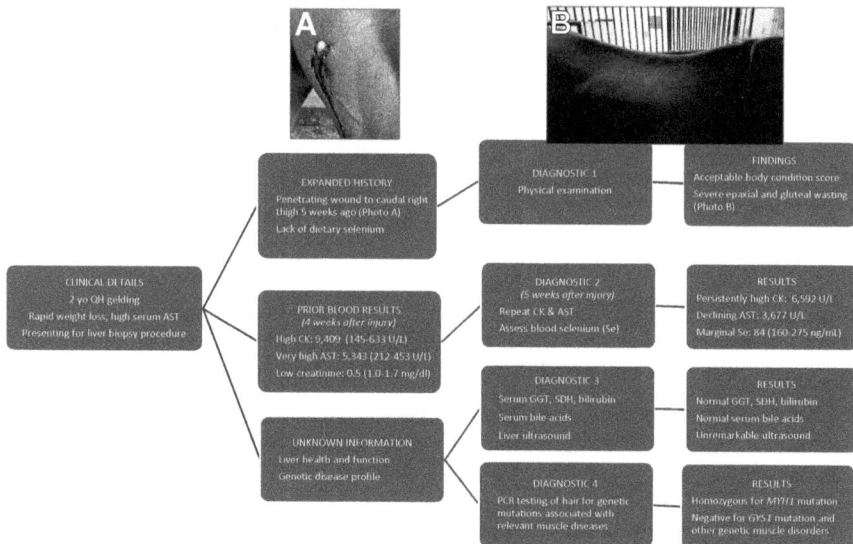

Fig. 1. (A,B) Case flow algorithm in a 2-year-old Quarter Horse gelding presenting for evaluation of weight loss. Ultimately the gelding was diagnosed with immune-mediated myositis linked to a homozygous genetic profile for the myosin heavy chain myopathy mutation and was found to have concurrent marginal selenium status. Treatment consisted of a tapering oral dexamethasone regimen and a single intramuscular injection of selenium followed by daily oral selenium supplementation (3 milligrams/day). See the section in this article on obtaining an effective clinical history for full details.

that was presented for liver biopsy because of perceptions by the owner of weight loss, and discovery of elevated serum aspartate transferase (AST) activity, suspected to be of hepatic origin. Conversing with the client revealed that a small penetrating wound had occurred to the horse's caudal thigh 5 weeks before, for which a photograph was available (**Fig. 1**A). The prior serum chemistry results were available and had been obtained at 4 weeks after injury with no preceding recent exercise. On retrospective evaluation, the serum AST appeared too high to align with hepatic origin and was accompanied by moderately elevated serum CK suggesting a non-exertional rhabdomyolysis disorder as the cause of these derangements. Additionally, the serum creatinine concentration was abnormally low for the patient's signalment, suggesting unusually low muscle mass (**Fig. 1** for relevant clinical pathology values in this case). Physical examination 5 weeks after injury identified that the apparent weight loss was attributable to severe symmetric atrophy of the epaxial and gluteal musculature (**Fig. 1**). Repeat clinical pathology showed decreasing AST activity, but lack of normalization of CK, indicating an ongoing non-exertional rhabdomyolysis process. Based on the horse's management (green pasture, with no additional supplements), whole blood selenium was also evaluated and found to be marginal, leading to selenium supplementation of the gelding and recommendations for supplementation of other horses and ruminants on the property. Because of the client's concerns about the gelding's liver health, appropriate steps were taken to evaluate the horse for liver disease with no abnormal findings in this regard (**Fig. 1**). Genetic testing for diseases that can cause epaxial and gluteal atrophy in Quarter Horses was recommended.[1,12–14] Immune-mediated myositis from myosin heavy chain myopathy was considered the primary differential given the horse's signalment, recent muscle trauma, and physical examination and clinical pathology findings.[13,14] The horse was found to be negative for the glycogen synthase 1 (GYS1) mutation associated with type 1 polysaccharide storage myopathy, and homozygous for the myosin heavy chain 1 (MYH1) mutation associated with immune mediated myositis.[4] Since the owner had breeding stock related to this gelding, other genetic disorders were concurrently tested for. The horse made a full recovery after treatment with a tapering corticosteroid regimen and selenium supplementation, although the owner was cautioned that because the horse is homozygous for the MYH1 mutation, relapse was likely.[14]

PERFORMING THE EXAMINATION

A competent and fruitful examination of the neuromuscular system occurs in a controlled environment and when the correct equipment is available.[15] A list of equipment that may be useful in a comprehensive examination is listed:

1. A bright light source that can be focused on a small area and that is bright enough to elicit a rapid pupillary light reflex in normal horses.
2. Direct ophthalmoscope to facilitate examination of the retina for relevant changes.[16]
3. A pair of forceps or similar instrument that can induce a response without injury when used to stroke or pinch selected parts of the body or periphery.
4. A large block to stand on to allow elevation above the horse's back for effective palpation and visualization.
5. A form for recording findings in a standardized manner and to avoid missing critical steps.
6. Capacity for photo or video recording of specific findings including muscle mass, asymmetry, gait abnormalities, and other findings to help with re-evaluation over

time, opinions from other clinicians, or as a backup when important information is not recorded correctly.

7. Specialized equipment for 3-dimensional scanning of muscle mass may also have utility.[17]

Examination is aided substantially by an experienced handler or owner willing to follow instructions, wearing safe footwear, and who is good at allowing the horse to move with relative freedom during testing. Ideally a quiet enclosed area should be available for thoracic auscultation and at-rest assessments, and also a firm runway available for gait assessment, in addition to an arena for any lunge-line or ridden work that might occur in the examination.

The clinician should develop a comprehensive but efficient routine that covers basic assessment of neuromuscular function on every horse examined, extending or enhancing the examination as needed depending on the clinical complaints and initial historical and physical findings. Comprehensive neuromuscular examination can be divided into different areas of emphasis: mentation, cranial nerve function, spinal reflexes, muscle evaluation, and the ambulatory gait and postural evaluation; excellent descriptions of sequential evaluation of the neurologic system of horses exist.[15,18,19] Revisiting the history or expanding assessment of historical records should also be pursued if it becomes relevant in the course of the examination. The neurologic component of the examination should be used to determine the presence of any ophthalmic or cranial nerve abnormalities, as well as the presence of paresis (reduced motor function) and ataxia that is reflected by proprioceptive deficits evident in abnormal positioning or placement of the limbs and body.[15] The muscle component of the evaluation seeks to determine the presence of abnormal responses of muscle to stimulation (eg, muscle pain, fasciculations, or contractions) or the presence of abnormal mass (eg, atrophy, hypertrophy, or asymmetry) or character (eg, mineralization, fibrosis, or defects).[1] Performing a standardized examination in a routine manner provides the highest chance of identifying anomalies, and a suggested routine is outlined:

1. Assess head and limb position, behavior, and response to interaction. Watch for fine tremors in the large muscles of the proximal limbs, the flanks, and the back, for intermittent weight shifting or other anomalies.
2. Perform visual inspection and palpation while the horse is standing squarely and determine body condition score and evaluate muscle symmetry and mass. Provide an assessment of muscle mass (such as a grade out of 3 or 4, or mild, moderate, or severe atrophy), describe muscle symmetry and specific locations where mass is abnormal (increased or decreased, asymmetric or misshapen).
3. Evaluate the eyes including the retinas with a direct ophthalmoscope, and perform organized cranial nerve assessment.
4. Palpate both masseter muscles and lift the forelock to assess the temporalis muscles for changes in size or character. Determine if the mouth can be readily opened to check for trismus. Consider offering feed to evaluate prehension and swallowing.
5. Check both sides of the neck for muscle symmetry (lift the mane) and determine willingness to flex the neck laterally to each side as well as to lift the head up and down.
6. Palpate limb muscles, and back and gluteal musculature to identify point sensitivity, bands or defects, abnormal tone, or fine or inducible tremors.
7. Evaluate willingness to dip and flex laterally when a pointed object is drawn over the back and to tuck when a pointed object is drawn over the croup (these responses may be stilted with back pain).

8. Assess muscle response to percussion, tapping sharply with bridged fingers or a neurologic percussion hammer over the large muscle groups (eg, gluteals, triceps, or biceps), particularly in horses with suspected myotonia, unusually large muscle mass, or fasciculations (**Fig. 2**).

9. Evaluate in motion for gait anomalies representing paresis and ataxia and where present, provide an ataxia grade independently for the fore- and hindlimbs. Other movement disorders (eg, shivers or stringhalt) should also be characterized and described.[20] Move the horse forwards and backwards, in a circle both directions, and if possible evaluate movement on hard and soft ground and slopes. Consider testing strength in a standing and walking tail pull maneuver, and ability to resist pushing against the shoulders while standing, for evidence of weakness.

10. Evaluate for lameness on a firm surface, and where present, provide a lameness grade for each affected limb. Apply additional physical diagnostics (eg, hoof testers, flexion tests, or limb palpation) to try to identify the potential site from which lameness derives.

Examination findings are summarized, including specific findings that aid neuroanatomic localization or support a specific origin for any lameness, and a determination made as to whether a muscle disorder is likely present. If present, whether a muscle disorder is the primary problem or secondary to another issue should be determined. A likely differential list is constructed, and diagnostic pathway planning commences in collaboration with the client.

Where significant weakness and/or lameness is evident in a single limb, examination is a critical first step to determine if an orthopedic issue such as fracture is the cause, or if neuropathy or muscle injury explain the signs. It is possible for all three to occur

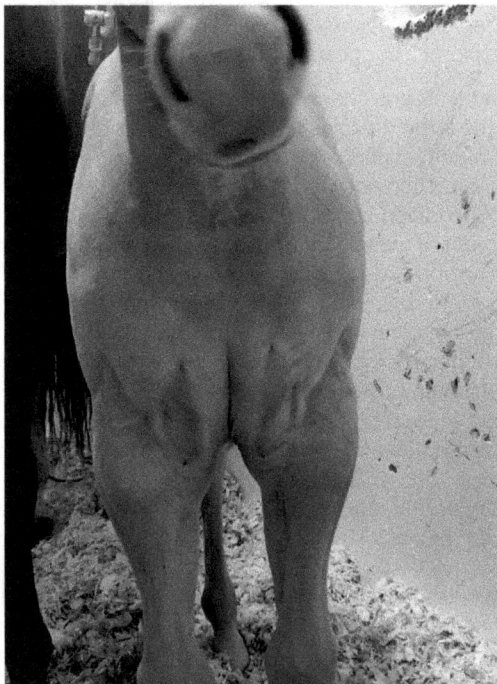

Fig. 2. Generalized unusually large muscle mass in a 3-week-old foal.

concurrently in a serious injury such as a humerus fracture. The appearance and rapid muscle atrophy associated with various peripheral neuropathies are described, as well as injuries to specific hind limb muscles that lead to characteristic abnormalities of voluntary and forced limb positioning:[18,21–23]

- Brachial plexus injury. Horse is unable to bear weight on the affected forelimb, with dropped elbow, and subluxation of shoulder. There is rapid atrophy of the supra- and infraspinatus, triceps, and extensor carpi radialis.
- Suprascapular n. injury. There is immediate lateral instability of the shoulder ('Sweeney') and rapid atrophy of the supraspinatus and infraspinatus muscles.
- Radial n. injury. This can be complete (dropped elbow, unable to normally advance and weight bear on limb, dorsal pastern on ground) or partial loss of function (can bear weight if limb held extended), or even milder signs (tendency to stumble). Atrophy depends on the level at which the lesion occurred. Triceps myopathy can generate a similar appearance, but there is often pain on palpation. Additionally, there may be heat and swelling initially evident in the muscle; similarly, fracture of the humerus must be excluded by appropriate imaging techniques (**Fig. 3**).
- Musculocutaneous n. injury. There are minimal gait anomalies with atrophy of the biceps brachii and brachialis. Autonomous zone of skin sensation over dorsomedial carpus and proximal cannon bone can aid injury diagnosis.
- Median and ulnar n. injury. There is hyperextension from the carpus down (stiff limb with toe dragging during advancement), loss of sensation over the caudal

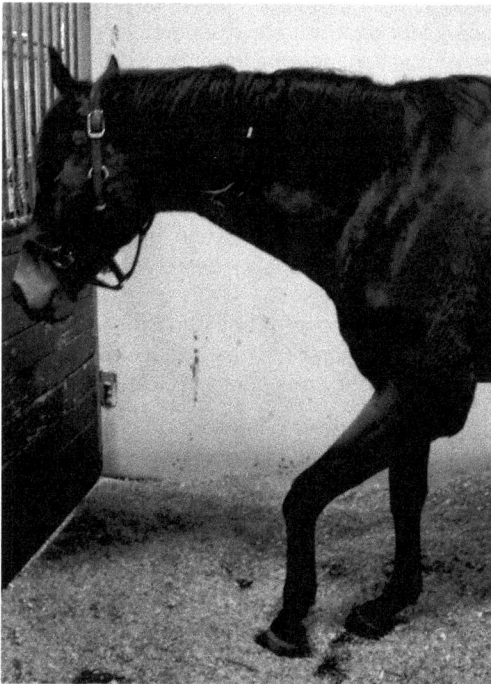

Fig. 3. A horse with dropped elbow appearance, which can arise from triceps muscle injury, radial neuropathy, proximal limb fractures, and other causes. This horse had an anesthetic myopathy event affecting the triceps mass.

proximal forelimb (ulnar n.), the lateral cannon (ulnar n.), and the medial pastern (median n.), as well as atrophy of the carpal and digital flexors.

- Femoral n. injury. Affected hindlimb is flexed, with foot flat on the ground, and buckling with weight bearing. Bilateral lesions may cause crouching or recumbency. High lesions, proximal to the saphenous branch, are associated with loss of sensation over the medial thigh and quadriceps atrophy.
- Obturator n. injury. There is inability to abduct; leg may splay. Bilaterally affected animals are often recumbent.
- Sciatic n. injury. The distal hind limb is flexed with the dorsal hoof wall on the ground with stifle and hock extended. Quadriceps and biceps femoris are used to protract the limb. Weight bearing is possible if the foot is placed correctly and there is wide loss of sensation except for the inner thigh.
- Gluteal n. injury. There is mild limb abduction, outward rotation of the stifle, and gluteal muscle atrophy.
- Peroneal n. injury. There is extension of the hock and flexion of distal limb with the dorsal hoof wall on the ground, as well as a toe drag during ambulation with weak protraction. Additionally, there is loss of sensation over the lateral cannon, and atrophy of the cranial tibial and long and lateral digital extensors.
- Tibial n. injury. The limb will be flexed with normal foot position and knuckling of the fetlock. Motion is associated with a gait that mimics stringhalt. Sensation is lost over the caudal cannon and heel bulbs. Flexor reflex (tested by skin pinch over dorsal fetlock) is reduced on the affected side, and gastrocnemius muscle atrophy can develop.
- Peroneus tertius rupture arises from overextension of the hock joint, and the hind limb can be pulled straight (both hock and stifle concurrently extended) behind the horse. These joints can operate independently of one another. The hock does not flex on protraction, and the lower limb is flaccid.
- Gastrocnemius rupture. There is dropped hock and extended stifle, inability to straighten the limb, or bear weight (if complete rather than partial rupture). There is usually notable swelling of the upper limb. Bilateral ruptures cause recumbency. Injury to the origin may cause lateral rotation of the calcaneus with medial rotation of the toe (**Fig. 4**).
- Adductor injury. Severe lameness may be evident with pronounced medial swelling of the inner thigh or palpable defects in the muscle. Bilateral lesions can cause recumbency.
- Fibrotic myopathy can affect one or both hindlimbs, resulting in fibrous or even mineralized changes in the semitendinosus muscles generating palpable abnormalities of the musculature, and a slapping gait with abruptly truncated protraction.

Definitive diagnosis of specific muscle injuries and disorders can require additional specialized techniques. Radiography, ultrasonography, thermography, and nuclear scintigraphy can be used in combination to differentiate, localize, and characterize orthopedic and muscle lesions.[9,22] (**Fig. 5**) Electromyography can be used to differentiate neurogenic from myogenic muscle atrophy and to elucidate disorders generating abnormal muscle tone or increased muscle mass such as myotonia congenita (see Aleman's article, "Disorders Of Muscle Mass And Tone," in this issue). Scientifically validated genetic testing assists the diagnosis of several exertional and non-exertional rhabdomyolysis disorders, in addition to hyperkalemic periodic paralysis[4,14] (see Finno's article, "Genetics of Muscle Disease," in this issue). Muscle biopsy is indicated where diagnosis cannot be readily achieved or excluded by other means (see Valberg and Porter's article, "Skeletal Muscle Biopsy," in this issue).

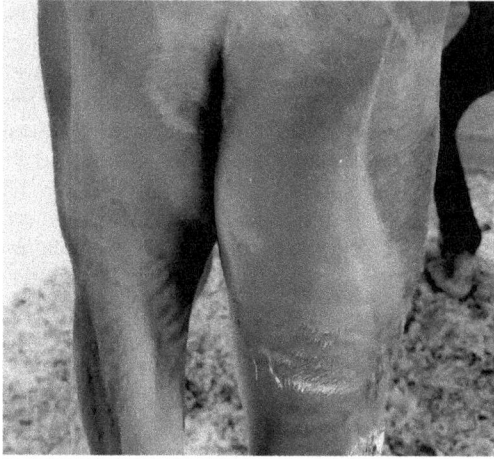

Fig. 4. Proximal limb swelling in a 2-week-old foal with complete unilateral gastrocnemius muscle rupture due to manual interventions during a dystocia birth.

CLINICAL PATHOLOGY

Clinical pathology is economic, convenient, and widely available. It is of substantial importance in the detection of exertional and non-exertional rhabdomyolysis, which both arise from a wide range of muscle disorders.[1–3] Reference intervals for hematologic and biochemical variables have been thoroughly described and cataloged for athletic horses, relevant to breed, age, and performance discipline.[24] To ensure quality results, samples for hematology and biochemistry analyses should be collected and transported carefully, and the timing and purpose of sampling considered. Hematologic evaluation should be considered wherever an inflammatory component is suspected, such as in rapid epaxial, and gluteal atrophy potentially related to immune-mediated myositis, where there is focal severe myositis at injection sites, and in horses with muscle manifestations of *Streptococcus equi* or *Corynebacterium*

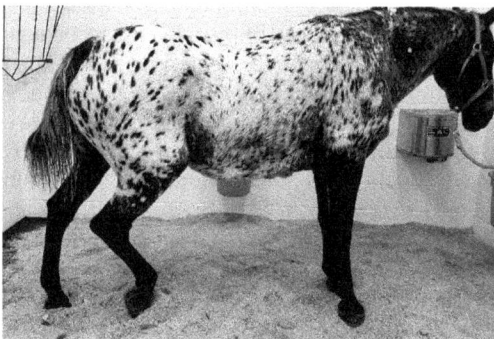

Fig. 5. A 20-year-old mare with severe lameness of the right hind limb and swelling of the semimembranosus and adductor regions. Abscessation of these areas of musculature was identified on ultrasound, and osteomyelitis of the femur was evident on radiographs. *Corynebacterium pseudotuberculosis* was identified from cytologic examination and bacterial culture of abscess aspirates.

pseudotuberculosis infections, for example.[10] Serum chemistry is essential to determine the presence and degree of muscle enzyme evaluations, which often correspond poorly to severity of clinical signs. Severe rhabdomyolysis can also provoke perturbations in acid-base and hydration status, and plasma electrolyte, mineral and even protein concentrations, and characterizing these changes is critical to diagnosis and treatment.[24] Triglyceride measurement should be considered in miniature horses, donkeys, and ponies where prolonged anorexia or unusually high peripheral total solids values are obtained on refractometry. Cardiac troponin measurement is indicated where muscle disease is accompanied by clinical indications of cardiac disease, or where a potentially cardiotoxic etiology is suspected such as in hypoglycin A or ionophore toxicity.[25,26] Similarly, serum and urine acylcarnitine profiles are indicated where specific plant toxicities including Box Elder (*Acer negundo*), Sycamore maple (*A. pseudoplatanus*), or Marsh Mallow (*Malva parviflora*) are possible causes of rhabdomyolysis with or without cardiac involvement.[27,28] Vitamin E should be measured in serum or plasma, and selenium on whole blood samples, where deficiencies in these nutrients are suspected.[4] (see Finno and McKenzie's article, "Vitamin E and selenium related manifestations of muscle disease," in this issue).

Creatine kinase (CK) activity measured in serum or plasma is the most accurate and specific indication of skeletal muscle necrosis (rhabdomyolysis) in the horse, which can arise from underlying myopathy disorders, muscle tears, and nutritional deficiencies, among other causes.[1–3,29] In horses, CK reflects purely skeletal muscle necrosis, and therefore appropriately timed cardiac troponin measurement is necessary to determine presence and severity of myocardial necrosis.[24] The serum or plasma activity of CK rises rapidly, peaking within 4 to 6 hours, and normalizes rapidly within 72 hours if rhabdomyolysis resolves.[29] Hence timing of measurement is important, and persistent increases, even if mild, indicate that ongoing skeletal muscle necrosis is occurring. Serum CK therefore provides a sensitive and useful test for evidence of rhabdomyolysis and can be used to assess response to treatment and resolution of rhabdomyolysis (**Fig. 6**). The immensity of increase also indicates the volume of muscle damaged, and values can measure tens to hundreds of thousands of units per liter in horses with severe, diffuse rhabdomyolysis associated with exertional rhabdomyolysis disorders and with non-exertional myopathies including ionophore toxicosis, malignant hyperthermia, toxic myopathies, nutritional myodegeneration, and myosin heavy chain myopathy. However, even mild elevations of a few thousand units per liter can be associated with severe disease if produced from a severe, focal muscle tear or if they reflect loss of a large proportion of muscle mass because of severe chronic damage over time such as in equine motor neuron disease or chronic selenium deficiency.[8,9] Mild changes that persist over time can also be suggestive of an underlying chronic hereditary myopathy, such as type 1 polysaccharide storage myopathy (PSSM1). However, many muscle disorders do not generate increases in serum CK and a normal baseline CK value is not reason to exclude the possibility of a myopathy. Short, controlled exercise tests consisting of 15 minutes of walk and trot exercise may provoke abnormal increases in serum CK of 2 to 3 times baseline in horses with specific disorders, particularly PSSM1, and can be a useful addition to clinical examination of the muscle system in some cases.[1]

Serum AST also increases within 18 to 24 hours with any cause of exertional or non-exertional rhabdomyolysis in horses, but elevations must be differentiated from hepatocellular disease. Very large increases (>4000 U/L) are a strong indicator of diffuse severe rhabdomyolysis since the equine muscle mass is large enough to generate such increases.[8,24] Elevations can persist for 10 to 14 days (see **Fig. 6**). Serum AST and CK should be interpreted with other hepatic enzymes, including

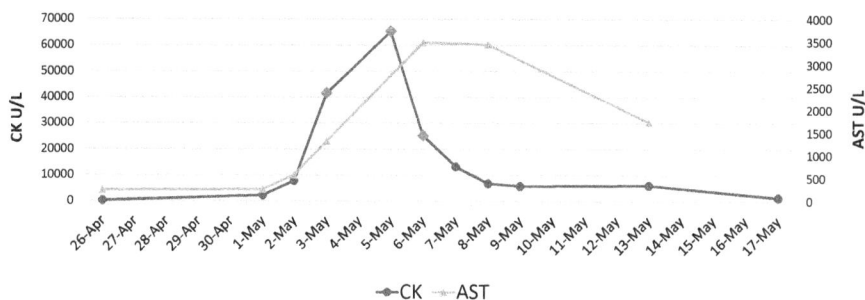

Fig. 6. Time course of changes in serum CK (left axis, *blue line*) and AST (right axis, *orange line*) in a 13-year-old Quarter Horse mare that developed signs of respiratory infection (rhinitis B virus positive) on April 24. Lymphopenia, neutrophilia, and elevation of plasma fibrinogen and serum globulins were reported, and rapid topline muscle atrophy also developed. Visible myoglobinuria was evident for 72 hours (red diamonds on the CK *line*). The mare tested homozygous positive for the equine myosin heavy chain myopathy (*MYH1*) mutation. Treatment with dexamethasone started May 3.

gammaglutamyltransferase (GGT), and if available, sorbitol dehydrogenase to determine if hepatocellular disease is the primary or a contributing entity to serum AST increases.[24] Elevated serum AST activity in a horse that has normal serum CK and GGT activities is strongly suggestive of muscle injury within the last 4 to 12 days.

In horses, short-to-moderate exercise events, even when intense, usually do not generate much change in muscle enzymes, and perturbations in these circumstances, such as after track racing, should be considered possible indicators of an underlying exertional rhabdomyolysis disorder.[24] However, prolonged endurance exercise can elevate serum CK sometimes several thousand units in apparently healthy horses. Larger increases in this population should be viewed with suspicion as indicators of potential myopathy including exhaustion-associated rhabdomyolysis and myofibrillar myopathy.[24,30,31]

In acute and severe rhabdomyolysis, whether exertional or non-exertional in nature, benchtop analyzers commonly cut off CK and AST values much below their actual value (**Table 1**). In such cases, dilutions should be performed to estimate absolute increases, and other evidence of severity of rhabdomyolysis monitored such as testing urine for pigmenturia. This ensures that optimal treatment plans are developed based on objective rather than subjective measures of severity, which can be variable. Acute severe rhabdomyolysis can also generate an artifactual increase in total carbon dioxide results produced by chemistry analyzers (and on specific analyzers, also potassium values) because of interference with the assays by accompanying massive elevations in serum lactate dehydrogenase.[32,33] Values generated by blood gas analyzers in these situations will be accurate and can be used as alternative assessments. Nonetheless, substantial perturbations of serum electrolytes and minerals can occur with severe rhabdomyolysis, and life-threatening abnormalities can include true hyperkalemia and hypocalcemia related to release of, and uptake by severely damaged muscle tissue. Hyponatremia and hypochloremia commonly accompany, and azotemia may also be apparent (see **Table 1**). Severe rhabdomyolysis causes release of myoglobin from muscle, which will be recognized as brown-to-red coloration of urine when the concentration is high enough, usually when serum CK exceeds 25,000 U/L (see **Fig. 6**). However, myoglobin is cleared rapidly by renal excretion and does not discolor serum or plasma.[34] Repeated incidences of myoglobinuria are a strong indicator of ongoing muscle necrosis and increase the risk of nephrotoxicity

Table 1
Selected presenting clinical pathology values from a 10-year-old Paint mare with tachycardia (heart rate 60 bpm), mild stiffness of gait, and brown urine (positive for 'blood' on dipstick)

Variable	Result	Interpretation	Reference Interval
CK	>2000 (diluted to 594,202)	Cut off, subsequent dilution proves very high CK	145–633 U/L
AST	364	Normal (acute muscle damage)	212–453 U/L
TCO_2 (chemistry)	78	Impossibly high (artifact)	22–31 mEq/L
Bicarbonate (blood gas)	21	Low normal	21–30 mEq/L
Sodium	128	Mildly low	133–142 mEq/L
Chloride	93	Mildly low	94–105 mEq/L
Total calcium	7.0	Severely low, check ionized calcium	11.5–13.3 mg/dL
Potassium	6.1	High, treatment indicated	3.2–4.2 mEq/L

Chemistry findings indicate severe, hyperacute rhabdomyolysis (based on very high CK with normal AST) with expected electrolyte disturbances, and artifactual interference with total CO_2 result from a chemistry analyzer (note the normal bicarbonate value for the same horse derived from a blood gas analyzer).

from pigmenturia. In horses with discolored urine, pigmenturia (bilirubin, myoglobin, hemoglobin) must be differentiated from hematuria (red cells in urine) or iatrogenic causes of urine discoloration (eg, rifampin, phenazopyridine, or other medications). A positive orthotolidine ('blood') reaction on urine dipstick analysis therefore requires differentiation of hematuria, myoglobinuria, and hemoglobinuria; a simple approach based on centrifugation of urine and common blood variables is laid out in **Fig. 7**. Urine

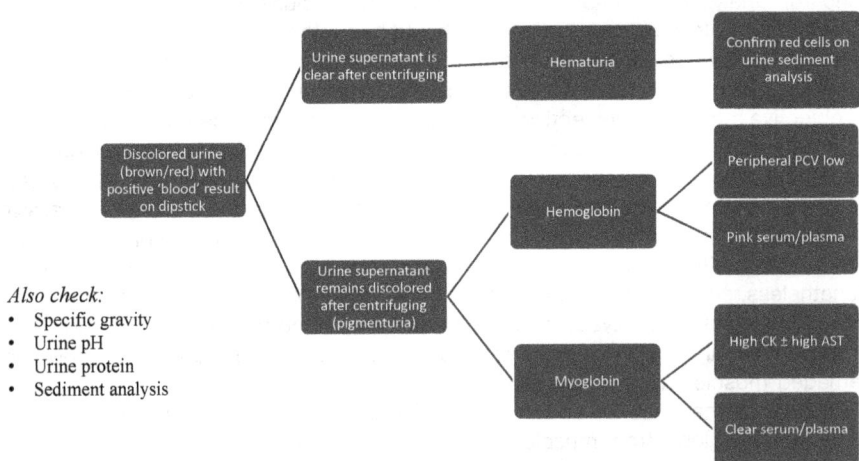

Also check:
- Specific gravity
- Urine pH
- Urine protein
- Sediment analysis

Fig. 7. A simple algorithm to differentiate the cause of a positive 'blood' result (hemoglobin, myoglobin or hematuria) on urine dipstick analysis using a combination of urine centrifugation and assessment of basic clinical pathology results.

samples should also be assessed for concentration (specific gravity) before influence of sedatives or intravenous or enteral fluids, and for the presence of an acidic pH, which increases the nephrotoxic potential of myoglobin and might promote alkalinization as part of the treatment plan. Horses should be assessed for concurrent azotemia. Persistence of azotemia despite appropriate fluid therapy, or azotemia with concurrently isosthenuric urine-specific gravity collected before intravenous or enteral fluid administration is suggestive of suboptimal renal function.[35]

CLINICS CARE POINTS

- Equine muscle disorders are a prevalent cause of disease in horses and arise from a range of genetic and acquired etiologies.

- Recognition and differentiation require careful history assessment and skilled physical examination.

- Clinical pathology is an essential adjunct in most cases to detect rhabdomyolysis and its severity, and to help distinguish likely differentials and to determine effective treatment plans.

DISCLOSURES

The authors have nothing to disclose.

REFERENCES

1. Valberg SJ. Muscle conditions affecting sport horses. Vet Clin N Am Equine Pract 2018;34(2):253–76.
2. Aleman M. A review of equine muscle disorders. Neuromuscul Disord 2008;18(4): 277–87.
3. Piercy RJ, Rivero JL. Muscle disorders of equine athletes. In: Hinchcliff KW, Kaneps AJ, Geor RJ, van Erck-Westergren E, editors. Equine sports medicine and surgery. 3rd edition. Elsevier; 2024. p. 178–219.
4. Valberg SJ. Genetics of equine muscle disease. Vet Clin N Am Equine Pract 2020;36(2):353–78.
5. McKenzie EC, Firshman AM. Optimal diet of horses with chronic exertional myopathies. Vet Clin N Am Equine Pract 2009;25(1):121–35, vii.
6. Urschel KL, McKenzie EC. Nutritional influences on skeletal muscle and muscular disease. Vet Clin N Am Equine Pract 2021;37(1):139.
7. Pitel MO, McKenzie EC, Johns JL, et al. Influence of specific management practices on blood selenium, vitamin E, and beta-carotene concentrations in horses and risk of nutritional deficiency. J Vet Intern Med 2020;34(5):2132–41.
8. Ludvikova E, Jahn P, Lukas Z. Nutritional myodegeneration as a cause of dysphagia in adult horses: three case reports. Vet Med 2007;52(6):267–72.
9. Cullen TE, Semevolos SA, Stieger-Vanegas SM, et al. Muscle tears as a primary cause of lameness in horses: 14 cases (2009-2016). Can Vet J 2020;61(4): 389–95.
10. Faccin M, Landsgaard KA, Milliron SM, et al. Myosin heavy-chain myopathy in 2 American quarter horses. Vet Pathol 2024;61(3):462–7.
11. Kilcoyne I, Nieto JE, Dechant JE. Predictive value of plasma and peritoneal creatine kinase in horses with strangulating intestinal lesions. Vet Surg 2019;48(2): 152–8.

12. McCue ME, Valberg SJ, Miller MB, et al. Glycogen synthase (*GYS1*) mutation causes a novel skeletal muscle glycogenosis. Genomics 2008;91:458–66.

13. Finno CJ, Gianino G, Perumbakkam S, et al. A missense mutation in MYH1 is associated with susceptibility to immune-mediated myositis in Quarter Horses. Skeletal Muscle 2018;8(1):7.

14. Aleman M, Scalco R, Malvick J, et al. Prevalence of genetic mutations in horses with muscle disease from a neuromuscular disease laboratory. J Equine Vet Sci 2022;118:104129.

15. Hahn C. Neurological examination of horses. Vet Clin N Am Equine Pract 2022; 38(2):155–69.

16. Finno CJ, Kaese HJ, Miller AD, et al. Pigment retinopathy in warmblood horses with equine degenerative myeloencephalopathy and equine motor neuron disease. Vet Ophthalmol 2017;20(4):304–9.

17. Valberg SJ, Borer Matsui AK, Firshman AM, et al. Dimensional photonic scans for measuring body volume and muscle mass in the standing horse. PLoS One 2020; 15(2):e0229656.

18. MacKay RJ. Diseases of the peripheral nerves, neuromuscular junction, or uncertain sites: relevant examination techniques and illustrative video segments. AAEP Proceedings 2011;57:363–6.

19. Johnson AL. How to perform a complete neurologic examination in the field and identify abnormalities AAEP. Proceedings 2010;56:331–7.

20. Draper AC, Trumble TN, Firshman AM, et al. Posture and movement characteristics of forward and backward walking in horses with shivering and acquired bilateral stringhalt. Equine Vet J 2015;47(2):175–81.

21. Emond AL, Bertoni L, Seignour M, et al. Peripheral neuropathy of a forelimb in horses: 27 cases (2000-2013). J Am Vet Med Assoc 2016;249(10):1187–95.

22. Walmsley EA, Steel CM, Richardson JL, et al. Muscle strain injuries of the hindlimb in eight horses: diagnostic imaging, management and outcomes. Aust Vet J 2010;88(8):313–21.

23. Swor TM, Schneider RK, Ross MW, et al. Injury to the origin of the gastrocnemius muscle as a possible cause of lameness in four horses. J Am Vet Med Assoc 2001;219(2):215–9.

24. McKenzie EC. Evaluation of clinicopathological abnormalities in athletic horses. In: Hinchcliff KW, Kaneps AJ, Geor RJ, et al, editors. Equine sports medicine and surgery. 3rd edition. Elsevier; 2024. p. 1052–72.

25. Kraus MS, Jesty SA, Gelzer AR, et al. Measurement of plasma cardiac troponin I concentration by use of a point-of-care analyzer in clinically normal horses and horses with experimentally induced cardiac disease. Am J Vet Res 2010; 71(1):55–9.

26. Verheyen T, Decloedt A, De Clercq D, et al. Cardiac changes in horses with atypical myopathy. J Vet Intern Med 2012;26(4):1019–26.

27. Bauquier J, Stent A, Gibney J, et al. Evidence for Marsh Mallow (Malva parviflora) toxicosis causing myocardial disease and myopathy in four horses. Equine Vet J 2017;49(3):307–13.

28. Sponseller B, Evans T. Plants causing toxic myopathies. Vet Clin N Am Equine Pract 2024;40(1):45–59.

29. Valberg S, Jönsson L, Lindholm A, et al. Muscle histopathology and plasma aspartate aminotransferase, creatine kinase and myoglobin changes with exercise in horses with recurrent exertional rhabdomyolysis. Equine Vet J 1993; 25(1):11–6.

30. Wilberger MS, McKenzie EC, Payton ME, et al. Prevalence of exertional rhabdo-myolysis in endurance horses in the Pacific Northwestern United States. Equine Vet J 2015;47:165–70.
31. Valberg SJ, McKenzie EC, Eyrich LV, et al. Suspected myofibrillar myopathy in Arabian horses with a history of exertional rhabdomyolysis. Equine Vet J 2016; 48(5):548–56.
32. Collins ND, LeRoy BE, Vap L. Artifactually increased serum bicarbonate values in two horses and a calf with severe rhabdomyolysis. Vet Clin Pathol 1998;27:85–90.
33. Valberg SJ, Clancey NP, Salinger A, et al. Pseudohyperkalemia in horses with rhabdomyolysis reported by an enzymatic chemistry analyzer. J Am Vet Med As-soc 2023;262(1):1–5.
34. Holmgren N, Valberg S. Measurement of serum myoglobin concentrations in horses by immunodiffusion. Am J Vet Res 1992;53(6):957–60.
35. Divers TJ. Acute kidney injury and renal failure in horses. Vet Clin N Am Equine Pract 2022;38(1):13–24.

Genetics of Muscle Disease

Carrie J. Finno, DVM, PhD

KEYWORDS

• Biopsy • DNA • Equine • Horse • Inherited • Myopathy

KEY POINTS

- Genetic testing should be included in any workup of recurring muscle disease.
- Validated genetic tests exist for the inherited muscle diseases hyperkalemic periodic paralysis, malignant hyperthermia, glycogen branching enzyme disease, type 1 polysaccharide storage myopathy, and myosin heavy chain myopathy.
- For diseases without validated genetic tests, diagnosis via clinical presentation, serum creatine kinase and aspartate aminotransferase activities, and muscle biopsy are warranted.

INTRODUCTION

In the field of equine muscle disorders, many conditions have a genetic basis. Thus, genetic testing is an important part of the diagnostic evaluation in these cases. Genetic testing is the only way to determine a specific genetic cause in horses with clinical signs of these conditions, which can lead to specific treatments and improved outcomes with some conditions. For others, genetic testing can guide breeding management practices and guard against creating foals with lethal conditions.

An important consideration with genetic testing is that it is testing for a specific mutation in a specific gene. Genetic heterogeneity can exist with some conditions and the DNA test is only testing for one of those conditions. For example, polysaccharide storage myopathy (PSSM) in horses is defined as the accumulation of abnormal glycogen in the skeletal muscle.[1] However, with the identification of the genetic mutation for Type 1 PSSM, it became evident that additional types of PSSM exist across horse breeds that may be due to another genetic cause.[2] This constitutes genetic heterogeneity, where different mutations can cause what appears to be the same disease.

Another important consideration is phenotypic heterogeneity. This is where the underlying DNA change, or genetic variation, is the same but affected animals present with different clinical signs. Other genetic, epigenetic, and environmental factors

Department of Veterinary Population Health and Reproduction, School of Veterinary Medicine, University of California Davis, Room 4206 Vet Med 3A One Shields Avenue, Davis, CA 95616, USA
E-mail address: cjfinno@ucdavis.edu

Vet Clin Equine 41 (2025) 17–29
https://doi.org/10.1016/j.cveq.2024.10.002   vetequine.theclinics.com
0749-0739/25/© 2024 Elsevier Inc. All rights reserved, including those for text and data mining, AI training, and similar technologies.

account for part of this heterogeneity. An example of phenotypic heterogeneity in the horse is myosin heavy chain myopathy (MYHM), where a horse can present with either nonexertional rhabdomyolysis or immune-mediated myositis.[2]

The genotype–phenotype relationship can be described by 3 terms: penetrance, expressivity, and pleiotropy (**Fig. 1**). Penetrance is the percentage of individuals carrying a particular mutation that exhibit certain detectable phenotypic traits (ie, clinical signs). For example, glycogen branching enzyme deficiency (GBED) is 100% penetrant, with all homozygous foals clinically affected by this lethal disease.[3] Expressivity is the degree of phenotype severity in an individual that exhibits detectable mutant phenotype. In horses, type 1 PSSM demonstrates variable expressivity, with some horses demonstrating severe signs of rhabdomyolysis and others may be subclinical.[2] Pleiotropy is defined by a gene that, when mutated, leads to multiple phenotypes, often in multiple tissues or organs.

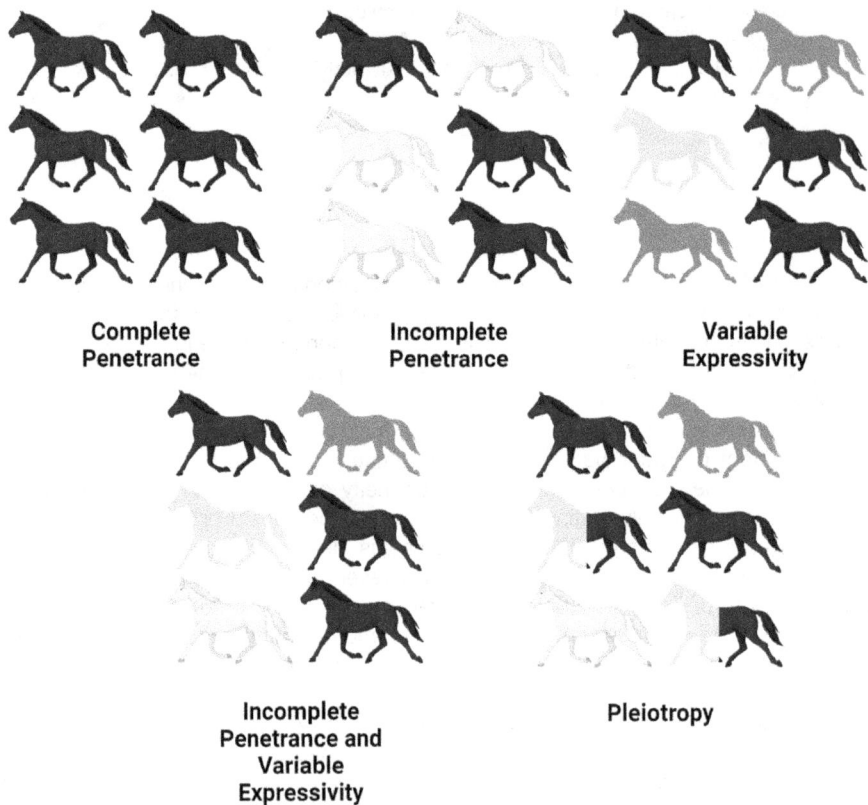

Complete Penetrance **Incomplete Penetrance** **Variable Expressivity**

Incomplete Penetrance and Variable Expressivity **Pleiotropy**

Fig. 1. Visual representation of the terms: (1) Complete penetrance, where all individuals with the DNA variant demonstrate the full phenotype; (2) incomplete penetrance, where a subset of individuals with the DNA variant demonstrate the full phenotype and a subset are subclinical (50% in this example); (3) variable expressivity, where all individuals with the DNA variant demonstrate a phenotype but the phenotype varies from mild to moderate to severe; (4) incomplete penetrance with variable expressivity, where a subset of individuals demonstrate a spectrum of the phenotype (mild to severe) and another subset are subclinical; and (5) pleiotropy, where the DNA variant has different effects in different tissues or organs.

Heritable muscle diseases in horses disrupt energy metabolism pathways, muscle contractility, and muscle structure. In the horse, many of the first genetic tests identified were for muscle disorders. From a breed registry perspective, the American Quarter Horse Association (AQHA) has mandated that all breeding stallions have a 5 panel genetic test on file prior to registration of foals resulting from breedings after January 1, 2015 (https://www.aqha.com/genetic-testing). This panel includes genetic tests for hyperkalemic period paralysis (HYPP), GBED, PSSM1, malignant hyperthermia (MH), and the nonskeletal muscle disease hereditary equine regional dermal asthenia. Since 2018, the American Paint Horse Association also required breeding stallions to have the 5 panel genetic disease test results on file, plus lethal white foal syndrome prior to the registration of their foals. In January of 2023, the AQHA added MYHM to the required testing panel for breeding stallions. However, any stallion that was registered before January 2023 is not required to add MYHM retroactively. This article focuses on the available genetic tests for inherited equine muscle disorders and discusses ongoing efforts for other myopathies.

EQUINE MUSCLE DISORDERS WITH DNA TESTS
Hyperkalemic Periodic Paralysis

Clinical signs
HYPP results in episodic weakness and paralysis. Episodes typically last between 15 and 60 minutes and horses may appear completely normal between episodes.[4,5] Muscle fasciculations and sweating in flanks, necks, and shoulders may be observed. During severe attacks, horses may dog sit or become recumbent.[4,5] Potassium concentrations are often elevated (5–9 mEq/L) during HYPP attacks but can return to normal shortly thereafter.[4] Serum creatine kinase (CK) activity may be normal or mildly increased during episodes.[4,5] Homozygous foals may demonstrate respiratory stridor, dysphagia, or respiratory distress.[6] Factors that can precipitate HYPP episodes include feeding diets high in potassium, anesthesia and stress, including transport.[4] When undergoing anesthesia, clinicians should inquire about the HYPP status of any Quarter Horse or related breed, especially if the horse displays the heavy muscling that is often observed with the HYPP phenotype.[7]

Genetic etiology
HYPP is inherited as an autosomal codominant trait.[8] HYPP was the first hereditary disease in horses for which the molecular defect was determined. The disease has only been reported in Quarter Horse and Quarter Horse-related breeds. The genetic etiology is a missense mutation (F1416 L) in the voltage-dependent skeletal muscle *sodium channel alpha-subunit* (SCN4A).[8] The mutation results in failure of a subpopulation of sodium channels to inactivate when serum potassium concentrations are increased. The excessive influx of sodium and efflux of potassium results in persistent depolarization of muscle cells followed by temporary weakness.[8] The designation for genotypes is heterozygous affected, N/H; homozygous affected, H/H; and normal unaffected, N/N.

HYPP affects Quarter Horses, American Paint Horses, and Quarter Horse-related breeds. The mutation was linked to the popular Quarter Horse sire, Impressive, whose offspring dominate the halter horse industry.[7] Since the disease is inherited as a codominant trait, homozygotes demonstrate more severe episodes.

Prevalence
Prevalence estimates demonstrate that approximately 1.5% of Quarter Horse breeds and 4.5% of the American Paint Horse breed are affected, when evaluated across all performance disciplines.[9] Within a discipline, however, HYPP affects 56% of the halter

horse population as of 2009.[9] The disease appears to be rare in cutting, reining, and racing Quarter Horses.[9] In a sampling of 296 horses that had muscle biopsies submitted to the University of California Davis (UC Davis), only one was identified to have HYPP and also had concurrent MYHM.[10] In Brazil, allele frequencies were evaluated in the bull-catching (vaquejada) Quarter Horse and found in 1 out of 126 horses tested (H/N; 0.8%).[11] The allele frequency of HYPP has not decreased over the years, despite available testing, due to the preferential selection of affected well-muscled horses by halter horse show judges.[7]

Treatment and Management of HYPP is covered in Dr Monica Aleman's article, "Disorders of Muscle Mass and Tone," in this issue.

Malignant Hyperthermia

Clinical signs

Rhabdomyolysis due to MH can follow exercise or anesthesia but can be very intermittent.[12–14] The unusual feature to distinguish MH as an underlying cause of exertional rhabdomyolysis is an increased body temperature during episodes.[13] Clinical signs during anesthesia include hyperthermia, lactic acidosis, and muscle rigidity.[14] Halothane anesthesia was first noted to induce episodes[14] but there is a risk with any type of anesthesia. Episodes are often fatal when triggered.[10]

Genetic etiology

MH is inherited as an autosomal dominant trait and only the heterozygous state has been described.[13] The disease has only been identified in Quarter Horse and Quarter Horse-related breeds. The genetic etiology is a missense mutation (R2455G, based on the most recent EquCab3.0 assembly) in the *ryanodine receptor type 1* gene (*RYR1*).[12] The mutation results in excessive release of calcium into the myoplasm and a hypermetabolic state. The designation for genotypes is heterozygous affected, M/N, and normal unaffected, N/N.

Prevalence

MH is rare, with the highest prevalence in halter and pleasure horse lines.[13] In the sampling of horses with muscle biopsies submitted to UC Davis, 6 horses were identified as M/N.[10] Of these, 2 had concurrent MYHM, 2 had concurrent PSSM1, and these 4 horses had presented for rhabdomyolysis and acute death. The one horse that only had MH on genetic testing was presented for anesthesia-associated myopathy. All 6 of these MH cases were fatal.[10] In Brazilian vaquejada Quarter Horses, there were no MH cases identified out of 126 horses.[11]

Treatment and management

To prevent an episode, pretreatment with dantrolene (4 mg/kg) 30 to 60 minutes prior to anesthesia is advised.[15] Repeated doses of dantrolene should be avoided since muscle weakness can occur with higher doses.[15] During an episode, hyperthermia and acidemia should be treated with alcohol, chilled intravenous fluids with sodium bicarbonate and mechanical ventilation. However, most cases are fatal once an episode is underway.[10]

Glycogen Branching Enzyme Deficiency

Clinical signs

Clinical signs of GBED include stillbirth, transient flexural limb deformities in neonatal foals, hypoglycemic seizures, and respiratory or cardiac failure (**Fig. 2**).[16,17] Genotyping of 190 Quarter Horse foals that were aborted, stillborn, or died near term of unknown causes identified that 4% were homozygous for GBED.[16–18]

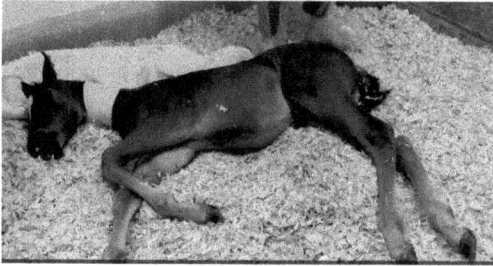

Fig. 2. A Quarter Horse foal affected with glycogen branching enzyme deficiency (GBED).

Genetic etiology

GBED is inherited as an autosomal recessive trait that affects Quarter Horse and Quarter Horse-related breeds.[3] GBED is caused by a nonsense mutation (Y34*) in the *glycogen branching enzyme* gene (*GBE1*).[3] The mutation results in the inability to create the branched structure of glycogen. As a result, cardiac and skeletal muscle, liver, and brain cannot store or mobilize glycogen to maintain normal glucose homeostasis. The designation for genotypes is heterozygous carrier, Gb/N, homozygous affected, Gb/Gb, and normal unaffected, N/N.

Carrier frequencies range from 8% to 11% in the Quarter Horse and 4% to 7% in Paint Horse breeds.[9,18] Within Quarter Horse disciplines, Western pleasure horses had the highest prevalence of carriers (26%), followed by cutting (14%) and working cow horses (10%).[9] In the sampling of horses with muscle biopsies submitted to UC Davis, 14 out of 296 horses were identified as Gb/N.[10] Nine of the 14 horses had other disease variants (MYHM, PSSM1, MH) that likely explained the disease findings, with the carrier status for GBED identified as an incidental finding.[10]

Treatment and management

There is no effective treatment. Despite the level of care, all affected foals died or were euthanized by 18 weeks of age.[16,17]

Type 1 Polysaccharide Storage Myopathy

Clinical signs

Clinical signs of PSSM are affected by environmental factors, such as diet and turnout, and by breed. Horses with PSSM may be asymptomatic or demonstrate signs of exertional rhabdomyolysis.[1] In Quarter Horses, clinical signs of PSSM develop at around the age of 5 years, with less than 20 minutes of slow exercise (walk and trot), especially if the horse has been rested for several days.[19] Acute episodes are associated with markedly increased serum CK activity and myoglobinuria.[19] In Draft breeds, muscle fasciculations and gait abnormalities can be evident,[20] with an average age diagnosis at 8 years.[21] Many Draft horses may be asymptomatic.[22] Despite a high incidence of both diseases in Belgian Draft horses, there is no association between the gait abnormality "shivers" and PSSM1.[21] In Warmbloods, clinical signs include reluctance to collect and engage the hindquarters, lumbosacral pain, gait abnormalities, and muscle atrophy, with an average of onset between the age of 8 and 11 years.[23,24] Serum CK activity is often increased from normal values by 2 fold or greater after 15 minutes of light exercise.[25] Older horses homozygous for the PSSM1 mutation can develop gradual pronounced topline atrophy.

Genetic etiology

PSSM1 is inherited as an autosomal dominant disease in Quarter Horses and Quarter Horse-related breeds, Draft horses, and Warmbloods, among other breeds.[26] The genetic mutation is a missense mutation (R309H) in the *glycogen synthase 1* gene (*GYS1*).[26] The mutation results in unregulated glycogen synthesis and potentially impaired aerobic glycogen metabolism. The designation for genotypes is heterozygous affected, P/N, homozygous affected, P/P, and normal unaffected, N/N.

In Quarter Horses and American Paint Horses, the prevalence of PSSM1 ranges between 6% and 10%.[9,27] The highest frequency was found in halter horses (28%) and the lowest in barrel racing Quarter Horses (1.4%).[9] The prevalence of PSSM1 in draft breeds ranges from 36% to 92% between North American and continental European draft breeds, respectively.[27,28] The mutation has been identified in over 20 breeds, including Irish drafts, Gypsy Vanner breeds, and Warmbloods.[2] It is not commonly found in lighter horse breeds, including Arabians, Standardbreds, and Thoroughbreds.[27,29] In the sampling of horses with muscle biopsies submitted to UC Davis, 33 out of 296 horses were identified as P/N.[10] Of these, 24 had histologic diagnosis of PSSM1, 6 had myonecrosis with no evidence of abnormal glycogen accumulation and variants at multiple loci (MYHM, GBED, MH), and 3 had normal histology.[10] In Brazilian vaquejada Quarter Horses, there were 3/129 PSSM1 horses identified.[11]

Treatment and Management of PSSM1 can be found in the article by Drs Anna M. Firshman and Stephanie J. Valberg, "Polysaccharide Storage Myopathy," in this issue and "The Role of Nutrition in Managing Muscle Disorders" by Dr Joe Pagan in this issue.

Myosin Heavy Chain Myopathy

Clinical signs

Myosin heavy chain myopathies include 2 distinct phenotypes that are due to the same underlying genetic mutation (ie, phenotypic heterogeneity).[30] The first is nonexternal rhabdomyolysis, which is not induced by exercise and presents as stiffness, muscle pain, weakness, and recumbency.[31] Serum CK and aspartate aminotransferase (AST) activities are often very high (>100,000 U/L) and myoglobinuria is common.[31] Muscle atrophy is a frequent sequala to these episodes (**Fig. 3**).[31] The second disease is immune-mediated myositis. Clinical signs are biphasic in the population, affecting young horses (≤8 years) or older horses (≥17 years).[32] Clinical signs, consisting of rapid muscle atrophy of the topline muscles, can occur following respiratory disease exposure, particularly with *Streptococcus equi equi*, *Streptococcus zooepidemicus*, or a respiratory virus.[32,33] Clinical signs can often develop after vaccination against influenza, equine herpes virus 4, or *S. equi equi*.[32,33] Serum CK and AST may be moderately elevated during the acute phase of the disease but can be normal in later phases.[2] In some horses with immune-mediated myositis, systemic calcinosis or calciphylaxis can occur.[34] This is a rare, but fatal syndrome of calcium accumulation in soft tissues and organs. Ventral edema is an early indicator of systemic calcinosis and additional signs include mild fever, stiffness, muscle atrophy, and multiple organ failure.[34] Hyperphosphatemia is evident with these cases, with a product of total calcium concentration (mg/dL) multiplied by phosphorus concentration greater than 65 g/dL (1 mg/dL of calcium = 0.25 mmol/L; 1 mg/dL of phosphorus = 3.1 mmol/L).[2]

Genetic etiology

MYHM is inherited as an autosomal codominant disease of Quarter Horses and Quarter Horse-related breeds with variable penetrance.[30] The genetic mutation is a missense mutation (E320G, based on the most recent EquCab3.0 assembly) in the

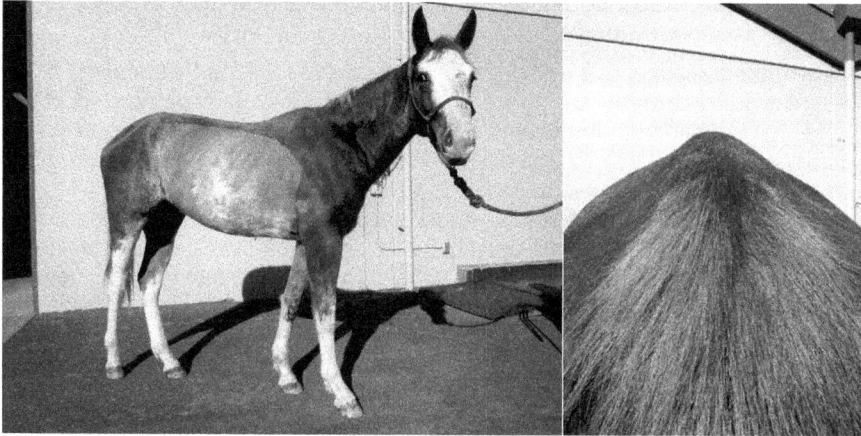

Fig. 3. A Paint Horse yearling that recovered from a pectoral abscess due to *Corynebacterium pseudotuberculosis* and subsequently developed immune-mediated myositis, due to the genetic mutation in myosin heavy chain 1 (MYH1, myosin heavy chain myopathy). Note the severe and widespread muscle atrophy.

myosin heavy chain 1 gene.[30] This genetic variant appears to result in a hypercontractile phenotype that could lead to the observed myopathy.[35] The mutation was initially discovered in horses with immune-mediated myositis[30] but later confirmed to also cause nonexertional rhabdomyolysis, as described earlier.[31] The designation for genotypes is heterozygous affected, N/My, homozygous affected, My/My, and normal unaffected, N/N. Homozygotes (My/My) typically demonstrate more severe clinical signs and recurrence of disease as compared with heterozygotes.[30,31]

In a recent retrospective study aimed at identifying potential triggers of atrophy and stiffness in horses with MYHM, atrophy occurred more frequently in My/My horses.[36] Additionally, fewer My/My horses fully recovered.[36] Three months before observed clinical signs, 47% of MYHM Quarter Horses had been vaccinated or had respiratory or gastrointestinal disease.[36] Inciting causes were not identified in over half the cases. While there did not appear to be a difference in performance success among My/My, My/N, and N/N horses, only 2 out of 10 My/My horses were still actively competing at the time of the study.[36]

Allele frequencies were estimated to be approximately 7% in the general Quarter Horse population and highest among reining (24%), working cow (17%), and halter horses (16%) and the allele was not detected in the barrel racing and racing Quarter Horse subpopulations studied.[37] In the sampling of horses with muscle biopsies submitted to UC Davis, 60 out of 296 horses were identified as having MYHM.[10] Of these 60 horses, 47 (78%) had histologic diagnosis of immune-mediated myositis. Within the 27 out of 60 homozygous (My/My horses), 16 had clinical signs and muscle enzyme activities consistent with severe rhabdomyolysis with myonecrosis on biopsy. Heterozygous horses (33 out of 60; My/N) were less likely to have this severe rhabdomyolysis, with only 6 out of 33 affected.[10] In Brazilian vaquejada Quarter Horses, 10 out of 122 (8%) MYHM horses were identified.[11]

Treatment and Management of MHYM can be found in the article by Drs Sian A. Durward-Akhurst and Stephanie J. Valberg, "Myosin Heavy Chain Myopathy and Immune-Mediated Muscle Disorders," in this issue.

INHERITED EQUINE MUSCLE DISORDERS WITH ONGOING RESEARCH EFFORTS
Type 2 Polysaccharide Storage Myopathy and Myofibrillar Myopathy

Following the discovery of the DNA mutation causative for PSSM1, the term PSSM2 was assigned to cases where clinical signs of exercise intolerance were identified, in addition to abnormal aggregates of polysaccharide in muscle fibers of horses that did not possess the GYS1 mutation.[38] PSSM2 was identified as the most common form of PSSM in the Warmblood and Arabian horses.[39]

Subsequent histologic analyses of muscle biopsies from Warmbloods and Arabians with PSSM2 identified abnormal aggregates of desmin, a cytoskeletal protein, in a small percentage of type 2A muscle fibers.[40,41] Glycogen appeared to pool between these disorganized myofibrils.[40,41] Thus, the subset of PSSM2 horses with these findings were reclassified as having a myofibrillar myopathy (MFM), with PSSM2 likely being an earlier manifestation of MFM in these horses.[29,40,41]

Commercial genetic testing is currently offered for PSSM2 and MFM using single nucleotide polymorphisms (SNPs) in the genes myotilin (MYOT: P2, corresponds to the SNP rs1138656462), filamin C (FLNC: P3a, rs1139799323 and P3b rs1142918816), and myozenin (MYOZ3: P4, rs1142544043; https://www.equiseq.com/). These variants were proposed as DNA tests for PSSM2 and MFM, based on the knowledge that various mutations in MYOT and FLNC have been associated with MFM-like disorders in humans.[42] However, careful assessment in well-phenotyped cases of PSSM2 and MFM in horses has completely refuted these commercial tests.[43]

In the Quarter Horse breed, PSSM2 does not appear to be associated with MFM.[44] Additionally, the P2, P3, and P4 variants offered commercially were not associated with PSSM2 in Quarter Horses.[44] In fact, 57% of healthy Quarter Horses, as diagnosed on muscle biopsy, would be misdiagnosed with PSSM2/MFM using this commercial test.[44] Thus, there are currently no validated genetic tests for PSSM2 or MFM and muscle biopsies are still required for diagnosis.

In Quarter Horses with PSSM2, amylase-resistant polysaccharide is apparent and muscle glycogen concentrations are higher than control horses, but lower than PSSM1 horses.[45] PSSM2 in Quarter Horses can be managed like PSSM1 and is detailed in Anna M. Firshman and Stephanie J. Valberg's article, "Polysaccharide Storage Myopathy," in this issue. PSSM2 does appear to be inherited in the Quarter Horse breed, and variants in 12 candidate genes impacting glycogen metabolism were recently excluded as being associated with the phenotype.[45] Thus, genetic investigations continue for PSSM2 in the Quarter Horse breed, but muscle biopsies are still required for diagnosis.

Recurrent Exertional Rhabdomyolysis

Recurrent exertional rhabdomyolysis (RER) occurs in approximately 7% of Thoroughbred racehorses, especially young nervous fillies, and in 6% of Standardbred racehorses.[46–48] RER may also occur in racing Quarter Horses, Arabian, and Warmblood horses.[49] Episodes of rhabdomyolysis occur intermittently and are associated with sudden increases in serum CK activity.[50] RER appears to be inherited,[51,52] with modifying environmental factors that affect the frequency and severity of these episodes. Using equine SNP genotyping arrays, heritability estimates ranged from 0.41 to 0.46 (Thoroughbreds) and 0.39 to 0.49 (Standardbreds), further supporting that RER is moderately heritable.[53]

With RER, increased sensitivity to potassium-induced, caffeine-induced, and halothane-induced muscle contracture in vitro suggested that altered myoplasmic calcium regulation may underlie this disease during exercise.[54] Genes that regulate

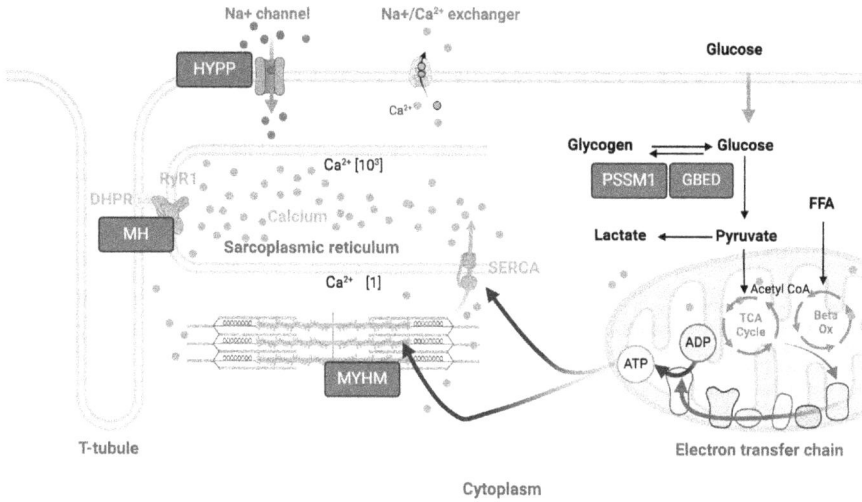

Fig. 4. Diagram outlining where each genetic mutation in the horse affects the resulting protein in skeletal muscle. Genetic disease abbreviations for equine specific diseases can be found in the text. DHPR, dihydropyridine receptor; FFA, free fatty acids; RyR1, ryanodine receptor 1; SERCA, sarcoendoplasmic reticulum calcium ATPase; TCA, tricarboxylic acid cycle. (*Created in* BioRender. Valberg, S. (2025) https://BioRender.com/l03e998.)

myoplasmic calcium, including *RYR1, ATP2A1*, and *CACNA1S*, were initially excluded as candidate genes using microsatellite markers.[55] The genes *sarcolipin (SLN), myoregulin*, and *dwarf open reading frame*, which are transmembrane regulators of the sarcoplasmic reticulum calcium transporting ATPase, were subsequently excluded as candidate genes.[56] However, it was uncovered that equine *SLN* encodes a uniquely truncated peptide that is specific to the horse and of evolutionary interest.[56] Subsequent studies revealed that horse skeletal muscle contractility and susceptibility to exertional rhabdomyolysis are promoted by enhanced sarcoplasmic reticulum calcium uptake and luminal calcium storage.[57] Thus, horses have evolved to have a delicate balance between optimal skeletal muscle performance and disease.

Attempts to identify a genetic cause for RER have continued.[58] However, to date, no causative single gene has been identified. Gene expression pathway analyses repeatedly support perturbation of pathways for calcium regulation and mitochondrial oxidative stress in Standardbreds[59] and Thoroughbreds.[60]

Treatment and management of RER can be found in Stephanie J. Valberg's article, "Sporadic and Recurrent Exertional Rhabdomyolysis," in this issue.

SUMMARY

A summary of where each genetic mutation affects skeletal muscle is provided in **Fig. 4**. With the continued advancement of genetic tools for investigation of genetic diseases in the horse, additional DNA tests are likely to become available for inherited muscle disorders across breeds. Appropriate validation of these tests is a critical step prior to commercialization to guard against misdiagnosis. Genetic and phenotypic heterogeneity should be considered during these genetic investigations, and genetic counseling will become an essential part of the equine practitioner's tool kit.

CLINICS CARE POINTS

- Many recurring muscle diseass have an underlying genetic basis.
- To date, DNA testing exists for five validated inherited muscle disorders.

DISCLOSURE

A portion of proceeds from the genetic testing for MYHM that is performed at the UC Davis Veterinary Genetics Laboratory is returned to Dr C.J. Finno's laboratory to support ongoing genetic research.

REFERENCES

1. Valberg SJ, Cardinet GH 3rd, Carlson GP, et al. Polysaccharide storage myopathy associated with recurrent exertional rhabdomyolysis in horses. Neuromuscul Dis 1992;2:351–9.
2. Valberg SJ. Genetics of equine muscle disease. Vet Clin N Amer Equine Pract 2020;36:353–78.
3. Ward TL, Valberg SJ, Adelson DL, et al. Glycogen branching enzyme (GBE1) mutation causing equine glycogen storage disease IV. Mamm Genome 2004;15:570–7.
4. Spier SJ, Carlson GP, Holliday TA, et al. Hyperkalemic periodic paralysis in horses. J Am Vet Med Assoc 1990;197:1009–17.
5. Naylor JM. Hyperkalemic periodic paralysis. Vet Clin N Amer Equine Pract 1997;13:129–44.
6. Carr EA, Spier SJ, Kortz GD, et al. Laryngeal and pharyngeal dysfunction in horses homozygous for hyperkalemic periodic paralysis. J Am Vet Med Assoc 1996;209:798–803.
7. Naylor JM. Selection of quarter horses affected with hyperkalemic periodic paralysis by show judges. J Am Vet Med Assoc 1994;204:926–8.
8. Rudolph JA, Spier SJ, Byrns G, et al. Periodic paralysis in quarter horses: a sodium channel mutation disseminated by selective breeding. Nat Genet 1992;2:144–7.
9. Tryon RC, White SD, Bannasch DL. Homozygosity mapping approach identifies a missense mutation in equine cyclophilin B (PPIB) associated with HERDA in the American Quarter Horse. Genomics 2007;90:93–102.
10. Aleman M, Scalco R, Malvick J, et al. Prevalence of genetic mutations in horses with muscle disease from a neuromuscular disease laboratory. J Equine Vet Sci 2022;118:104129.
11. Sperandio LMS, Lago GR, Albertino LG, et al. Allele frequency of muscular genetic disorders in bull-catching (vaquejada) quarter horses. J Equine Vet Sci 2024;136:105052.
12. Aleman M, Riehl J, Aldridge BM, et al. Association of a mutation in the ryanodine receptor 1 gene with equine malignant hyperthermia. Muscle Nerve 2004;30:356–65.
13. Aleman M, Nieto JE, Magdesian KG. Malignant hyperthermia associated with ryanodine receptor 1 (C7360G) mutation in Quarter Horses. J Vet Intern Med 2009;23:329–34.
14. Aleman M, Brosnan RJ, Williams DC, et al. Malignant hyperthermia in a horse anesthetized with halothane. J Vet Intern Med 2005;19:363–6.

15. Valverde A, Boyd CJ, Dyson DH, et al. Prophylactic use of dantrolene associated with prolonged postanesthetic recumbency in a horse. J Am Vet Med Assoc 1990;197:1051–3.
16. Valberg SJ, Ward TL, Rush B, et al. Glycogen branching enzyme deficiency in quarter horse foals. J Vet Intern Med 2001;15:572–80.
17. Render JA, Common RS, Kennedy FA, et al. Amylopectinosis in fetal and neonatal quarter horses. Vet Path 1999;36:157–60.
18. Wagner ML, Valberg SJ, Ames EG, et al. Allele frequency and likely impact of the glycogen branching enzyme deficiency gene in Quarter Horse and Paint horse populations. J Vet Intern Med 2006;20:1207–11.
19. Firshman AM, Valberg SJ, Bender JB, et al. Epidemiologic characteristics and management of polysaccharide storage myopathy in Quarter Horses. Am J Vet Res 2003;64:1319–27.
20. Valentine BA, Credille KM, Lavoie JP, et al. Severe polysaccharide storage myopathy in Belgian and Percheron draught horses. Equine Vet J 1997;29:220–5.
21. Firshman AM, Baird JD, Valberg SJ. Prevalences and clinical signs of polysaccharide storage myopathy and shivers in Belgian draft horses. J Am Vet Med Assoc 2005;227:1958–64.
22. Valentine BA, Habecker PL, Patterson JS, et al. Incidence of polysaccharide storage myopathy in draft horse-related breeds: a necropsy study of 37 horses and a mule. J Vet Diag Invest 2001;13:63–8.
23. Quiroz-Rothe E, Novales M, Aguilera-Tejero E, et al. Polysaccharide storage myopathy in the M. longissimus lumborum of showjumpers and dressage horses with back pain. Equine Vet J 2002;34:171–6.
24. McCue ME, Ribeiro WP, Valberg SJ. Prevalence of polysaccharide storage myopathy in horses with neuromuscular disorders. Equine Vet J Suppl 2006;36:340–4.
25. Valberg SJ, Mickelson JR, Gallant EM, et al. Exertional rhabdomyolysis in quarter horses and thoroughbreds: one syndrome, multiple aetiologies. Equine Vet J Suppl 1999;30:533–8.
26. McCue ME, Valberg SJ, Miller MB, et al. Glycogen synthase (GYS1) mutation causes a novel skeletal muscle glycogenosis. Genomics 2008;91:458–66.
27. McCue ME, Anderson SM, Valberg SJ, et al. Estimated prevalence of the type 1 polysaccharide storage myopathy mutation in selected North American and European breeds. Anim Genet 2010;41(Suppl 2):145–9.
28. Baird JD, Valberg SJ, Anderson SM, et al. Presence of the glycogen synthase 1 (GYS1) mutation causing type 1 polysaccharide storage myopathy in continental European draught horse breeds. Vet Rec 2010;167:781–4.
29. McKenzie EC, Eyrich LV, Payton ME, et al. Clinical, histopathological and metabolic responses following exercise in Arabian horses with a history of exertional rhabdomyolysis. Vet J 2016;216:196–201.
30. Finno CJ, Gianino G, Perumbakkam S, et al. A missense mutation in MYH1 is associated with susceptibility to immune-mediated myositis in Quarter Horses. Skelet Muscle 2018;8:7.
31. Valberg SJ, Henry ML, Perumbakkam S, et al. An E321G MYH1 mutation is strongly associated with nonexertional rhabdomyolysis in Quarter Horses. J Vet Intern Med 2018;32:1718–25.
32. Lewis SS, Valberg SJ, Nielsen IL. Suspected immune-mediated myositis in horses. J Vet Intern Med 2007;21:495–503.
33. Hunyadi L, Sundman EA, Kass PH, et al. Clinical implications and hospital outcome of immune-mediated myositis in horses. J Vet Intern Med 2017;31:170–5.

34. Tan JY, Valberg SJ, Sebastian MM, et al. Suspected systemic calcinosis and cal-ciphylaxis in 5 horses. Can Vet J 2010;51:993–9.

35. Ochala J, Finno CJ, Valberg SJ. Myofibre hyper-contractility in horses expressing the myosin heavy chain myopathy mutation, MYH1(E321G). Cells 2021;10(12): 3428.

36. Valberg SJ, Schultz AE, Finno CJ, et al. Prevalence of clinical signs and factors im-pacting expression of myosin heavy chain myopathy in Quarter Horse-related breeds with the MYH1(E321G) mutation. J Vet Intern Med 2022;36:1152–9.

37. Gianino GM, Valberg SJ, Perumbakkam S, et al. Prevalence of the E321G MYH1 variant for immune-mediated myositis and nonexertional rhabdomyolysis in per-formance subgroups of American Quarter Horses. J Vet Intern Med 2019;33: 897–901.

38. McCue ME, Armien AG, Lucio M, et al. Comparative skeletal muscle histopatho-logic and ultrastructural features in two forms of polysaccharide storage myop-athy in horses. Vet Path 2009;46:1281–91.

39. Lewis SS, Nicholson AM, Williams ZJ, et al. Clinical characteristics and muscle glycogen concentrations in warmblood horses with polysaccharide storage myopathy. Am J Vet Res 2017;78:1305–12.

40. Valberg SJ, McKenzie EC, Eyrich LV, et al. Suspected myofibrillar myopathy in Arabian horses with a history of exertional rhabdomyolysis. Equine Vet J 2016; 48:548–56.

41. Valberg SJ, Nicholson AM, Lewis SS, et al. Clinical and histopathological features of myofibrillar myopathy in Warmblood horses. Equine Vet J 2017;49:739–45.

42. Fichna JP, Maruszak A, Zekanowski C. Myofibrillar myopathy in the genomic context. J Appl Genet 2018;59:431–9.

43. Valberg SJ, Finno CJ, Henry ML, et al. Commercial genetic testing for type 2 poly-saccharide storage myopathy and myofibrillar myopathy does not correspond to a histopathological diagnosis. Equine Vet J 2021;53:690–700.

44. Valberg SJ, Henry ML, Herrick KL, et al. Absence of myofibrillar myopathy in Quarter Horses with a histopathological diagnosis of type 2 polysaccharide stor-age myopathy and lack of association with commercial genetic tests. Equine Vet J 2023;55:230–8.

45. Valberg SJ, Williams ZJ, Finno CJ, et al. Type 2 polysaccharide storage myopathy in Quarter Horses is a novel glycogen storage disease causing exertional rhab-domyolysis. Equine Vet J 2023;55:618–31.

46. Isgren CM, Upjohn MM, Fernandez-Fuente M, et al. Epidemiology of exertional rhabdomyolysis susceptibility in standardbred horses reveals associated risk factors and underlying enhanced performance. PLoS One 2010;5:e11594.

47. MacLeay JM, Sorum SA, Valberg SJ, et al. Epidemiologic analysis of factors influ-encing exertional rhabdomyolysis in Thoroughbreds. Am J Vet Res 1999;60: 1562–6.

48. McGowan CM, Fordham T, Christley RM. Incidence and risk factors for exertional rhabdomyolysis in thoroughbred racehorses in the United Kingdom. Vet Rec 2002;151:623–6.

49. Hunt LM, Valberg SJ, Steffenhagen K, et al. An epidemiological study of myopa-thies in Warmblood horses. Equine Vet J 2008;40:171–7.

50. Valberg S, Haggendal J, Lindholm A. Blood chemistry and skeletal muscle meta-bolic responses to exercise in horses with recurrent exertional rhabdomyolysis. Equine Vet J 1993;25:17–22.

51. MacLeay JM, Valberg SJ, Sorum SA, et al. Heritability of recurrent exertional rhabdomyolysis in Thoroughbred racehorses. Am J Vet Res 1999;60:250–6.

52. Dranchak PK, Valberg SJ, Onan GW, et al. Inheritance of recurrent exertional rhabdomyolysis in thoroughbreds. J Am Vet Med Assoc 2005;227:762–7.
53. Norton EM, Mickelson JR, Binns MM, et al. Heritability of recurrent exertional rhabdomyolysis in standardbred and thoroughbred racehorses derived from SNP genotyping data. J Hered 2016;107:537–43.
54. Lentz LR, Valberg SJ, Herold LV, et al. Myoplasmic calcium regulation in myotubes from horses with recurrent exertional rhabdomyolysis. Am J Vet Res 2002;63: 1724–31.
55. Dranchak PK, Valberg SJ, Onan GW, et al. Exclusion of linkage of the RYR1, CAC-NA1S, and ATP2A1 genes to recurrent exertional rhabdomyolysis in Thorough-breds. Am J Vet Res 2006;67:1395–400.
56. Valberg SJ, Soave K, Williams ZJ, et al. Coding sequences of sarcoplasmic retic-ulum calcium ATPase regulatory peptides and expression of calcium regulatory genes in recurrent exertional rhabdomyolysis. J Vet Intern Med 2019;33:933–41.
57. Autry JM, Svensson B, Carlson SF, et al. Sarcoplasmic reticulum from horse gluteal muscle is poised for enhanced calcium transport. Vet Sci 2021;8(12):289.
58. Fritz KL, McCue ME, Valberg SJ, et al. Genetic mapping of recurrent exertional rhabdomyolysis in a population of North American Thoroughbreds. Anim Genet 2012;43:730–8.
59. Valberg SJ, Velez-Irizarry D, Williams ZJ, et al. Enriched pathways of calcium regulation, cellular/oxidative stress, inflammation, and cell proliferation charac-terize gluteal muscle of standardbred horses between episodes of recurrent ex-ertional rhabdomyolysis. Genes (Basel) 2022;13:1853.
60. Aldrich K, Velez-Irizarry D, Fenger C, et al. Pathways of calcium regulation, electron transport, and mitochondrial protein translation are molecular signatures of sus-ceptibility to recurrent exertional rhabdomyolysis in Thoroughbred racehorses. PLoS One 2021;16:e0244556.

Skeletal Muscle Biopsy

Stephanie J. Valberg, DVM, PhD[a],*, Amy Porter, HT (ASCP) QIHC[b]

KEYWORDS

- Myopathy • Diagnosis • Frozen sections • Staining • Sampling

KEY POINTS

- Selection of the appropriate muscle to biopsy is key to obtaining an accurate diagnosis.
- Open surgical and percutaneous needle biopsy techniques can be used.
- Samples that are shipped fresh and subsequently frozen are ideal for research laboratories to diagnose and discover new diseases.
- Formalin-fixed samples can be used to diagnose known diseases if laboratories utilize special tinctorial and immunohistochemical stains.
- An accurate diagnosis requires that an experienced histopathologist combines signalment, history, and clinical signs with histopathologic findings.

INTRODUCTION

A window into the world of equine muscle physiology opened when Arne Lindholm[1] and David Snow[2] adapted the percutaneous needle biopsy technique for use in horses. A modified 6 mm Bergström needle (**Fig. 1**) made it possible to repeatedly sample gluteal muscle from horses and to characterize the properties of equine muscle. Knowledge from other species could be integrated with equine studies to obtain a clear picture of the structure and function of equine muscle. Dr George Cardinet III established the first neuromuscular diagnostic laboratory that provided routine diagnostic services in veterinary medicine at the University of California, Davis, in the late 1970s. Dr Cardinet's training in human neuromuscular disease and his close collaboration with neurologist Dr Terryl Holliday provided a unique, clinically focused platform to investigate muscle diseases in veterinary medicine.[3] Equine neuromuscular diagnostic laboratories sprung from this platform, which provided unique opportunities to assimilate muscle biopsy samples and clinical input from thousands of equine veterinarians and identified pathognomonic features of specific neuromuscular diseases, and led to the development of diagnostic genetic tests.

[a] Large Animal Clinical Sciences, College of Veterinary Medicine, Michigan State University, East Lansing, MI, USA; [b] Investigative HistoPathology Laboratory, Department of Physiology, Division of Pathology, Michigan State University, 567 Wilson Road, Room 2133, East Lansing, MI 48824, USA
* Corresponding author. 833 Blacksmith Trail, Williamston, MI 48895.
E-mail address: valbergs@msu.edu

Vet Clin Equine 41 (2025) 31–45
https://doi.org/10.1016/j.cveq.2024.10.003
0749-0739/25/© 2024 Elsevier Inc. All rights are reserved, including those for text and data mining, AI training, and similar technologies.

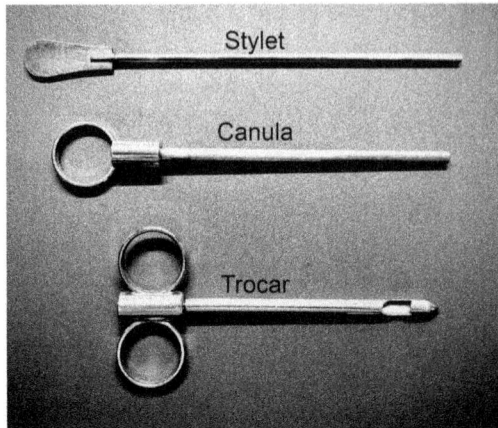

Fig. 1. The components of the modified Bergström muscle biopsy needle. The trocar contains the cutting window. The canula has a cutting end that slices off muscle in the cutting window after which the sample migrates up the hollow core of the canula. After the biopsy is taken, the stylet is placed into the canula to express the muscle sample.

SELECTION OF A MUSCLE TO BIOPSY

The selection of the muscle to biopsy is determined by differential diagnoses derived from the history and clinical signs. A muscle biopsy is not necessary to obtain a diagnosis for myopathies that have validated genetic tests. Validated genetic tests are currently available for equine muscle disorders including hyperkalemic periodic paralysis, malignant hyperthermia, glycogen branching enzyme deficiency, type 1 polysaccharide storage myopathy, and myosin heavy chain myopathy (MYHM; see the articles "Myosin heavy chain myopathy and immune mediated muscle disorders" by Durward-Akhurst and "Polysaccharide storage myopathy" by Firshman in this issue for the current state of knowledge on these conditions).[4,5] In cases where genetic testing is negative, or another myopathy is suggested by signalment and clinical signs, a muscle biopsy can be critical for obtaining a diagnosis. To make an accurate diagnosis, care must be taken to select the appropriate muscle for biopsy based on the patient's history and clinical signs.

- For exertional myopathies, the gluteal or semimembranosus muscles are preferred because they are actively recruited during exercise and more likely to exhibit pathology.[6,7] In human medicine, quadriceps muscle is often biopsied, but in horses, this muscle does not provide optimal diagnostic material.
- For nonexertional rhabdomyolysis, the gluteal or semimembranosus muscles are sampled due to the ease of obtaining these biopsies. With MYHM, a gluteal muscle biopsy is optimal, although genetic testing provides the most accurate diagnosis.[8] If horses have died, it is ideal to obtain samples shortly after death to prevent depletion of muscle glycogen from occurring. In such cases, myocardium, semimembranosus, gluteal, and adductor muscles should be sampled shortly after death and placed in formalin. At necropsy, the deep muscles surrounding the hip joint, the diaphragm, loin muscles adjacent to the caudal aorta, and any pale or hemorrhagic areas are sampled and the specific muscle labeled.
- For horses with generalized weakness and muscle atrophy, the sacrocaudalis dorsalis medialis muscle is ideal because it contains a high proportion of oxidative type 1 fibers that are most frequently affected in equine motor neuron disease or vitamin E responsive myopathy.[9,10] For acute symmetric rapid onset

atrophy in Quarter Horse-related breeds, genetic testing for MYHM provides a definitive diagnosis.[8,11]

- For focal or asymmetric muscle atrophy, the affected muscle should be sampled. For masseter muscles, the facial nerve must be avoided, and to identify lesions, the sample should be obtained deep in the muscle rather than superficially under the fascia.[12] If focal atrophy is prolonged and severe, end-stage muscle may be encountered where loss of myofibers is severe, muscle tissue is replaced by fibrovascular and adipose tissue.[13] In such cases, a more moderately affected muscle should also be sampled.
- Ultrasonography can be used to select the specific site for muscle biopsy if the affected area is not immediately apparent or the depth to sample is uncertain.

BIOPSY TECHNIQUE
Open Muscle Biopsy

The open technique is usually performed on the semimembranosus, semitendinosus, or sacrocaudalis dorsalis medialis muscles under sedation with the tail wrapped. It is important to avoid areas near the myotendinous junction because this introduces artifacts. Muscle is evaluated in cross-section, so the objective is to make a skin incision that is parallel to the muscle fibers and longer in length than width. Frequently, muscle fibers run in the same direction as the haircoat lays, so if anatomy books are unavailable, cutting parallel to the way the haircoat lies is an option. It is very important to avoid squeezing or crushing the central portion of the biopsy during the sampling process because this creates artifactual acute necrosis, atrophy, and glycogen aggregation, clouding an accurate diagnosis.

Semimembranosus or semitendinosus biopsy

The author prefers to sample the semimembranosus muscle versus the semitendinosus muscle in adult horses because any potential scarring is hidden by tail hair. In foals, if an open biopsy is performed, the semitendinosus muscle is preferred because fecal contamination of the site is less likely.

- The site for the semimembranosus and semitendinosus muscles is midpoint between the tuber ischium and Achilles tendon origin (**Fig. 2**).
- The site is clipped and surgically sterilized. The author prefers to avoid using povidone iodine because it can cause a skin reaction in some horses.
- Five to 7 mL of local anesthetic such as lidocaine is injected subcutaneously. It is important not to infiltrate the muscle with lidocaine to avoid artifacts.
- A 4 to 6 cm incision is made through the skin, subcutaneous tissue, and fascia. The fascia should be preserved, and muscle exposed by making 1 cm dissections between the fascia and muscle on either side of the incision. This will allow the fascia to be preserved and sutured upon closure to prevent herniation of muscle and an unsightly appearance.
- Two parallel incisions 1 to 2 cm apart are made in the muscle parallel to the axis of the limb.
- Holding the muscle sample at one end with forceps, the muscle is transected proximally with a scalpel or scissors and dissected out at a depth of 1 cm and length of 2 cm (**Fig. 3**).
- The fascia and subcutaneous tissue are sutured, which prevents muscle from herniating and protruding under the skin as well as dehiscence.
- Interrupted skin sutures or continuous sutures with two interrupted sutures distally (to permit drainage should seromas occur) are placed and removed 10 to 14 days later.

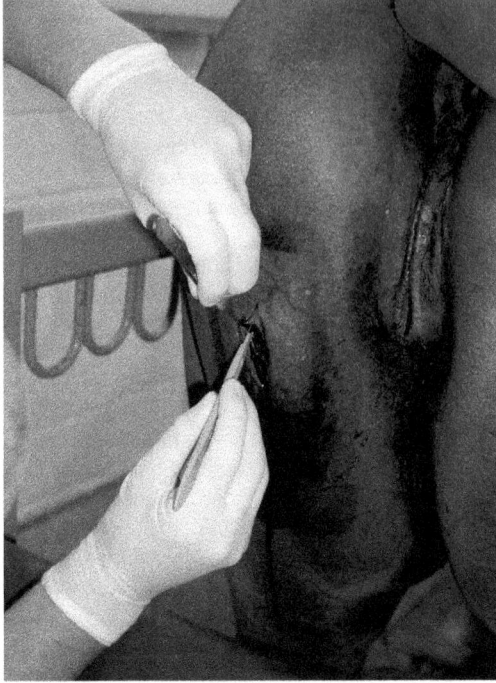

Fig. 2. The site for the semimembranosus muscle biopsy is midway between the tuber ischii and the origin of the Achilles tendon. The skin and fascia are incised, and a dissection is made between the fascia and the underlying muscle to preserve the fascia so it can be sutured during closure to prevent muscle herniation.

- Horses usually require 7 to 10 days rest after the procedure to allow the tissue to heal without dehiscence.

Rare complications from the procedure include muscle herniation through the fascia, hematoma formation, wound dehiscence, and infection. The advantage of the open technique is that it provides ample sample size with well-aligned fibers, the sample can be divided for snap freezing for later biochemical or genetic analysis as well as shipped fresh to the laboratory or placed in formalin for histology.

Sacrocaudalis dorsalis medialis muscle biopsy

Because of the sensitivity of this area, and location of the operator, for safety, horses should be heavily sedated for this procedure.

- The site for the sacrocaudalis medialis muscle is 1 cm off midline and 2 to 5 cm cranial to the tailhead (**Fig. 4**).
- The site is clipped and surgically sterilized.
- This region is well supplied with sensory nerves and often requires subcutaneous injection of 7 to 10 mL of lidocaine.
- The skin is not very pliable at this site making a larger ($\sim$6 cm) incision necessary.
- The skin and subcutis are incised parallel to the spine, often revealing a thin superficial muscle with transversely aligned fascicles that should also be incised.
- The fascia overlying the sacrocaudalis dorsalis medialis muscle is then incised.
- Weitlaner retractors are placed under the fascia to properly visualize the field (see **Fig. 4**).

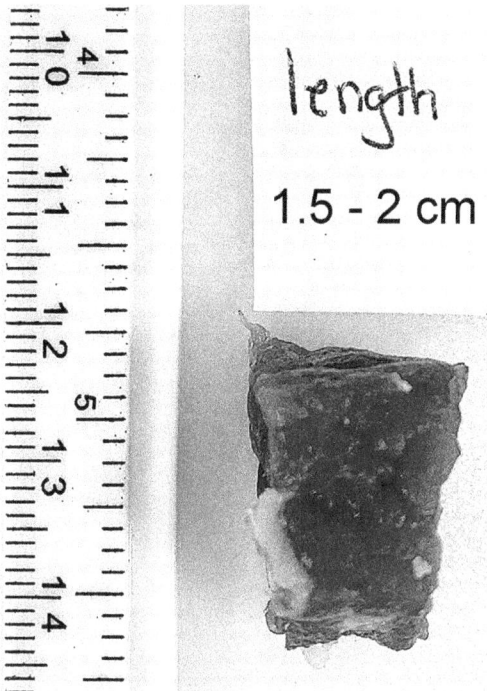

Fig. 3. The semimembranosus muscle sample is ideally 2 to 3 cm in length and 1 to 1.5 cm in depth and width.

- Two parallel incisions 1 to 2 cm apart are made in the muscle parallel to the axis of the spine.
- The muscle sample is grasped at one end with forceps and transected proximally with a scalpel or scissors then dissected out at a depth of 1 to 1.5 cm and length of 2 cm (see **Fig. 4**).
- The sacrocaudalis medialis procedure is more painful than the semimembranosus biopsy and provision of a nonsteroidal anti-inflammatory drug is recommended immediately after and for up to 3 days after the procedure.
- The area should be well protected from flies.

Rare complications include wound dehiscence, infection, or sampling of fat and connective tissue rather than muscle.

Percutaneous Needle Biopsy

Needle biopsy is performed using a 6 mm modified Bergström needle (see **Fig. 1**) that is made by Kruuse A/S (Jorgen Kruuse A/S, Langeskov, Denmark) (www.Kruuse.com). Cutting needle samples (such as Tru-cut - Merit Medical, South Jordan, UT) are too small to obtain meaningful diagnostic results. The needle biopsy technique is ideal for gluteal muscle and can also be used, but is more difficult to perform, on semimembranosus, triceps or other limb muscles. It is imperative for diagnostic purposes that an adequate sample size be obtained. Whether through one insertion of the needle or several insertions, a sample 2.5 to 3 cm long is required to make a definitive histologic diagnosis. The advantage of the needle biopsy is that it is less traumatic than the open biopsy and involves much less rest time. The human literature indicates that during the

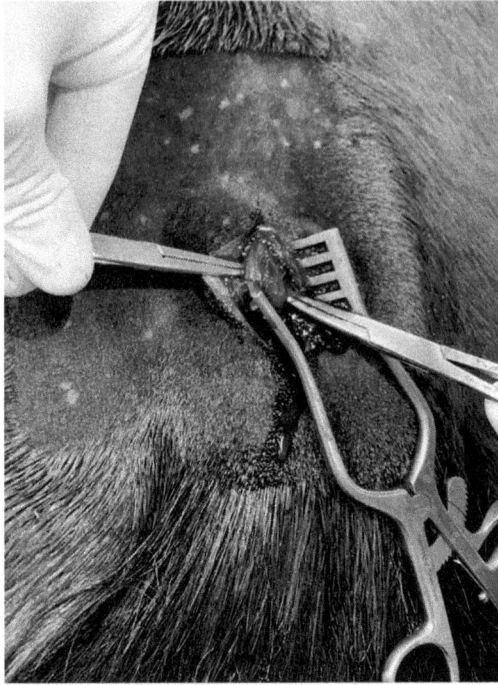

Fig. 4. The site for the sacrocaudalis dorsalis medialis biopsy is 1 cm off midline and 2 to 5 cm cranial to the tailhead. Weitlaner retractors are placed under the fascia to properly visualize the field and 2 parallel incisions 1 to 2 cm apart are made in the muscle parallel to the axis of the spine. The muscle sample is grasped at one end with forceps and transected proximally with a scalpel or scissors then dissected out at a depth of 1 cm and length of 1.5 to 2 cm.

procedure, the patient feels deep pressure, and sometimes, if the muscle is not relaxed, they can complain of a muscle cramp sensation.[14] The disadvantage of the needle biopsy for fresh samples is that the sample must be received in the laboratory the same day. Too much artifact is introduced when fresh needle biopsy samples are shipped to the laboratory for this technique to be diagnostic for fresh-shipped samples. The needle biopsy technique is ideal for shipping formalin-fixed samples.

Needle biopsy procedure

- A line is drawn from the highest point of the tuber coxae to the tailhead over the middle gluteal muscle. The biopsy site is 20 cm (8 in) from the tuber coxa along this line (**Fig. 5**A, B).
- A 3 cm (1.5 in) square is clipped. On show horses, scissors can be used to hand clip a small area (0.5 cm wide and 1 cm long).
- The area is surgically sterilized. The author avoids povidone iodine because it can cause skin irritation in some horses.
- The subcutaneous tissue is infiltrated with 3 mL of local anesthetic.
- A stab incision through the skin, subcutaneous tissue, and fascia (#11 scalpel blade preferred) is made, and the skin incision is extended to 1 cm (0.25 in).
- The cutting canula is placed into the trocar.

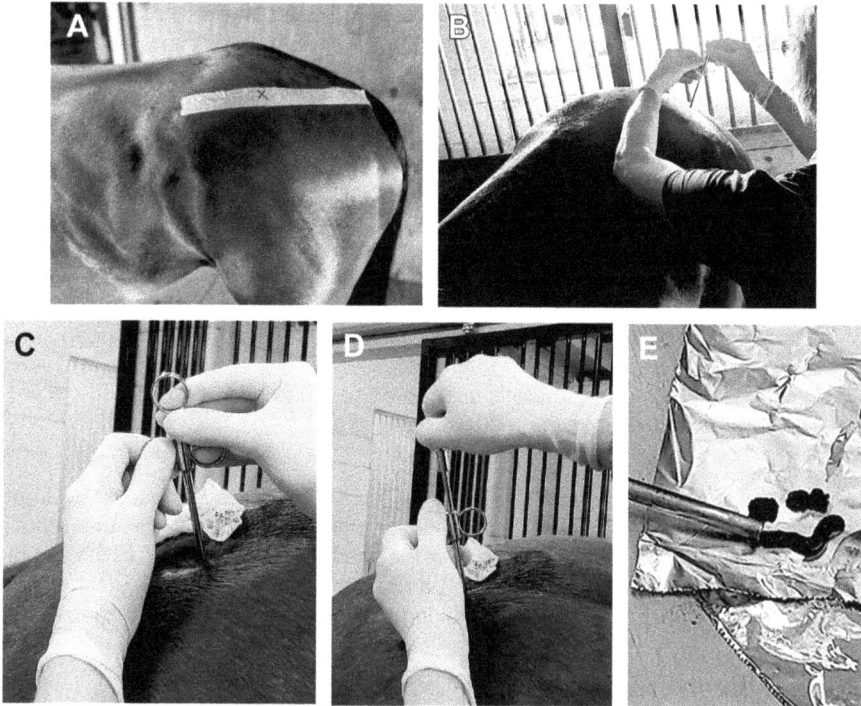

Fig. 5. (*A*) The site for percutaneous needle biopsy of the gluteal muscle is 20 cm along a line from the highest point of the tuber coxa to the point of the tail. (*B*) After surgical skin preparation, local anesthetic and stab incision through skin and subcutis, the canula is placed into the trocar and keeping the canula down in the trocar, the trocar is inserted through the skin. (*C*) With the cutting window pointing toward the operator, the fascia is penetrated with pressure. Once at a depth of 6 cm, the window is turned toward the tuber coxa on the same side as the operator. (*D*) The window is wedged into the muscle by pushing the rings of the trocar away from the operator. The middle finger placed on the needle can be used to maintain the pressure. The trocar is kept still, and the inner canula slid halfway up and pushed down quickly, repeating the cutting motion 5 to 10 times while wedging the window into the muscle. (*E*) The canula is pulled out of the trocar, placed over the foil or cassette, and the stylet inserted into the canula to express the sample.

- Keeping the canula down in the trocar, the trocar is inserted through the skin and, with pressure, through the fascia keeping the cutting window pointing toward the operator (**Fig. 5**C).
- The depth to which the needle is inserted depends upon the size of the horse, in adults the point of the needle is inserted 6 to 8 cm and in foals approximately 3 cm.
- The needle is turned slightly so the cutting window faces the tuber coxa on the same as the operator.
- The window is wedged into the muscle by pushing the rings of the trocar away from the operator. It helps to put the middle finger on the needle to put pressure on the lower part of the needle wedged into the muscle (**Fig. 5**D).
- The trocar is kept still, and the inner canula slid halfway up the length of the trocar and pushed down quickly, repeating the cutting motion 5 to 10 times while

wedging the window into the muscle (see **Fig. 5**D). The needle can be turned slightly to establish pressure against the window, and the cutting motion repeated. The sample moves up into the canula as it is cut.

- The canula is then kept fully inserted in the trocar and the needle removed from the muscle.
- On a table that has tin foil or a tissue cassette, the canula is quickly pulled out of the trocar, placed over the foil or cassette and the stylet inserted into the canula to express the sample (**Fig. 5**E).
- If the sample is not sufficient, the procedure can be repeated through the same incision changing the angle slightly as it is inserted into the muscle. Samples after the initial sample should be checked for appearance to ensure they contain muscle tissue rather than being composed primarily of coagulated blood.
- One simple or cruciate suture is used to close the skin incision site.
- The suture can be removed in 3 to 5 days.
- Horses can go back to work the next day.

Complications are extremely rare with the percutaneous technique and largely comprise hemorrhage from the skin or when an artery is sampled within the muscle. If this happens pressure can be placed over the site and the site sutured. If the sample size is not adequate, the procedure can be repeated in the opposite gluteal muscle using a site 1 cm more medial or cranial along the line used to identify the biopsy site.

SAMPLE PREPARATION FOR SHIPPING SAMPLES
Fresh Samples

Fresh samples should be wrapped in saline moistened (damp but not dripping wet) gauze, put in a sealed nondeformable plastic container, placed on ice packs (ensuring no direct contact of sample with the ice pack), and shipped overnight to arrive in the laboratory within 24 hours. It is vital that samples be kept chilled until they arrive at the laboratory because substrates and enzymes degrade up until the time samples are frozen. If there absolutely must be a delay in shipping the sample, it should be stored in the refrigerator and shipped as soon as possible.

Formalin-Fixed Samples

The muscle sample is left in the air for 5 minutes after biopsy to allow contraction to take place. This avoids contraction artifacts from forming in the fixed tissue.

- Open biopsy samples are trimmed to 1 cm thick cross-sections for adequate penetration of formalin. If adequate sample size is obtained, the sample can be divided and one retained prior to shipping in case of loss during shipping.
- Ideally, percutaneous needle biopsy samples are placed in tissue cassettes prior to formalin-fixation to maintain structural integrity.
- The volume of formalin fixative to use is 10 to 20 times the volume of tissue.
- Samples are placed in 10% neutral buffered formalin that had been purchased within the last 6 months. Fresh formalin is required for adequate immunohisto-chemical staining.
- Formalin containers are sealed with tape, placed in a sealable plastic bag with paper towel to absorb leaks and then that bag is placed into another sealable plastic bag.
- Samples are shipped at room temperature and do not require overnight shipping. Ice packs delay the needed fixation time of approximately 4 days.

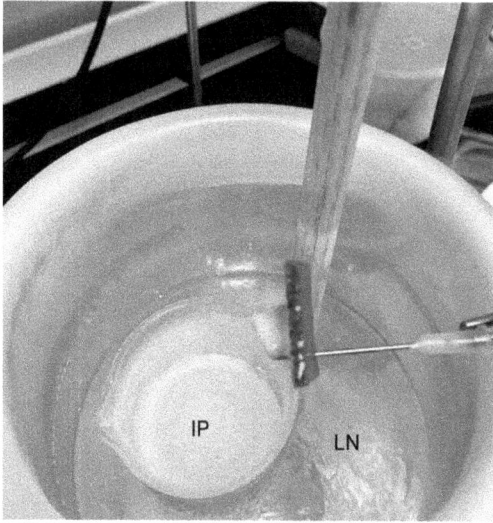

Fig. 6. A muscle sample mounted on cork with OCT media is plunged into isopentane (IP) that has been chilled in liquid nitrogen (LN) when the isopentane reaches a temperature of −155°C.

LABORATORY PREPARATION AND ANALYSIS

There are, in general, 3 means by which muscle tissue can be fixed for evaluation: frozen, formalin-fixed, and fixed for electron microscopy.

Frozen Specimens

Many neuromuscular diagnostic laboratories, particularly those engaged in research, prefer examination of fresh samples that are frozen in the laboratory.[13,15,16]
   Samples for research are usually divided into portions.

- As soon as possible after biopsy, samples for biochemical analysis are plunged directly into liquid nitrogen using forceps and, once completely frozen, placed in chilled cryovials and stored at −80°C.
- Muscle samples for genetic investigations can either be frozen as described earlier or 0.5 cm cubes can be placed in RNAlater (Thermo Fisher Scientific, Walthan, MA),[a] which can be stored at room temperature for up to a week before RNA extraction.
- Samples for histologic analysis are ideally frozen within minutes to hours of sampling the horse. While this is viable if the neuromuscular laboratory is within the same hospital as the patient, more often, fresh samples are shipped on ice packs to neuromuscular laboratories and arrive the following day. Proper freezing and storage of histologic specimens is crucial to avoid producing ice crystal artifacts that create large vacuoles in cells and make interpretation difficult to impossible.[16,17] Samples placed directly in liquid nitrogen even if coated in optimal cutting (OCT) media are not suitable for histopathology because of extensive ice crystal formation in a tissue that contains 80% water.

---

[a] Thermo Fisher Scientific 168 Third Avenue. Waltham, MA, USA 02451.

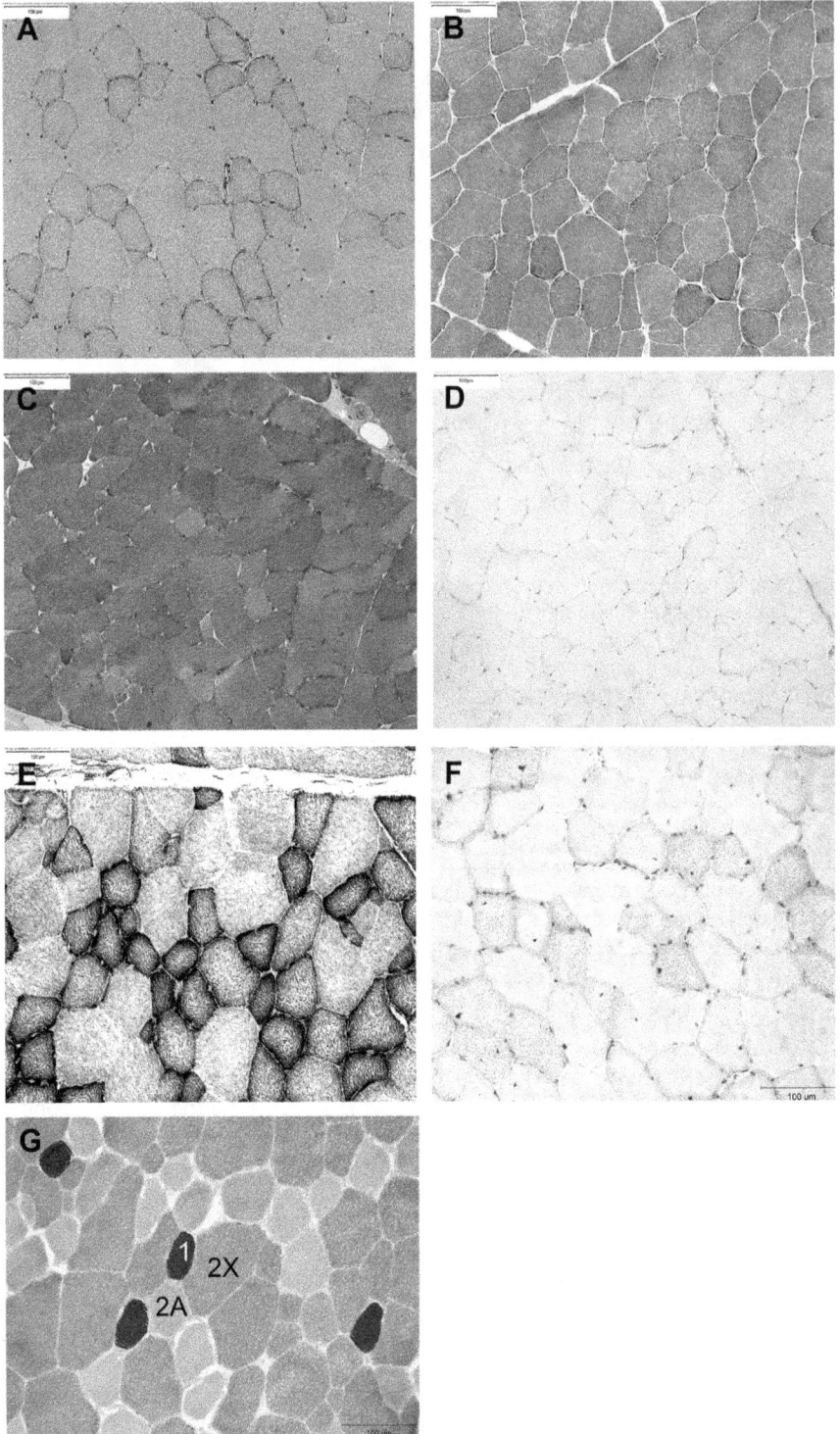

Fig. 7. The battery of stains commonly used on frozen muscle samples (20×). (*A*) Hematoxylin and eosin (HE) is used to evaluate basic tissue organization, cellular structure, and inflammatory infiltrates. (*B*) Modified Gomori trichrome stain is used to identify

Freezing samples

In the laboratory, fresh samples are trimmed, and cross-sectioned muscle is mounted on cork using OCT to cover the bottom of the sample (**Fig. 6**). Isopentane (2-methyl butane) at the appropriate temperature is crucial for freezing samples for histopathology. A beaker containing 50 to 100 mL of isopentane is suspended in a liquid nitrogen-filled Dewar (see **Fig. 6**). When the isopentane reaches $-155°C$ to $-160°C$, reflected by the formation of 0.5 to 1 cm of solid isopentane around the edges of the beaker, the muscle is submerged in the isopentane (see **Fig. 6**). The sample is then placed in a cryostat to allow emersion liquid to completely evaporate and stored in airtight containers at $-80°C$ until sectioned in the cryostat.

Staining of frozen sections

Frozen cryostat cross-sections (5–8 μm) are cut for histologic, histochemical, and immunohistochemical analyses. A battery of stains is routinely performed including[13]

1. Hematoxylin and eosin (HE) for the evaluation of basic tissue organization, cellular structure, and inflammatory infiltrates (**Fig. 7**A).
2. Modified Gomori trichrome stain to identify mitochondrial abnormalities, inclusion bodies and myelin integrity in nerve branches (**Fig. 7**B).
3. Periodic acid–Schiff (PAS) reaction to stain glycogen and other polysaccharides (**Fig. 7**C).
4. Amylase-PAS is used to identify abnormal polysaccharides (**Fig. 7**D).
5. Oil-red-O to identify the amount and distribution of lipid (**Fig. 7**E).
6. Nicotinamide adenine dinucleotide tetrazolium reductase (**Fig. 7**F) or succinate dehydrogenase activity to assess mitochondria and endoplasmic reticulum.
7. Myosin adenosine triphosphatase stain at multiple pH levels to demonstrate contractile fiber types, type 1, 2A, and 2X (**Fig. 7**G).

The advantages of receiving fresh muscle samples are that biochemical and genetic analysis can be performed on snap frozen muscle and frozen sections can be used for a wide variety of histochemical, immunofluorescent, and immunohistochemical stains including those using monoclonal antibodies. The disadvantages of frozen sections are the limited availability of neuromuscular laboratories that cryopreserve samples, the expense of running nonautomated procedures to maintain such laboratories, the expense of shipping chilled samples overnight, and the amount of artifact introduced by shipping fresh samples to the laboratory. It can be difficult to determine if acute myonecrosis, glycogen depletion, and aggregation of glycogen are real or artifacts in fresh-shipped samples.

Formalin-Fixed Specimens

Formalin-fixed paraffin-embedded specimens are used by most traditional pathology laboratories because formalin-fixation maintains more cytologic details than frozen sections and because sectioning and staining can be automated. Further advantages of fixed specimens are that they are not impacted by artifacts introduced by shipping,

---

mitochondrial abnormalities, inclusion bodies, and myelin integrity in nerve branches. (*C*) Periodic acid–Schiff (PAS) stain is used to examine glycogen. (*D*) Amylase-PAS is used to identify abnormal polysaccharides. (*E*) Nicotinamide adenine dinucleotide tetrazolium reductase (NADH-TR) is used to assess mitochondria and endoplasmic reticulum. (*F*) Oil-red-O is used to identify the amount and distribution of lipid. (*G*) Myosin adenosine triphosphatase (ATPase) stain at pH 4.6 is used to identify contractile fiber types, type 1, 2A, and 2X.

they do not require overnight shipping or ice packs, and percutaneous needle biopsy samples can be used. Disadvantages of fixed specimens are that many of the stains described earlier cannot be performed on fixed tissue and they do not provide an opportunity for biochemical, genetic, or monoclonal antibody investigations, thereby hampering the identification of new diseases. Rather than the traditional HE examination used by most pathology services, a neuromuscular diagnostic service using formalin-fixed tissue must routinely use specific tinctorial and immunohistochemical stains to identify known equine muscle disorders.

Preparation of formalin-fixed specimens

Muscle is fixed at room temperature in formalin for 4 days and then trimmed to provide cross-sectioned muscle. Samples are processed on a vacuum infiltrating tissue processor with standard 1 hour incubations in each station at 25°C followed by paraffin embedment. In this process, the tissue is dehydrated to enable embedding with paraffin, which is water insoluble. Paraffin is typically heated to 60°C and then allowed to harden overnight.

Staining of formalin-fixed sections

A microtome is used to section muscle biopsies 4 μm thick. The embedding process must be reversed to remove the paraffin wax from the tissue and to allow water-soluble dyes to

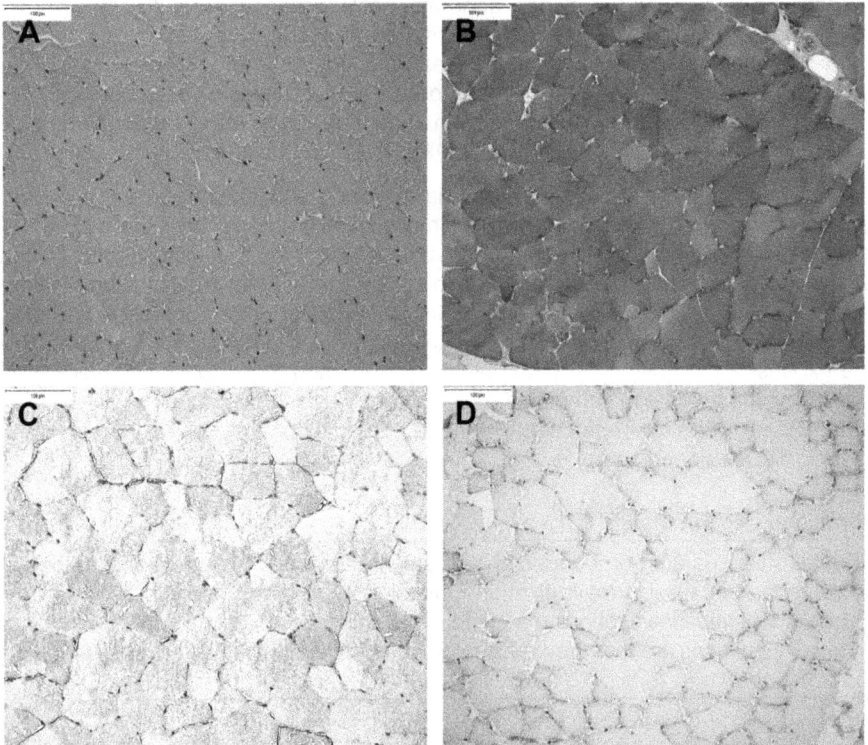

Fig. 8. The battery of stains used to evaluate paraffin-embedded formalin-fixed muscle (20×). (*A*) Hematoxylin and eosin (HE) stain. (*B*) Periodic acid–Schiff (PAS) stain for glycogen. (*C*) Immunohistochemical stain for desmin. (*D*) Immunohistochemical stain for mitochondrial succinate dehydrogenase demonstrating darker staining oxidative fibers and lighter staining low oxidative fibers.

penetrate the sections. Before staining, the slides are "deparaffinized" by running them through xylenes (or substitutes), then alcohols, and then water. Stains used by equine neuromuscular diagnostic laboratories that evaluate formalin-fixed sections include

1. HE for basic tissue organization, cellular structure, and inflammatory infiltrates (**Fig. 8**A).
2. PAS to identify glycogen storage disorders (**Fig. 8**B).
3. Amylase-PAS for the identification of abnormal polysaccharide.
4. Desmin immunohistochemical staining for regenerative fibers, desmin aggregation (**Fig. 8**C).
5. Succinate dehydrogenase A immunohistochemical staining for mitochondria (**Fig. 8**D).

Electron Microscopy

Investigation of new disease may be advanced through ultrastructural evaluation. For electron microscopy, small cubes of muscle (5 mm^2) should be prepared, left in the air for 5 minutes, and then placed in 2.5% glutaraldehyde in 0.1 mol/L sodium cacodylate buffer.

INTERPRETATION OF HISTOPATHOLOGY

Much of the interpretation of muscle histopathology is based on the examiner's previous experience and the recognition of similarities between the histopathology in biopsy sample and known diseases.[16] A systematic approach is required involving the assessment of muscle fiber sizes, fiber shapes, degeneration, inflammation, regeneration, presence of vacuoles, inclusions, and staining for glycogen, lipid, desmin, and mitochondrial morphology.[16] Acute myodegeneration is evident as pale, vacuolated fibers, and chronic myodegeneration as macrophage infiltration of degenerating fibers. Lymphocytic infiltrates are more typical of an inflammatory/immune-mediated disorder. Myogenic atrophy is evident as anguloid atrophied fibers that have concavity on one or more sides and neurogenic atrophy is characterized by angular atrophied fibers that are compressed into angular shapes (**Fig. 9**A, B). The number of fibers with inclusions is assessed and the type of inclusion

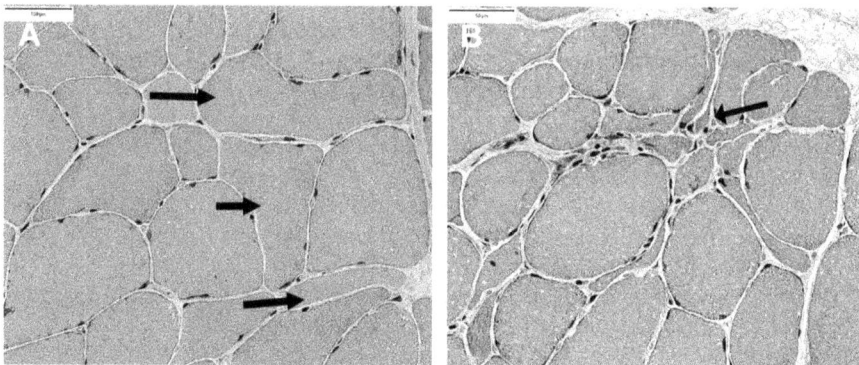

Fig. 9. Hematoxylin eosin stain of cross-sections of skeletal muscle. (*A*) Anguloid atrophy (*arrows*) of muscle fibers showing indentation of one or more sides by adjacent fibers rather than a normal rounded shape. This is common with myogenic forms of muscle atrophy. (*B*) Angular atrophy of muscle fibers (*arrow*) showing extensive loss of myofilaments resulting in a pointed, angular appearance of the muscle fibers. This is common with neurogenic atrophy.

characterized by their staining for glycogen, lipid, desmin, mitochondria, or endoplasmic reticulum. The pattern of staining for mitochondria across fibers and within fibers is assessed. A diagnosis is made by interpreting and correlating histopathologic findings with the signalment, history, and clinical features. The more information the histopathologist is given about the case from the attending veterinarian, the more accurate the final diagnosis will be.

CLINICS CARE POINTS

- The selection of the muscle biopsy site is important for the diagnosis.
- For exertional myopathies, gluteal and semimembranosus sites are best.
- For generalized atrophy, the sacrocaudalis site is best.
- For focal atrophy, that atrophied muscle is best.

DISCLOSURE

S.J. Valberg directs the Valberg Neuromuscular Disease Laboratory (ValbergNMDL.com) and receives remuneration for analyzing muscle biopsies. Her Web site is sponsored by Kentucky Equine Research, and she receives royalties from the type 1 polysaccharide storage myopathy (PSSM1) genetic test and the feed products Releve (Kentucky Equine Research, Versailes, KY) and MFM pellet developed in association with Kentucky Equine Research.

REFERENCES

1. Lindholm A, Piehl K. Fibre composition, enzyme activity and concentrations of metabolites and electrolytes in muscles of standardbred horses. Acta Vet Scand 1974;15:287–309.
2. Snow D, Guy P. Percutaneous needle muscle biopsy in the horse. Equine Vet J 1976;8:150–5.
3. Cardinet GH, Holliday TA. Neuromuscular diseases of domestic animals: a summary of muscle biopsies from 159 cases. Ann N Y Acad Sci 1979;317:290–331.
4. Durward-Akhurst SA. Myosin heavy chain myopathy and immune mediated muscle disorders. In: McKenzie EC, Valberg SJ, editors. Muscle disorders of horses: Veterinary Clinics of North America: equine practice. 2025. p. 61–75.
5. Firshman AC, Valberg SJ. Polysaccharide storage myopathy. In: McKenzie EC, Valberg SJ, editors. Muscle Disorders of horses: an issue of Veterinary Clinics of North America: equine practice. 2025. p. 125–37.
6. Valberg SJ, Mickelson JR, Gallant EM, et al. Exertional rhabdomyolysis in quarter horses and thoroughbreds: one syndrome, multiple aetiologies. Equine Vet J Suppl 1999;30:533–8.
7. Valentine B, Credille K, Lavoie JP, et al. Severe polysaccharide storage myopathy in Belgian and Percheron draught horses. Equine Vet J 1997;29:220–5.
8. Valberg SJ, Henry ML, Perumbakkam S, et al. An E321G MYH1 mutation is strongly associated with nonexertional rhabdomyolysis in Quarter Horses. J Vet Intern Med 2018;32:1718–25.
9. Valentine BA, Divers T, Murphy D, et al. Muscle biopsy diagnosis of equine motor neuron disease and equine polysaccharide storage myopathy. Equine Vet Educ 1998;10:42–50.

10. Bedford HE, Valberg SJ, Firshman AM, et al. Histopathologic findings in the sacrocaudalis dorsalis medialis muscle of horses with vitamin E–responsive muscle atrophy and weakness. J Am Vet Med Assoc 2013;242:1127–37.
11. Finno CJ, Gianino G, Perumbakkam S, et al. A missense mutation in MYH1 is associated with susceptibility to immune-mediated myositis in Quarter Horses. Skelet Muscle 2018;8:7.
12. Aleman M. Brief review of masseter muscle disorders. Equine Vet Educ 2023;35: 305–10.
13. Dubowitz V, Sewry CA, Oldfors A. Muscle biopsy: a practical approach. Philadelphia, PA: Elsevier Health Sciences; 2020.
14. Derry KL, Nicolle MN, Keith-Rokosh JA, et al. Percutaneous muscle biopsies: review of 900 consecutive cases at London Health Sciences Centre. Can J Neurol Sci 2009;36:201–6.
15. Celio MR. Calbindin D-28k and parvalbumin in the rat nervous system. Neuroscience 1990;35:375–475.
16. Meola G, Bugiardini E, Cardani R. Muscle biopsy. J Neurol 2012;259:601–10.
17. Nix JS, Moore SA. What every neuropathologist needs to know: the muscle biopsy. J Neuropathol Exp Neurol 2020;79:719–33.

Disorders of Muscle Mass and Tone

Monica Aleman, MVZ Cert, PhD

KEYWORDS

- Atrophy • Channelopathy • Equine • Myotonia • Paralysis • Sarcopenia

KEY POINTS

- Either primary muscle disease or neurogenic disorders can result in muscle atrophy in horses.
- Primary muscle disease, disuse, metabolic or endocrine disease, chronic administration of corticosteroids, and aging are examples of non-neurogenic muscle atrophy.
- Lower motor neuron disease, nerve root disease, and neuropathies are examples of causes of neurogenic muscle atrophy.
- Causes of muscle tone disorders can be primary (genetic, such as channelopathies) or acquired (eg, electrolytes derangements, ear-tick-associated myotonia).
- Myotonia congenita, myotonic dystrophy, and ear-tick-associated myotonia are myotonic disorders characterized by persistent muscle contraction and delayed relaxation.

INTRODUCTION

Successful locomotion and performance require healthy skeletal muscle in terms of mass, tone, and function.[1] Skeletal muscle comprises about 55% of the horse's body weight.[1] Muscle disorders are an important cause of poor performance and impairment of overall well-being. Breeding for desirable traits such as muscle mass, strength, speed, and endurance has also inadvertently increased the frequency of undesirable traits (muscle disease) particularly in the Quarter Horse and related breeds.[2,3] Clinical manifestations of muscle disorders vary and depend on the etiology ranging from exertional to non-exertional rhabdomyolysis, myalgia, myotonia, myasthenia, fasciculations, stiffness, exercise intolerance, poor performance, postural and gait deficits, and alterations in muscle mass such as atrophy or hypertrophy.[1–3] This article will review disorders causing muscle atrophy and altered tone.

MUSCLE ATROPHY

Normal myofibers have a polygonal shape (**Fig. 1**A) and their size is regulated and influenced by several growth factors such as insulin-like growth factor, myostatin,

SVM: Department of Medicine and Epidemiology, University of California, Davis, Tupper Hall 2108, One Shields Avenue, Davis, CA 95616, USA
E-mail address: mraleman@ucdavis.edu

Vet Clin Equine 41 (2025) 47–60
https://doi.org/10.1016/j.cveq.2024.10.004
0749-0739/25/© 2024 Elsevier Inc. All rights reserved, including for text and data mining, AI training, and similar technologies.

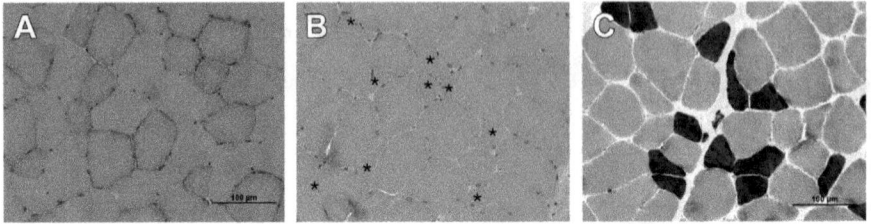

Fig. 1. Skeletal muscle histology. (*A*) Normal muscle tissue. Note myofibers' polygonal shape with multiple nuclei at the periphery on hematoxylin and eosin (H&E) stain in this formalin-fixed specimen. (*B*) Neurogenic muscle atrophy. Note angular myofibers* (sharp pointy edges) in H&E in this fresh-frozen muscle section. (*C*) Selective type 2 myofiber atrophy in a horse due to long-term corticosteroid therapy. Note smaller size of type 2 (*brown*) than type 1 myofibers (*pink*). Some type 2 myofibers display anguloid atrophy. Myofibrillar ATPase preincubation pH 9.8 in fresh-frozen muscle.

signaling pathways, innervation, and workload.[4] Non-neurogenic and neurogenic disorders can result in myofiber atrophy in which the myofiber loses its normal shape due to a reduction in diameter and cross-sectional area.[4] Depending of the underlying cause, both types of myofibers (types 1 and 2) can be affected.[4] Regenerating myofibers are small and must not be confused with atrophy on histologic examination.[4] Non-neurogenic muscle atrophy can occur with disuse, malnutrition, metabolic or endocrine disease, primary muscle disorders, and use of corticosteroids, among others.[4,5] Neurogenic muscle atrophy occurs secondary to a denervating process.[4,6] The distribution of large and small myofibers in a muscle biopsy helps in the distinction of a primary muscle disorder from a denervating process.[4] Atrophy can occur in single myofibers or in clusters.[4] The distribution of large and small myofibers is random and diffuse in myopathies, whereas in denervation atrophy occurs in clusters or large groups.[4] Clusters of small myofibers, characteristic of denervation, are called small group atrophy.[4,6] Similarly, large clusters of small myofibers are called large group atrophy.[4,6]

Changes in myofiber size might affect one or both fiber types (types 1 and 2).[4] A random pattern of atrophic and hypertrophic myofibers of both types might be seen in myopathic disorders, whereas groups of atrophy of both myofiber types and groups of hypertrophic type 1 myofibers are seen in neurogenic disorders.[4] Furthermore, atrophic myofibers adopt an angular shape (with sharp borders like an arrow or star, **Fig. 1**B) in neurogenic processes.[6] Atrophy of type 2 (both 2A and 2B, most commonly 2B, **Fig. 1**C) myofibers occurs in disuse, corticosteroid therapy, aging, and impaired muscle strength secondary to non-myopathic conditions.[4,7] Anguloid type 2 myofibers can be observed in these cases.[5,7] Selective type 1 fiber atrophy has been reported in several congenital myopathies and myotonic dystrophy in humans.[4]

Sarcopenia is a multifactorial geriatric syndrome resulting in loss of muscle mass, tone, and strength due to aging and immobility.[8] Sarcopenia is different to cachexia which is a complex metabolic syndrome associated with chronic illness resulting in loss of muscle mass with or without fat loss, and characterized by inflammation (cytokine-mediated).[8] Causes of muscle atrophy such as vitamin E responsive myopathy,[9] immune-mediated myositis, and neurogenic causes (eg, equine motor neuron disease, nerve root disease, neuropathies) are discussed in other articles in this issue.

MUSCLE TONE DISORDERS

Alterations in muscle tone can be of neurogenic and non-neurogenic origin. Neurologic causes will not be discussed in this article except for neuromyotonia. Myotonic disorders, an important cause of altered muscle tone, are characterized by delayed relaxation after muscle contraction from voluntary movement or following mechanical stimulation such as muscle percussion.[10] Acquired (eg, electrolyte derangements,[11] tick myotonia[12,13]) or primary (eg, genetic[2]) alterations in muscle membrane potential result in changes in cell excitability, which is the main feature of myotonic disorders.[10] In humans, dystrophic and non-dystrophic myotonias with an underlying genetic cause have been documented.[10] Dystrophic myotonias characterized by progressive alterations in muscle tone and atrophy result from nucleotide repeat expansions in different genes; whereas non-dystrophic myotonias (non-progressive with preservation of muscle mass) involve disease variants in sodium and chloride channels.[10] Both, dystrophic and non-dystrophic myotonias have been reported in horses but genetic variants associated with disease have not been identified except for a single case discussed in the following sections.[14–16] The following sections will review disorders affecting muscle function and tone.

MYOTONIC DISORDERS
Myotonia Congenita

Myotonia congenita is usually detected in foals and characterized by prominent musculature with mild to moderate pelvic limb stiffness, a stiff, stilted gait that is more apparent in the pelvic limbs ("bunny hop gait") and more profound at the initiation of exercise.[17] Thigh muscle dimpling can be observed with exercise or percussion upon which muscles remain contracted for a minute or more, followed by delayed relaxation.[17] This form of myotonia is usually not progressive beyond 6 to 12 months of age.[17] An underlying genetic cause is suspected in these foals. A 7-month-old New Forest pony colt with episodes of stiffness, recumbency, and myotonic discharges on electromyography (EMG) was found to have an autosomal recessive missense mutation in the chloride channel (*CLCN1*) gene.[16] This mutation resulted in a substitution of aspartic acid for alanine in codon 592 (c.1775 A>C,p.D592 A) of the C-terminal cytoplasmic domain of the chloride channel.[16] The affected colt was homozygous for this variant.[16] Genetic testing for this specific variant of myotonia is available at the Veterinary Genetics Laboratory at the University of California Davis (https://vgl.ucdavis.edu/). This variant was investigated in Quarter horse foals with non-progressive myotonia but was not found to be responsible for their disease.[3]

Histologic findings in a muscle biopsy from affected horses can vary from normal to showing myofiber size variation with intermixed hypotrophy and hypertrophy and myofibers that are larger than those from age-matched healthy foals.[17] Myotonic discharges ("dive bomber" sound) are a characteristic EMG finding.[17]

Myotonic Dystrophy

A severe progressive myotonic disorder that resembles myotonic dystrophy (DM) in humans has been reported in Quarter Horse, Thoroughbred, and Anglo-Arabian-Sardinian foals.[14,18–22] An underlying genetic etiology is suspected in foals, but this has not been determined. There is a single report of myotonic dystrophy in a Warmblood mare.[23] Myotonic dystrophies are the most common muscular dystrophies in adult humans with two genetically distinct types: type 1 (DM1) and type 2 (DM2) resulting from nucleotide repeat expansions in different genes.[24] DM1 results from CTG repeat expansions in the dystrophia myotonica protein kinase (*DMPK*) gene on chromosome 19, and DM2 from CCTG repeat expansions in the cellular nucleic acid-binding protein (*CNBP*) gene on chromosome 3.[24] Both types are autosomal dominant systemic diseases that generate disease in multiple organs in addition to skeletal muscle with substantial overlap in clinical manifestations.[24] Myotonic dystrophies are characterized by progressive weakness, myotonia, and cardiac conduction abnormalities.[25] Congenital DM1 has severe progressive manifestations including behavior and cognitive alterations, multisystem dysfunction, and reduced life expectancy.[24] Glucose metabolism dysregulation resulting in diabetes mellitus is common,[24] although hypoglycemia can also occur in infants.[26]

In foals, the predominant signs include weakness, generalized myotonia (**Fig. 2**A), percussion myotonia, stiffness, impaired ambulation, retinal dysplasia, lenticular opacities, and testicular hypoplasia in males.[14,18–22] A mixture of hypertrophy and hypertonicity with stiffness of proximal and paraspinal muscles precedes weakness and muscle atrophy as the disease progresses.[14] Myotonic discharges ("dive bomber" sound) resulting from waxing and waning of action potentials in muscle are the classic EMG finding. Histopathological findings include marked myofiber size variation, multiple internal nuclei, loss of myofibers, increased fibrous tissue, fat infiltration, sarcoplasmic masses, and ringbinden, moth-eaten, and whorled fibers.[14,22] A mixture of myofiber atrophy (sometimes in clusters) and hypertrophy is also commonly observed.[14,19,22] Myofiber type grouping and atrophy of both types might be observed. Inflammation is not a feature of myotonic dystrophy.[22] Ultrastructural findings include disruption of Z bands, sarcolemmal loss with glycogen accumulation, and dilation of the sarcotubular system.[19] Sensory and motor nerve conduction studies were reported to be normal in a single case.[19] Prognosis is poor in affected foals.[14,18–22]

Neuromyotonia

Neuromyotonia is a rare progressive nerve disorder characterized by hyperexcitability that causes muscle twitching at rest (myokymia), cramps, impaired muscle relaxation, and spontaneous single motor unit discharges with doublet, triplet, or multiplet morphology on EMG.[27] The etiology in humans can be genetic or acquired (autoimmune).[27] In acquired forms, antibodies bind to potassium channels on the motor nerve. Neuromyotonic and myokymic discharges seen on EMG are abnormal electrical muscular discharges caused by ectopic discharges from motor axons.[28] A 19-month-old colt Quarter Horse cross that presented with stiffness, muscle asymmetry of pelvic limbs of more than 6 months duration, and myokymia of sacrococcygeal,

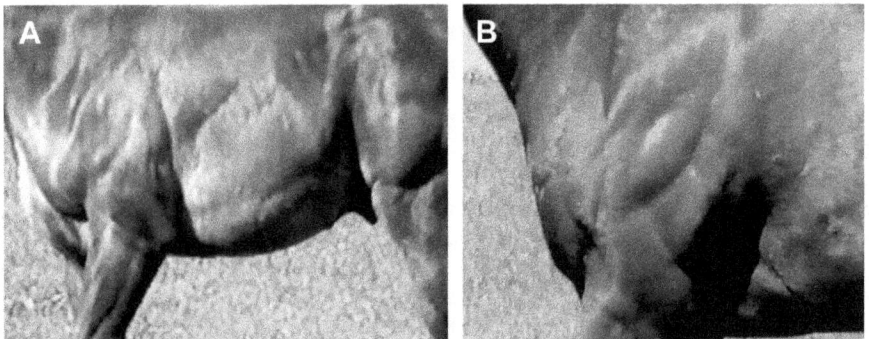

Fig. 2. Myotonic disorders. (A) Foal with myotonic dystrophy. Note marked diffuse sustained muscle contraction. (B) Adult horse with ear-tick-associated myotonia. Note marked sustained contraction of triceps muscle. ([A] *Courtesy of* Dr. Sharon J. Spier, DVM, PhD, Diplomate ACVIM.)

paravertebral, and gluteal muscles was diagnosed with neuromyotonia.[29] Myokymia manifests as a continuous undulating or wave-like movement of the overlying skin.[27,29] Spontaneous fibrillation potentials, positive sharp waves, fasciculation potentials, and complex repetitive discharges were observed on EMG in muscles at rest.[29] Muscle biopsy revealed mixed neurogenic and myopathic alterations.[29] Variations in myofiber size, hypertrophy, small anguloid myofibers in groups, myofiber splitting, internal nuclei, and increased endomysial connective tissue were seen in this single case.[29] Neuromyotonia has been suspected in horses.[30,31] Long-term follow-up of these cases is not available.

Tick Myotonia

Tick myotonia is an acquired myotonic disorder in horses caused by infestation with the ear tick *Otobius megnini*.[12] Intermittent painful spontaneous or induced (eg, movement, percussion) muscle contractions of various muscles including pectoral, triceps (**Fig. 2**B), abdominal, semitendinosus, semimembranosus, and quadriceps can occur.[12] Signs mimic those of colic (eg, pawing, sweating, flank-watching), and in severe cases, recumbency can occur.[12] Episodes can last a few minutes to hours. Mild to moderate rhabdomyolysis is often seen with serum creatine kinase activities ranging from 4000 to 170,000 IU/L.[12] Treatment consists of removing ear ticks and treating the ear canals topically with pyrethrins and piperonyl butoxide. Relief of clinical signs occurs within hours to a couple of days.

Channelopathies

Ion channels are transmembrane glycoproteins located in the surface of the cell or intracellular organelles (eg, mitochondria, endoplasmic, or sarcoplasmic reticulum) formed by functional subunits that aggregate to form an aqueous pore that allows passage of ions.[32,33] Depending on their mode of activation, channels can be classified as non-gated and gated channels.[33] The non-gated channels allow the passive flux of ions through a concentration gradient which include Na^+, K^+, and Cl^- channels.[33] The gated channels are further subdivided into voltage-gated, ligand-gated, proton-gated, mechanically-gated, and second messenger-gated.[33] Channels can have three different states which include opened (activated) when triggered, and two closed states: inactivated and resting.[33] The inactivated state is a refractory period that occurs immediately after opening and during which ions will not pass through.[33] The voltage-gated ion channels are activated and inactivated by changes in membrane action potential. These channels are named according to the principal ion conducted: Na^+, K^+, Ca^{2+}, or Cl^-.[33]

Channelopathies are a heterogenous group of disorders of ion channels that lead to abnormal cell excitability (decrease, increase) usually manifesting as episodic events.[34–36] Channelopathies can involve various body organs/systems (eg, nervous, skeletal and cardiac muscle, gastrointestinal, and others). The focus in this section is on skeletal muscle. Skeletal muscle channelopathies can be primary (genetic) or secondary (acquired).[22,34] Channelopathies causing delayed muscle relaxation result in dysfunction characterized by myotonia, whereas those causing transient membrane inactivation result in periodic weakness (periodic paralysis).[34] In humans, non-dystrophic myotonias include myotonia congenita, paramyotonia congenita, and sodium-channel myotonia, among others.[34] Periodic paralysis disorders include hyperkalemic, normokalemic, hypokalemic, or late-onset periodic paralyses.[34] It is important to mention that for the diagnosis of diseases with a genetic basis, tissue samples must be submitted to licensed laboratories which use strictly validated tests of confirmed genetic variants associated with or causing disease (https://vgl.ucdavis.edu/).

Hyperkalemic Periodic Paralysis

Hyperkalemic periodic paralysis (HYPP), a channelopathy resembling hyperkalemic periodic paralysis in humans,[37] is an inherited autosomal dominant disease of horses caused by a missense mutation of the skeletal muscle sodium channel gene (*SCN4A*, **Fig. 3**A).[38,39] The first clinical descriptions of HYPP in Quarter Horses were made in the 1980s, but a genetic variant causing disease was not identified until 1992.[40–42] Since then, related breeds such as Paints, Appaloosas, and Quarter Horse-crossbreds have been documented with HYPP. A prevalence of 4% has been estimated for this condition in the Quarter Horse breed with most of the affected horses being of halter lineage.[38,43] Carrying even a single copy of the allele can impart susceptibility to disease.[44,45] The base-pair missense mutation (C to G) results in a phenylalanine/leucine substitution in the alpha subunit of the voltage-dependent sodium channel of skeletal muscle in chromosome 11.[39] This mutation causes failure of inactivation following activation of the sodium channel, leading to persistent depolarization with inward flux of sodium and outward flux of potassium manifested as muscle fasciculations and eventually paralysis from loss of membrane electrical excitability.[46]

Clinical signs range from asymptomatic to episodes of tachycardia, tachypnea, and diffuse or patchy muscle fasciculations (commonly neck, shoulders, flank), changes in muscle tone, sweating, weakness, collapse, and recumbency.[46] Horses with mild episodes remain standing, while those with severe signs might stagger, sway, and collapse.[40] Laryngeal paralysis and death can occur in severe cases.[44] Episodes usually last a few minutes to an hour and horses remain relatively bright and alert, except during severe episodes in which horses appear distressed.[44] Both heterozygous (N/H) and homozygous (H/H) animals display signs with homozygotes having a more severe phenotype in terms of severity and frequency of signs.[44,46] Age at onset of first signs can range from the neonatal period in homozygous foals to 2 or 3 years of age, often at a time when training has been initiated.[41,44,47] Dysphagia, dysphonia, dyspnea, laryngopalatal edema and displacement, respiratory stridor, and periodic laryngeal collapse due to paralysis causing respiratory distress can be observed as early as the neonatal period and in older homozygous foals.[44] Heterozygous foals are less severely affected and usually do not show signs until they are weaned.[44] General anesthesia can also induce episodes of paralysis. Protrusion of the third eyelids during clinical episodes has been reported more often in homozygous horses.

Clinical manifestations can occur spontaneously or can be associated with fasting, sudden changes in diet, stress, transportation, exposure to extreme environmental temperatures, and general anesthesia, among other factors. Diets providing greater than 1.1% potassium dry matter (DM) on a daily basis can precipitate episodes.[48] High-potassium diets include alfalfa, molasses, kelp-based supplements, and other supplements containing potassium.[48]

The definitive diagnosis of HYPP is achieved through the identification of the genetic variant causing disease in whole blood or hair roots by a licensed laboratory (https://vgl.ucdavis.edu/). Electromyography reveals fibrillation potentials, complex repetitive discharges (**Fig. 3**B), and occasionally myotonic discharges with trains of doublets between episodes.[46,49,50] Although the most common EMG finding between and during episodes is complex repetitive discharges[46,49], this abnormality is not exclusively found in cases of HYPP and other possible causes must be ruled out. Creatine kinase is usually normal or mildly to moderately elevated following an episode.[46] Histologic findings can range from normal to non-specific abnormalities such as vacuolation of type 2B

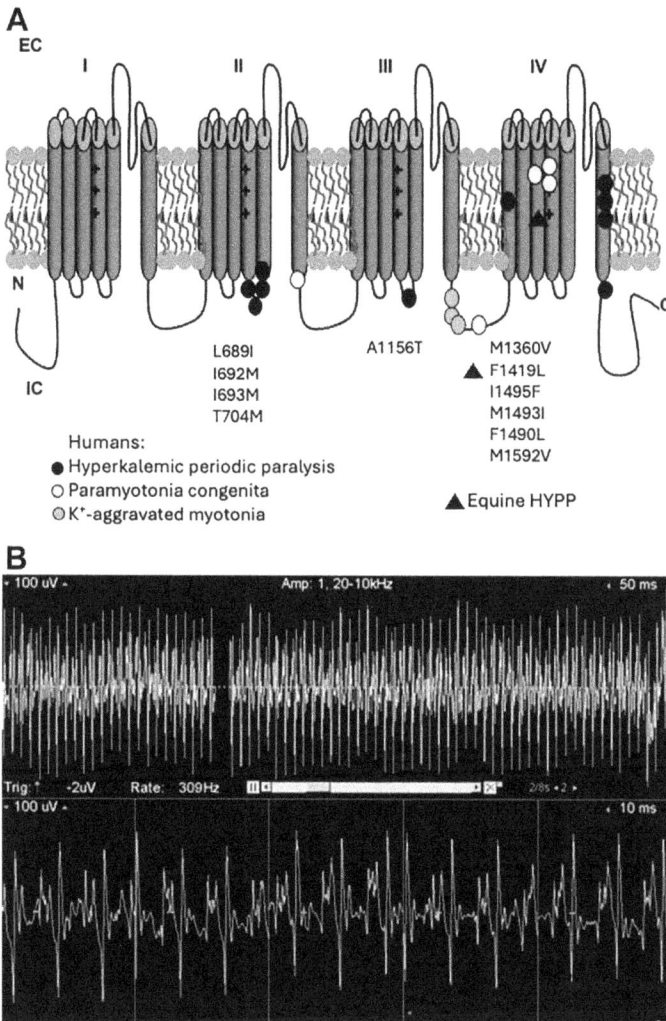

Fig. 3. Hyperkalemic periodic paralysis. (*A*) Representation of the voltage-gated sodium channel of skeletal muscle displaying the various regions of the channel with variants causing disease in humans (*circles: black* indicating hyperkalemic periodic paralysis). The equine variant is represented by a black triangle in the alpha subunit of the channel. EC, extracellular space, IC, intracellular space, I, II, III, IV = 4 functional subunits that form the sodium channel. Black circle = human hyperkalemic periodic paralysis (HYPP), yellow circle = human paramyotonia congenita, green circle = potassium-aggravated myotonia, black triangle = equine HYPP. (*B*) EMG showing complex repetitive discharges. (M. Aleman, A review of equine muscle disorders, Neuromuscular Disorders, 18 (4), 2008, 277-287, https://doi.org/10.1016/j.nmd.2008.01.001.)

myofibers and myodegeneration.[46] Marked hyperkalemia ranging from 5 to 9 mmol/L during an episode can be found.[46] Electrocardiogram shows absent or low-amplitude P waves, wide QRS complex, and tall T waves during episodes of hyperkalemia.[46]

Dietary modification to reduce potassium content such as utilizing late cuts of Timothy or Bermuda grass hay, grains (oat, corn, barley, wheat), beet pulp, or adding lite karo syrup (60–120 mL a day) to stimulate insulin-mediated movement of potassium might be beneficial to prevent occurrence of episodes.[51] Soaking hay can effectively reduce potassium by 40%.[52] Avoid feeds high in potassium such as alfalfa hay, soybean, and molasses. Horses with recurrent episodes should be fed balanced diets with <33 g of potassium/day.[51] Mild exercise might alleviate mild episodes of paralysis.[51] Pasture or access to a corral or turnout time with regular exercise, along with dietary modification might help in preventing episodes.[51]

During episodes, the administration of 5% dextrose solution intravenous (IV) (6 mL/kg) alone or followed by sodium bicarbonate IV (1–2 mmol/kg) can provoke potassium to move intracellularly.[51] Calcium gluconate 20 to 23% IV (0.2–0.4 mL/kg) diluted in 1 L of 5% dextrose often provides rapid improvement.[51] Loop diuretics such as furosemide (0.5–1 mg/kg IV, Salix, Merck Animal Health) to enhance potassium excretion can be used in moderate to severe cases (ensure hydration is maintained). In urgent situations, epinephrine (3 mL of 1:1000/500 kg) can be administered intramuscularly (IM) followed by solutions that will mobilize potassium into the cell. For cases with repeated episodes, acetazolamide orally (3 mg/kg q8-12h) or hydrochlorothiazide PO (0.5–1 mg/kg q12h) might be required in addition to dietary modification.[51] In cases of dyspnea or laryngeal paralysis, an emergency tracheostomy is indicated.[44,51] Breeding horses should be tested for the variant to prevent producing affected offspring and to ensure the overall long-term health of the Quarter Horse and related breeds.[41,42,51]

Malignant Hyperthermia

Malignant hyperthermia (MH) is a life-threatening pharmacogenetic disorder of skeletal muscle triggered by halogenated anesthetics, depolarizing muscle relaxants, and stress.[53] A genetic basis has been reported in humans, pigs, dogs, and horses.[53–57] An autosomal dominant single missense point mutation (C7360 G) in exon 46 of the ryanodine receptor 1 (RyR1) gene, generating a R2454 G amino acid substitution has been identified in Quarter horses and Paints with MH.[3,57,58] The ryanodine receptor 1 is the calcium release channel of the sarcoplasmic reticulum of skeletal muscle. Dysfunction of this receptor results in excessive release of calcium into the myoplasm which triggers a cascade of serial events that lead to a hypermetabolic state and hyperthermia, ultimately leading to cell death. Other co-variants can occur with the RyR1 variant.[3] These include those causing polysaccharide storage myopathy 1 (GYS1 gene), myosin heavy chain myopathy (MYH1), and glycogen branching enzyme deficiency (GBE1).[3] Genetic testing for MH is offered at https://vgl.ucdavis.edu/ and will aid in responsible breeding practices and prevention of fatal events.

In horses, both anesthetic-triggered and non-anesthetic-triggered forms of MH can occur.[59] Anesthetic triggers include halogenated anesthetics such as halothane (no longer under routine use and not commercially available) and isoflurane, and depolarizing muscle relaxants (succinylcholine).[60–62] Non-anesthetic triggers include stress including environmental stress (heat), exercise, breeding, and concurrent illnesses and myopathies.[59] Clinical and laboratory abnormalities are similar in both forms.[59] Triggered clinical manifestations include hyperacute rhabdomyolysis, muscle rigidity, stiffness, sweating, recumbency, and death.[59] Historically, some fatal cases had intermittent or persistent mild elevations of creatine kinase activity.[59]

Under anesthesia, the first signs noted are contracted pinnae, flared nostrils, third eyelid protrusion, severely retracted eye globe, trismus, tachycardia, rapidly progressive increase in body temperature (>40–45°C [>104–113°F]), followed by rapid generalized muscle contracture.[59,63] The most common abnormalities during an anesthetic-triggered MH episode include acidemia (pH 6.5–6.9, reference range 7.35–7.42) due to combined respiratory and metabolic acidosis (PaCO$_2$ > 69–274 mm Hg, base deficit >

8 mmol/L), severe hypoxemia despite mechanical ventilation with 100% oxygen (PaO_2 <122 mm Hg, reference range 400–500 mm Hg), and hypertension (mean arterial pressure >100–130 mm Hg).[59] Laboratory abnormalities include increased hematocrit, hyperproteinemia, hyperglycemia, azotemia, electrolyte derangements, and mildly elevated serum creatinine activities.[59] Similar abnormalities are found in non-anesthetic-triggered MH with hyperlactatemia (12–30 mmol/L, reference range <2 mmol/L) and higher creatine kinase activities. Necropsy reveals generalized rhabdomyolysis and adrenal hyperplasia.[59] Myopathic alterations include myonecrosis, hypercontracted myofibers, glycogen depletion, and edema.[59]

Avoiding anesthesia with halogenated anesthetics in horses with known MH susceptibility based on genetic testing is advisable. If anesthesia is required, treatment with oral dantrolene at 2 to 4 mg/kg one to two hours prior to anesthesia might aid in the prevention of MH (but also requires the provision of some food to aid intestinal absorption of this drug). If MH is triggered, discontinuation of anesthesia, administration of 100% oxygen, and rapid cooling (eg, IV fluids, cold hosing, and ice packs) is recommended. Administration of dantrolene sodium IV is the emergency drug of choice in human medicine but not readily available in veterinary hospitals.

Electrolyte Derangements

Electrolyte derangements can alter membrane potentials and function of ion channels at the neuromuscular junction at multiple levels, including the presynaptic membrane (nerve ending), synaptic space, and postsynaptic membrane (muscle membrane).[11] Derangement can impair conduction of nerve impulses, muscle contraction, regulation of cell volume, and cell signaling, resulting in alterations in muscle function and tone. Fasciculations, weakness or rigidity, hypertonia or hypotonia might be observed depending on the electrolyte(s) abnormality. Electrolyte analysis must include sodium, potassium, chloride, and the physiologically active ionized calcium and magnesium fractions which are essential for the function of muscle. Because hydrogen ions compete with ionized calcium and magnesium for binding sites on albumin and other proteins, alterations in pH can alter concentrations of these ions.[64,65] Critically ill patients such as those with septicemia, endotoxemia, and severe gastrointestinal disease are more likely to develop calcium and magnesium dysregulation.[66]

Hypocalcemia

Severe hypocalcemia also referred as hypocalcemic tetany due to its clinical similarities to tetanus,[67] results from the loss or lack of available calcium, particularly ionized calcium. Clinical hypocalcemia manifests as muscle fasciculations, tremors, colic and abdominal distension due to ileus, colic-like signs due to muscle pain, and diaphragmatic flutter, sweating, arrhythmias, dysphagia, salivation, and high-stepping gait.[68] Trismus, tetanic spasms, and rigidity ("tetany") have been observed with serum total calcium concentrations of 5 to 8 mg/dL.[68] Seizure-like activity, seizures, staggering, ataxia, and recumbency leading to death have been observed with serum total calcium less than 5 mg/dL.[68] Total serum calcium does not reflect ionized hypocalcemia; however, moderately to profoundly low total serum calcium (4–6 mg/dL) with normal total protein and albumin support hypocalcemia as the clinical diagnosis.

Hypocalcemia has been reported in heavily lactating mares, late pregnancy, horses in hard or prolonged work or undergoing prolonged transportation, excessive sweating, acute renal failure, gastrointestinal disease, primary hypoparathyroidism, oxalate toxicity, ingestion of blister beetle, and administration of tetracyclines, magnesium, rectal enemas with high content of phosphorus, and bisphosphonates.[69–77] Recently, a nonsense variant in Rap guanine nucleotide exchange factor 5 (*RAPGEF5* c.2624 C>A,p.Ser875*) was found to be associated with equine familial isolated hypoparathyroidism in Thoroughbred foals.[78] This disease variant causes tetany and seizures and is invariably fatal.[78] Pedigree analysis supported an autosomal recessive mode of inheritance and fatal cases were homozygous for the variant.[78]

Spontaneous muscle activity such as positive sharp waves, fibrillation potentials, doublets, triplets, and multiplets, and complex repetitive discharges can be seen in hypocalcemic horses on EMG.[31] Treatment of hypocalcemia consists of slow IV administration of calcium solutions such as 20 to 23% calcium gluconate at 0.5 to 1 mL/kg (eg, 250–500 mL/500 kg), ideally diluted 1:4 with saline or dextrose. A second dose 15 to 30 minutes later can be administered if signs persist.

SUMMARY

Neurogenic and non-neurogenic disorders, and genetic versus acquired causes of alterations in muscle mass and tone must be considered in horses with compatible clinical signs. Diagnosis of causes of altered muscle tone and atrophy requires careful clinical examination and appropriate diagnostic modalities to accurately determine etiology, treatment if available, and prognosis.

CLINICS CARE POINTS

- Neurogenic (neuropathies) and non-neurogenic (disuse, myopathies) disorders can result in muscle atrophy.
- Genetic (channelopathies) and acquired (tick myotonia) disorders can result in alterations of muscle tone.

DISCLOSURES

Nothing to disclose.

REFERENCES

1. Valberg SJ. Muscle conditions affecting sport horses. Vet Clin North Am Equine Pract 2018;34:253–76.
2. Valberg SJ. Genetics of equine muscle disease. Vet Clin North Am Equine Pract 2020;36:353–78.
3. Aleman M, Scalco R, Malvick J, et al. Prevalence of genetic mutations in horses with muscle disease from a neuromuscular disease laboratory. J Equine Vet Sci 2022;118:104129.
4. Dubowitz V, Sewry CA, Oldfors A. Histological and histochemical changes. In: Dubowitz V, Sewry CA, Oldfors A, editors. Muscle biopsy: a practical approach. 5th ed. China: Elsevier; 2021. p. 46–77.
5. Aleman M, Watson JL, Williams DC, et al. Myopathy in horses with pituitary pars intermedia dysfunction (Cushing's disease). Neuromuscul Disord 2006;16:737–44.
6. Dickinson PJ, LeCouteur RA. Muscle and nerve biopsy. Vet Clin North Am Small Anim Pract 2002;32:63–102.
7. Aleman M, Nieto JE. Gene expression of proteolytic systems and growth regulators of skeletal muscle in horses with myopathy associated with pituitary pars intermedia dysfunction. Am J Vet Res 2010;71:664–70.

8. Rolland Y, Abellan van Kan G, Gillette-Guyonnet S, et al. Cachexia versus sarcopenia. Curr Opin Clin Nutr Metab Care 2011;14:15–21.

9. Bedford HE, Valberg SJ, Firshman AM, et al. Histopathologic findings in the sacrocaudalis dorsalis medialis muscle of horses with vitamin E-responsive muscle atrophy and weakness. J Am Vet Med Assoc 2013;242:1127–37.

10. Montagnese F, Schoser B. [Dystrophic and non-dystrophic myotonias]. Fortschr Neurol Psychiatr 2018;86:575–83.

11. Aleman M. Miscellaneous neurologic or neuromuscular disorders in horses. Vet Clin North Am Equine Pract 2011;27:481–506.

12. Madigan JE, Valberg SJ, Ragle C, et al. Muscle spasms associated with ear tick (Otobius megnini) infestations in five horses. J Am Vet Med Assoc 1995; 207:74–6.

13. Miller SM. Putative Otobius megnini-associated clinical signs in horses in South Africa (2012-2018). J S Afr Vet Assoc 2020;91:e1–6.

14. Reed SM, Hegreberg GA, Bayly WM, et al. Progressive myotonia in foals resembling human dystrophia myotonica. Muscle Nerve 1988;11:291–6.

15. Steinberg S, Botelho S. Myotonia in a horse. Science 1962;137:979–80.

16. Wijnberg ID, Owczarek-Lipska M, Sacchetto R, et al. A missense mutation in the skeletal muscle chloride channel 1 (CLCN1) as candidate causal mutation for congenital myotonia in a New Forest pony. Neuromuscul Disord 2012;22:361–7.

17. Schooley EK, MacLeay JM, Cuddon P, et al. Myotonia congenita in a foal. J Equine Vet Sci 2004;24:483–8.

18. Hegreberg GA, Reed SM. Skeletal muscle changes associated with equine myotonic dystrophy. Acta Neuropathol 1990;80:426–31.

19. Montagna P, Liguori R, Monari L, et al. Equine muscular dystrophy with myotonia. Clin Neurophysiol 2001;112:294–9.

20. Shirakawa T, Ide M, Taniyama H, et al. Muscular dystrophy-like disease in a thoroughbred foal. J Comp Pathol 1989;100:287–94.

21. Jamison JM, Baird JD, Smith-Maxie LL, et al. A congenital form of myotonia with dystrophic changes in a quarterhorse. Equine Vet J 1987;19:353–8.

22. Aleman M. A review of equine muscle disorders. Neuromuscul Disor 2008;18: 277–87.

23. Ludvikova E, Lukas Z, Vondracek P, et al. Histopathological features in subsequent muscle biopsies in a warmblood mare with myotonic dystrophy. Vet Quarterly 2012;32:187–92.

24. Soltanzadeh P. Myotonic dystrophies: a genetic overview. Genes 2022;13.

25. Liao Q, Zhang Y, He J, et al. Global prevalence of myotonic dystrophy: an updated systematic review and meta-analysis. Neuroepidemiology 2022;56: 163–73.

26. Thomas MT, Shah S, Popat H, et al. Hypoglycaemia and myotonic dystrophy. J Paediatr Child Health 2022;58:713–4.

27. Zandi MS. Neuromyotonia. Handb Clin Neurol 2024;203:205–10.

28. Katirji B. Peripheral nerve hyperexcitability. Handb Clin Neurol 2019;161:281–90.

29. Zakia LS, Palumbo MIP, Teixeira RBC, et al. Neuromyotonia in a horse. J Vet Intern Med 2019;33:287–91.

30. Wijnberg ID, Franssen H, Jansen GH, et al. Quantitative electromyographic examination in myogenic disorders of 6 horses. J Vet Intern Med 2003;17:185–93.

31. Wijnberg ID, van der Kolk JH, Franssen H, et al. Electromyographic changes of motor unit activity in horses with induced hypocalcemia and hypomagnesemia. Am J Vet Res 2002;63:849–56.

32. Spillane J, Kullmann DM, Hanna MG. Genetic neurological channelopathies: molecular genetics and clinical phenotypes. J Neurol Neurosurg Psychiatry 2016;87: 37–48.

33. Bernard G, Shevell MI. Channelopathies: a review. Pediatr Neurol 2008;38:73–85.

34. Vicino A, Brugnoni R, Maggi L. Diagnostics in skeletal muscle channelopathies. Expert Rev Mol Diagn 2023;23:1175–93.

35. Vivekanandam V, Jayaseelan D, Hanna MG. Muscle channelopathies. Handb Clin Neurol 2023;195:521–32.

36. Vivekanandam V, Munot P, Hanna MG, et al. Skeletal muscle channelopathies. Neurol Clin 2020;38:481–91.

37. Sekhon DS, Vaqar S, Gupta V. Hyperkalemic periodic paralysis. StatPearls. Treasure Island (FL): StatPearls Publishing LLC.; 2024.

38. Bowling AT, Byrns G, Spier S. Evidence for a single pedigree source of the hyperkalemic periodic paralysis susceptibility gene in quarter horses. Anim Genet 1996;27:279–81.

39. Spier SJ, Carlson GP, Harrold D, et al. Genetic study of hyperkalemic periodic paralysis in horses. J Am Vet Med Assoc 1993;202:933–7.

40. Cox JH, De Bowes RM. Episodic weakness caused by hyperkalemic periodic paralysis in horses. Equine Vet Educ 1990;12:83–9.

41. Rudolph JA, Spier SJ, Byrns G, et al. Linkage of hyperkalaemic periodic paralysis in quarter horses to the horse adult skeletal muscle sodium channel gene. Anim Genet 1992;23:241–50.

42. Rudolph JA, Spier SJ, Byrns G, et al. Periodic paralysis in quarter horses: a sodium channel mutation disseminated by selective breeding. Nat Genet 1992;2: 144–7.

43. Tryon RC, Penedo MC, McCue ME, et al. Evaluation of allele frequencies of inherited disease genes in subgroups of American Quarter Horses. J Am Vet Med Assoc 2009;234:120–5.

44. Carr EA, Spier SJ, Kortz GD, et al. Laryngeal and pharyngeal dysfunction in horses homozygous for hyperkalemic periodic paralysis. J Am Vet Med Assoc 1996; 209:798–803.

45. Finno CJ, Spier SJ, Valberg SJ. Equine diseases caused by known genetic mutations. Vet J 2009;179:336–47.

46. Spier SJ, Carlson GP, Holliday TA, et al. Hyperkalemic periodic paralysis in horses. J Am Vet Med Assoc 1990;197:1009–17.

47. Naylor JM, Robinson JA, Bertone J. Familial incidence of hyperkalemic periodic paralysis in quarter horses. J Am Vet Med Assoc 1992;200:340–3.

48. Reynolds JA, Potter GD, Green LW, et al. Genetic-diet interactions in the hyperkalemic periodic paralysis syndrome in Quarter horses fed varying amounts of potassium: III. The relationship between plasma potassium concentration and HYPP symptoms. J Equine Vet Sci 1998;18:731–5.

49. Naylor JM. Equine hyperkalemic periodic paralysis: review and implications. Can Vet J 1994;35:279–85.

50. Naylor JM, Robinson JA, Crichlow EC, et al. Inheritance of myotonic discharges in American quarter horses and the relationship to hyperkalemic periodic paralysis. Can J Vet Res 1992;56:62–6.

51. Spier S. Hyperkalemic periodic paralysis: 14 years later52. San Antonio: Proceeding 69th Annual Convention of the American Association of Equine Practitioners; 2006. p. 347–50.

52. Owens TG, Barnes M, Gargano VM, et al. Nutrient content changes from steaming or soaking timothy-alfalfa hay: effects on feed preferences and acute glycemic response in Standardbred racehorses1. J Anim Sci 2019;97:4199–207.
53. McCarthy TV, Healy JM, Heffron JJ, et al. Localization of the malignant hyperthermia susceptibility locus to human chromosome 19q12-13.2. Nature 1990;343: 562–4.
54. Fujii J, Otsu K, Zorzato F, et al. Identification of a mutation in porcine ryanodine receptor associated with malignant hyperthermia. Science 1991;253:448–51.
55. Haluskova J, Holeckova B, Kokulova L, et al. Detection of the T1640C RYR1 mutation indicating malignant hyperthermia in dogs. Vet Med 2023;68:428–34.
56. Roberts MC, Mickelson JR, Patterson EE, et al. Autosomal dominant canine malignant hyperthermia is caused by a mutation in the gene encoding the skeletal muscle calcium release channel (RYR1). Anesthesiology 2001;95:716–25.
57. Aleman M, Riehl J, Aldridge BM, et al. Association of a mutation in the ryanodine receptor 1 gene with equine malignant hyperthermia. Muscle Nerve 2004;30: 356–65.
58. McCue ME, Valberg SJ, Jackson M, et al. Polysaccharide storage myopathy phenotype in quarter horse-related breeds is modified by the presence of an RYR1 mutation. Neuromuscul Disor 2009;19:37–43.
59. Aleman M, Nieto JE, Magdesian KG. Malignant hyperthermia associated with ryanodine receptor 1 (C7360G) mutation in Quarter Horses. J Vet Intern Med 2009;23:329–34.
60. Hildebrand SV, Howitt GA. Succinylcholine infusion associated with hyperthermia in ponies anesthetized with halothane. Am J Vet Res 1983;44:2280–4.
61. Riedesel DH, Hildebrand SV. Unusual response following use of succinylcholine in a horse anesthetized with halothane. J Am Vet Med Assoc 1985;187:507–8.
62. Hildebrand S. Neuromuscular blocking agents in equine anesthesia. Vet Clin North Am Equine Pract 1990;6:587–606.
63. Aleman M, Brosnan RJ, Williams DC, et al. Malignant hyperthermia in a horse anesthetized with halothane. J Vet Intern Med 2005;19:363–6.
64. Wang S, McDonnell EH, Sedor FA, et al. pH effects on measurements of ionized calcium and ionized magnesium in blood. Arch Pathol Lab Med 2002;126: 947–50.
65. Eatough DJ, Jensen TE, Hansen LD, et al. The binding of Ca2+ and Mg2+ to human serum albumin: a calorimetric study. Thermochim Acta 1978;25:289–97.
66. Hurcombe SD, Toribio RE, Slovis NM, et al. Calcium regulating hormones and serum calcium and magnesium concentrations in septic and critically ill foals and their association with survival. J Vet Intern Med 2009;23:335–43.
67. Kay G, Knottenbelt DC. Tetanus in equids: a report of 56 cases. Equine Vet Educ 2007;19:107–12.
68. Barreto-Junior RA, Minervino AH, Rodrigues FA, et al. Clinical presentation and biochemical profile of horses during induction and treatment of hypocalcemia. Austral J Vet Sci 2017;1:9–14.
69. Yocom A, Contino E, Kawcak C. Review of the mechanism of action and use of bisphosphonates in horses. J Equine Vet Sci 2023;127:104503.
70. Bischoff K. Cantharidin. Vet Clin North Am Equine Pract 2024;40:113–9.
71. Baird JD. Lactation tetany (eclampsia) in a Shetland pony mare. Aust Vet J 1971; 47:402–4.
72. Herbert EW, Dittmer KE. Acute and chronic oxalate toxicity in Miniature horses associated with soursob (Oxalis pes-caprae) ingestion. Equine Vet Educ 2017; 29:549–57.

73. Bowen JM, McMullan WC. Influence of induced hypermagnesemia and hypocalcemia on neuromuscular blocking property of oxytetracycline in the horse. Am J Vet Res 1975;36:1025–8.
74. Toribio RE. Disorders of calcium and phosphate metabolism in horses. Vet Clin North Am Equine Pract 2011;27:129–47.
75. Thompson AC, Mochal-King C. Primary hypoparathyroidism and recurring hypocalcemia in a quarter horse gelding-a case report. J Equine Vet Sci 2021;99: 103398.
76. Durie I, van Loon G, Hesta M, et al. Hypocalcemia caused by primary hypoparathyroidism in a 3-month-old filly. J Vet Intern Med 2010;24:439–42.
77. Beyer MJ, Freestone JF, Reimer JM, et al. Idiopathic hypocalcemia in foals. J Vet Intern Med 1997;11:356–60.
78. Rivas VN, Magdesian KG, Fagan S, et al. A nonsense variant in rap guanine nucleotide exchange factor 5 (RAPGEF5) is associated with equine familial isolated hypoparathyroidism in Thoroughbred foals. PLoS Genet 2020;16: e1009028.

Myosin Heavy Chain Myopathy and Immune-Mediated Muscle Disorders

Sian A. Durward-Akhurst, BVMS, MS, PhD, MRCVS[a],*,
Stephanie J. Valberg, DVM, PhD[b]

KEYWORDS

- Inflammatory • Muscle disease • Atrophy • Rhabdomyolysis • Infectious

KEY POINTS

- Infectious disease and vaccination appear to play an important inciting role in inflammatory myopathies.
- Myosin heavy chain myopathy (MYHM) is a codominantly inherited myopathy in Quarter Horse-related breeds.
- MYHM has 3 forms: nonexertional rhabdomyolysis, immune-mediated myositis, and systemic calcification or calciphylaxis.
- Infarctive purpura hemorrhagica causes firm, painful, focal muscle infarctions and progresses to infarction of multiple organs.
- There are other less well-characterized inflammatory myopathies associated with sarcocytosis, piroplasmosis, and viruses.

INTRODUCTION

Inflammatory myopathies are a heterogenous group of muscle disorders characterized by infiltration of leukocytes into skeletal muscle and around blood vessels.[1–3] Neutrophils, eosinophils, or lymphocytes predominate depending on the inciting cause, which is in stark contrast to most exertional myopathies that have macrophage infiltration of myofibers.[4,5] Inflammatory myopathies are less well characterized than in other species, with extensive overlap between myopathies with apparent infectious and immune-mediated components.[1,6–12] This review focuses on myosin heavy chain myopathy (MYHM), infarctive purpura hemorrhagica (IPH), and other inflammatory myopathies with a strong immune-mediated component.

[a] Department of Veterinary Clinical Sciences, University of Minnesota, C339 VMC, 1352 Boyd Avenue, St Paul, MN 55115, USA; [b] Large Animal Clinical Sciences, College of Veterinary Medicine, Michigan State University, East Lansing, MI, USA
* Corresponding author.
E-mail address: durwa004@umn.edu
Twitter: @sian.akhurst (S.A.D.-A.)

Vet Clin Equine 41 (2025) 61–75
https://doi.org/10.1016/j.cveq.2024.10.005
0749-0739/25/© 2024 Elsevier Inc. All rights reserved, including those for text and data mining, AI training, and similar technologies.

MYOSIN HEAVY CHAIN MYOPATHY

MYHM occurs in Quarter Horse-related breeds.[7,9,13,14] Prior to the identification of the genetic variant responsible for MYHM, it was termed equine immune-mediated myositis (IMM).[1,9] Subsequent research showed that MYHM exhibits pleiotropy with 3 clinical presentations: IMM, calciphylaxis, and nonexertional rhabdomyolysis.[6,10,13,15,16] There is evidence that a specific genetic background combined with infectious agents and the resulting immune response plays a role in MYHM development.[7,9]

Genetic Basis

The cause of MYHM is a missense variant (E321G) in the myosin heavy chain 1 (*MYH1*) gene, leading to an amino acid change from a negatively charged glutamic acid to a nonpolar glycine in the myosin-type 2X heavy chain.[6] The variant is in a highly conserved region of subfragment-1 of the myosin globular head and is predicted to markedly reduce protein stability.[6] MYHM follows an autosomal codominant mode of inheritance with variable penetrance, meaning that a single copy of the disease-allele is sufficient to cause disease and horses with 2 copies of the disease-allele are more severely affected.[6] Specifically, 80% of homozygous horses and 20% of heterozygous horses develop clinical signs of MYHM.[13,17] At least 50% of homozygous horses exhibit more frequent recurrence of clinical signs, compared to heterozygous horses.[6,13,18]

Prevalence

The prevalence of the *MYH1* variant in the general equine population is estimated to be 1.6% with clinical disease only reported in Quarter Horse-related breeds.[19] In Quarter Horses, the prevalence of the *MYH1* variant is 7% to 8%,[19–22] with reining (allele frequency: 22%–24%), working cow (allele frequency: 17%), and halter (allele frequency: 6%–16%) horse stallions having a higher prevalence.[22,23] The variant has not been reported in barrel or racing Quarter Horse stallions in the United States.[20] However, it is present in the Brazilian Quarter Horse barrel (allele frequency: 10%) and racing (allele frequency: 6%) populations.[22] Until recently, the variant had only been documented in Quarter Horse and related breeds (Appaloosa, Appendix horse, and Paints) but recently an unphenotyped MYHM heterozygous Belgian was reported.[19] Horses with the *MYH1* variant may also possess causative variants for other muscle diseases, including polysaccharide storage myopathy type 1, glycogen branching enzyme deficiency, malignant hyperthermia, and hyperkalemic periodic paralysis.[17,18,22]

Triggers Leading to the Development of Myosin Heavy Chain Myopathy Clinical Signs

Overall, 25% to 46% of horses with MYHM have a history of an environmental trigger, including respiratory diseases, for example, *Streptococcus equi equi* or *Streptococcus equi zooepidemicus*, concurrent *Corynebacterium pseudotuberculosis, Anaplasma phagocytophilum* or vaccination for influenza, equine herpes virus 4, and/or *S. equi equi*.[7,14,17,18,24] In hospitalized cases, 78% of severely affected horses have a history that includes these triggers.[14] There is also a report of a Quarter Horse filly with concurrent active *S. equi equi* infection, MYHM IMM, and purpura hemorrhagica.[16] Notably, in over half of cases, an inciting agent for the development of clinical signs is absent.

The 3 MYHM clinical phenotypes are IMM, calciphylaxis, and nonexertional rhabdomyolysis with some clinical overlap occurring among these.

MYOSIN HEAVY CHAIN MYOPATHY IMMUNE-MEDIATED MYOSITIS
Clinical Signs

Horses have a biphasic age range, with most cases at the age of 8 years or less and 17 years or more.[7] There is no sex predilection.[7] Profound rapid atrophy of the epaxial and gluteal muscles is the primary clinical sign (**Fig. 1**A).[7] Atrophy can be severe with some horses losing 40% of their affected muscle mass within 48 hours and the atrophy can persist for months.[7] Horses with pronounced atrophy may become weak and have frequent episodes of recumbency.[1] A concurrent fever is present in 44% of horses with the MYHM form of IMM.[14,17] Homozygotes develop rapid onset muscle atrophy more often than heterozygous horses (odds ratio: 136.0).[6,18] During acute muscle atrophy, serum creatine kinase (CK) and aspartate transaminase (AST) are moderately to severely increased, but during chronic atrophy, serum CK and AST activities may be normal.[20] Hematology is usually within normal limits unless concurrent infection is present.[9]

Diagnosis

Diagnosis is based on identification of the *MYH1* variant in horses of Quarter Horse-related breeds with severe muscle atrophy.[6] Trucut samples fixed in formalin or fresh frozen Bergstrom needle biopsies of the epaxial and/or gluteal muscles were the mainstay of diagnosis prior to the development of a genetic test.[1] Horses with the acute IMM form of MYHM have lymphocyte infiltration of type 2X myofibers without glycogen depletion and lymphocytic cuffing of small blood vessels (**Fig. 1**B).[6,9,13,14] Horses in the chronic stages of IMM, when atrophy has been present for several weeks, frequently have nonspecific myogenic atrophy and regeneration on muscle biopsy, without the characteristic lymphocytic inflammation.[1] Semimembranosus and semitendinosus muscles are often mildly affected or normal.[7]

Pathophysiology

MYHM IMM has similarities with human and canine immune-mediated myopathies.[25] This includes restriction to specific muscle groups, predominance of CD4+ T cells in affected muscles, and major histocompatibility class I and II expression on myofibers.[25] Lymphocyte populations in IMM are predominantly CD4+ T cells in 48% of cases and CD8+ T cells in 28% of cases.[9,17] Other cell types include CD20+ B cells and macrophages.[9] Immunoglobulin G staining of the sarcolemma is not a consistent feature of IMM.[7] In the acute phase of MYHM IMM, major histocompatibility type I

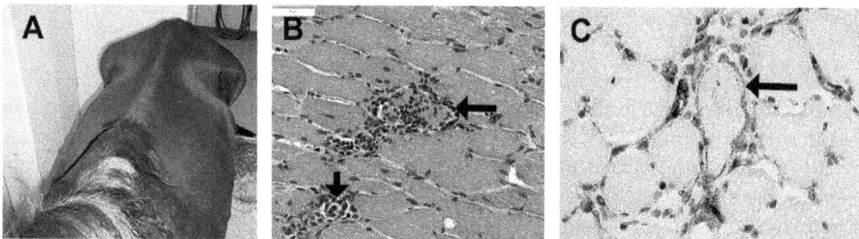

Fig. 1. (*A*) Quarter Horse with the immune-mediated myositis form of myosin heavy chain myopathy showing marked gluteal and epaxial muscle atrophy. (*B*) Cross section of gluteal muscle showing lymphocytic infiltration of myofibers (*horizontal arrow*) and vasculitis (*vertical arrow*, hematoxylin-eosin stain, 20X magnification). (*C*) Major histocompatibility complex (MHC) I staining of the sarcolemma in a selective myofiber (*arrow*). Immunohistochemical stain for MHC I 40X. ([*A*] *Courtesy of* Prof. Beatrice Sponseller, Dr. med. vet., DABVP (Equine).)

and/or II staining is present on scattered myofibers in 81% and 71% of horses, respectively (see **Fig. 1**C).[9] Major histocompatibility complex class I and II are not normally detectable on healthy mature myofibers and class II expression is highly specific for immune-mediated myopathies in humans.[26] Major histocompatibility complex expression develops in the presence of cytokines, but the reason it is upregulated on the sarcolemma of these horses is incompletely understood.[6,25,27]

The working hypothesis for the development of MYHM IMM is that damage to the myofibers, for example, by vaccination or trauma, leads to release of the altered myosin heavy chain form and activation of the innate immune response directed toward type 2X myofibers.[13,14,20,28] Horses with the MYHM variant and signs of IMM have fewer type 2X myofibers compared to controls likely as a result of type 2X fiber destruction.[6] It is thought that loss of hydrogen bonds in the altered myosin heavy chain protein leads to a myosin confirmation change and activation of toll-like receptors and autoimmunity.[6,29] Cardiac myosin fragments in humans can activate toll-like receptors, which are important for driving reactivity to self-epitopes supporting this hypothesis.[9,29,30] It is also hypothesized that the adaptive immune response may be triggered by shared epitopes between bacteria, such as the *Streptococcus* M protein and myosin, which is seen in some forms of human immune-mediated myocarditis.[6,30]

Treatment

Anti-inflammatory doses of corticosteroids tapered over 1 month are the mainstay of treatment. For example, intravenous dexamethasone at 0.05 to 0.07 mg/kg/day for 3 days, then oral prednisolone at 1 mg/kg/day for 7 to 10 days tapered by 100 mg/week, if serum CK remains stable.[7,20] Early corticosteroid treatment can reduce potential atrophy and time for muscle mass recovery.[7] Treatment of concurrent infection is indicated and supportive care may be necessary, especially in horses with frequent episodes of recumbency.[3] Muscle mass usually recovers over a period of weeks to months depending on the initial atrophy severity.[7] Horses can make full recoveries; however, recurrence occurs in 50% of MYHM homozygous horses, which also have more frequent and severe episodes and are less likely to return to normal muscle mass.[7,20]

MYOSIN HEAVY CHAIN MYOPATHY AND CALCIPHYLAXIS

Calciphylaxis or systemic calcinosis occurs in horses homozygous or heterozygous for the *MYH1* variant that are often less than 9 years of age and have clinical signs of IMM (*SJ Valberg, personal observation*).[8,15,31] In these horses, calcification of muscle fibers and multiple other organs develops and is frequently fatal.[8,10,15,31]

Clinical Signs

Common clinical signs include malaise, mild fever, stiffness, muscle atrophy, and mild ventral edema (**Fig 2**A).[1,2,8,10,31] One horse also had polyuria, polydipsia, and paroxysmal multiform ventricular tachycardia.[10] Rapid progression due to multiple organ failure occurs and can include respiratory distress, colic, and laminitis.[8,10,15,31] Half of reported cases have a history of recent infection, including *S. equi equi* or *Actinobacillus equuli*, *A. phagocytophilum*, Salmonella, a reaction to an immune stimulant, and being treated for IMM prior to the onset of calciphylaxis.[8,15,31]

Diagnosis

Genetic testing for the MYHM variant and the pathognomic biochemical finding of hyperphosphatemia, with the product of total calcium concentrations (mg/dL)

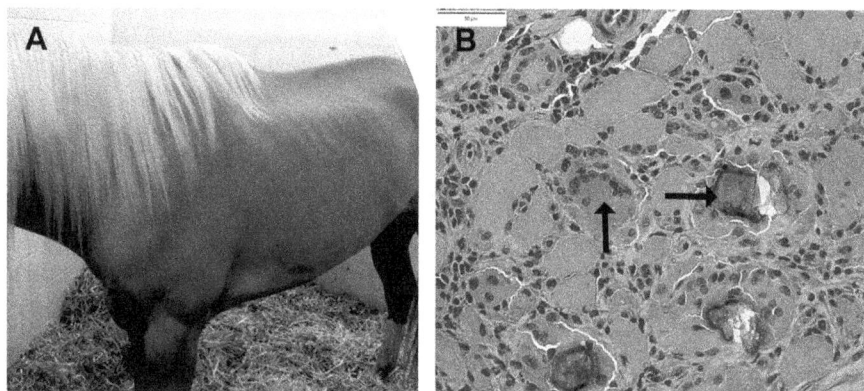

Fig. 2. (*A*) Quarter Horse with calciphylaxis with prominent epaxial and gluteal atrophy. (*B*) Cross section of gluteal muscle showing lymphocytic and macrophage infiltration of myofibers, calcification of myofibers (*horizontal arrow*) and multinucleated giant fibers (*vertical arrow*).

multiplied by phosphorous concentrations greater than 65 mg/dL, are the mainstay of diagnosis.[1,8] Other biochemical findings relate to the organs that are affected by calcification and include azotemia, hypoalbuminemia, elevated cardiac troponin I, and severely increased CK and AST activities.[8,10,31] On hematology, leukocytosis with neutrophilia and hyperfibrinogenemia are usually present.[8,31] Three of the 5 reported cases of *S equi equi* rhabdomyolysis had a product of serum total calcium (mg/dL) multiplied by phosphorous greater than 65 mg/dL (range: 65.3–82.8 mg/dL) and a fourth case had markedly elevated total phosphorous (12.2 g/gL, reference range: 1.7–3.9 g/dL) suggesting overlap between MYHM nonexertional rhabdomyolysis secondary to *S. equi equi* and calciphylaxis.[11,32]

Gluteal muscle biopsies show diffuse anguloid atrophy, centrally located myonuclei, and scattered myofibers with acute necrosis and severe dystrophic calcification (**Fig. 2**B).[8,10,15] Some horses have marked macrophage infiltration of myofibers, multinucleated giant cells, and mononuclear vasculitis (see **Fig. 2**B).[8,15] Findings are milder in the semimembranosus muscle.[8] Necropsy findings include pallor of multiple organs, including skeletal muscle, kidneys, heart, and lungs.[8,31] Dystrophic calcification of several muscles is frequently present and other tissues have varying degrees of calcification including the renal glomeruli, tubules, and/or collecting ducts, the aorta, aortic sinus endothelium, and surrounding connective tissue, and in the lungs, the primary bronchioles, alveoli, bronchiolar muscle, cartilage, and alveolar walls.[8,15,31] Less frequently, there is necrosis of the renal tubules, coagulative necrosis of the renal cortex and medulla, thrombosis of vessels, and renal interstitial infiltration with macrophages, lymphocytes, and plasma cells.[8]

Pathophysiology

It is thought that calciphylaxis has an immune-mediated component related to the MYHM variant (*SJ Valberg, personal observation*).[8,10,31] During inflammation, cytokines including tumor necrosis factor alpha and interleukin 6 can lead to enhanced bone resorption secondary to activation of Receptor Activator of Nuclear Factor Kappa-B (RANK).[33] The RANK ligand–RANK signaling pathway receptor activator is important for regulation of multinucleated osteoclast formation, activation, and survival as part of normal bone remodeling.[20] This may lead to hyperphosphatemia, and dystrophic calcification due to deposition of calcium phosphate secondary to blood phosphate "supersaturation." This promotes conversion of smooth muscle fibers into osteogenic cell types and causes increased parathyroid hormone secretion and reduced renal production of 1,25-dihydroxyvitamin D.[8] It is possible that the recent or concurrent diseases present in horses that developed calciphylaxis trigger the inflammation leading to the development of hyperphosphatemia and dystrophic calcification.[8,10] Other causes for calciphylaxis in people include end-stage renal failure and vitamin D toxicosis. Both are unlikely in MYHM with calciphylaxis. Most horses with calciphylaxis were healthy prior to disease onset, and horses with chronic renal failure typically develop hypophosphatemia in contrast to the hyperphosphatemia seen in humans.[8,10,15,31,34] Additionally, compared to calciphylaxis cases, horses with vitamin D toxicosis have hypercalcemia and gastrointestinal hemorrhage.[8,10,15,31]

Treatment

Treatment resembles that for horses with MYHM IMM and includes supportive care with fluid therapy and appropriate antimicrobial therapy.[1,10] Corticosteroid therapy is controversial because in humans, there are concerns about worsening bone resorption that exacerbates the hyperphosphatemia.[35] The prognosis is grave with only one report of an affected horse surviving.[8,10,15,31] The surviving horse was treated with dexamethasone (0.04–0.08 mg/kg intravenous every 24 hours), aluminum hydroxide (30 mg/kg oral every 24 hours), and slow administration of intravenous sodium thiosulfate (50 mg/kg diluted to 10% in 5% dextrose, intravenous every 48 hours) to combat tissue calcification.[10]

MYOSIN HEAVY CHAIN MYOPATHY NONEXERTIONAL RHABDOMYOLYSIS
Clinical Signs

MYHM horses can exhibit nonexertional rhabdomyolysis that is not triggered by exercise.[13] The *MYH1* variant is a common cause of nonexertional rhabdomyolysis in Quarter Horse-related breeds. Overall, 67% of Quarter Horses with nonexertional rhabdomyolysis have at least one MYHM allele compared to just 5% of the general Quarter Horse population.[13] Affected horses are usually young, may be febrile, have firm epaxial and hindquarter muscles, and show marked signs of pain, stiffness, and myoglobinuria with many horses showing a rapid progression to recumbency (**Fig 3A**).[11,13,32] Horses

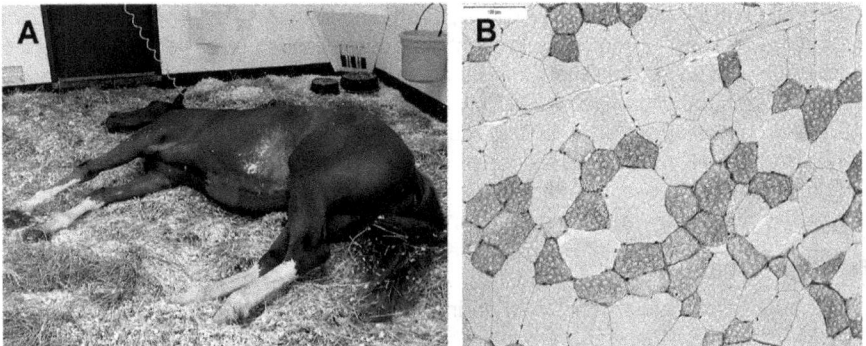

Fig. 3. (A) Young Quarter Horse with nonexertional rhabdomyolysis from myosin heavy chain myopathy showing signs of muscle pain, stiffness, and recumbency. (B) Cross section of gluteal muscle showing glycogen depletion of large myofibers in a 1 year old intact Paint colt with MYHM nonexertional rhabdomyolysis and serum CK of 13,440 U/L. The horse was down and unable to rise. Periodic acid Schiff's stain 20X magnification.

frequently die or require euthanasia due to pain and inability to stand within 24 to 48 hours of becoming recumbent. Recent *S. equi equi* or influenza/rhinopneumonitis vaccination or concurrent *S. equi equi* infection precedes clinical signs in 40% of cases.[13] MYHM nonexertional rhabdomyolysis has many similarities with the previously named *S. equi equi* associated myopathy, with 2 published cases (one heterozygous and one homozygous) known to have the *MYH1* variant (*SJ Valberg, personal observation*) and *Streptococcus equi equi* myopathy is likely to be a subtype of MYHM nonexertional rhabdomyolysis.[11,13,32]

Diagnosis

Identification of the *MYH1* variant in horses of Quarter Horse-related breeds with clinical signs of nonexertional rhabdomyolysis is diagnostic. Gluteal muscle biopsies show myofiber necrosis with macrophage infiltration and glycogen depletion in 30% of muscle fibers (see **Fig. 3**B). Less than 18% of cases have myofiber lymphocytic infiltrates.[13] Marked elevations in serum CK (>100,000 U/L) and AST are present.[13] Horses with concurrent *S. equi equi* infection typically have marked neutrophilia and hyperfibrinogenemia, guttural pouch empyema and may be culture and/or polymerase chain reaction (PCR) positive for *S. equi equi*.[11,32] *S. equi* M protein titer is positive in some cases.[11,32]

Pathophysiology

The lack of myofiber lymphocytic infiltration suggests that rhabdomyolysis may not be immune mediated.[13] MYHM nonexertional rhabdomyolysis is thought to occur due to readily induced and persistent calcium activation of actomyosin interaction from a hypercontractile phenotype, somewhat similar to the hypercontraction that occurs in horses with malignant hyperthermia.[13,36]

The severity and rapid deterioration of horses with concurrent *S. equi equi* is similar to humans with streptococcal toxic shock syndrome relating to streptococcal superantigens.[1,2,37,38] Superantigens can simultaneously bind major histocompatibility class II and T-cell receptors with a specific V-β region leading to massive T cell and antigen-presenting cell activation causing massive cytokine release and toxic shock.[32] Alternatively, it is possible that infiltration of skeletal muscle by *S. equi* and release of streptococcal proteases leads to myodegeneration.[11,39] Identification of remnants of *S. equi* bacteria in the muscle of affected horses is consistent with this.[11] It is also possible that the immune response to the *Streptococcus equi* M protein attacks muscle fibers due to similarities between the *Streptococcus equi* M protein and myosin.[30]

Treatment

Early diagnosis and implementation of treatment are critical. Treatment includes dantrolene (2–4 mg/kg orally three times daily) until serum CK activity has markedly declined.[20,40] Intravenous and/or oral fluid therapy to protect the kidneys may be necessary due to the severity of the myoglobinuria. If bacterial infection is suspected, then appropriate antimicrobials should be used.[2] Corticosteroids may be indicated depending on the severity of concurrent infectious disease.[2,7,14] Constant rate infusions of lidocaine or detomidine or butorphanol can be helpful as these horses are frequently profoundly painful. Prolonged recumbency can be life-threatening due to compressive myopathy and/or neuropathy, pressure necrosis, reduced gastrointestinal motility, and difficulty urinating.[14] Treated horses can recover but 35% develop acute muscle atrophy as described in MYHM IMM cases, which requires corticosteroid therapy.[13]

PREVENTION OF MYOSIN HEAVY CHAIN MYOPATHY EPISODES

Prevention of clinical signs is challenging but should focus on minimizing exposure to infectious agents, avoiding immunostimulants, and avoiding vaccination for Strangles.[7,14,20] If MYHM horses develop clinical signs after any vaccines, to identify the culprit, splitting up and using the minimum number of necessary vaccines is recommended in the subsequent year. Spacing out each of these vaccines by 4 to 6 weeks is recommended to find the inciting agent, for example, tetanus (wait 4–6 weeks), Eastern Equine Encephalitis virus (EEE), Western Equine Encephalitis virus (WEE) and Venezuelan Equine Encephalisis virus (VEE, wait 4–6 weeks), West Nile virus (wait 4–6 weeks), and rabies. If no muscle damage or atrophy is triggered, then it may be safe to combine vaccines the next year. If owners notice atrophy after vaccination, then a discussion about the risks or benefits of that specific vaccine is warranted. Because influenza is a common trigger of MYHM, influenza vaccination should be avoided or an intranasal formulation used.[7,14] Early administration of prednisolone is recommended if atrophy is observed after vaccination. To avoid producing horses most likely to develop a myopathy, breeding homozygous horses, or mating *MYH1* heterozygous horses with heterozygotes is not recommended.

INFARCTIVE PURPURA HEMORRHAGICA

Most horses with purpura hemorrhagica (72%) have a history of *S. equi equi* infection or vaccination, although infections with *Streptococcus equi zooepidemicus, Staphylococcus aureus, C. pseudotuberculosis*, equine influenza virus, equine viral arteritis virus, and equine herpesvirus type 1 are reported.[41,42] In IPH, a severe vasculitis develops that results in infarction of muscles initially, followed by infarction of other organs.[12,42]

Clinical Features

Although any breed of horse can be affected with IPH, Quarter Horses are overrepresented, with 72% of cases aged 10 years or younger.[41] Pectoral, hind limb adductor, and gaskin muscles that are compressed during recumbency develop focal firm and painful swellings (**Fig. 4**A).[12] Horses are usually stiff or lame with depression, petechiation, and well-demarcated limb edema.[12,41] As multiple organs become infarcted, oral ulcerations, colic, laminitis, and hemorrhagic gastric reflux often arise.[12,41] One horse with IPH secondary to *S aureus* had concurrent myocarditis and immune-mediated hemolytic anemia.[42]

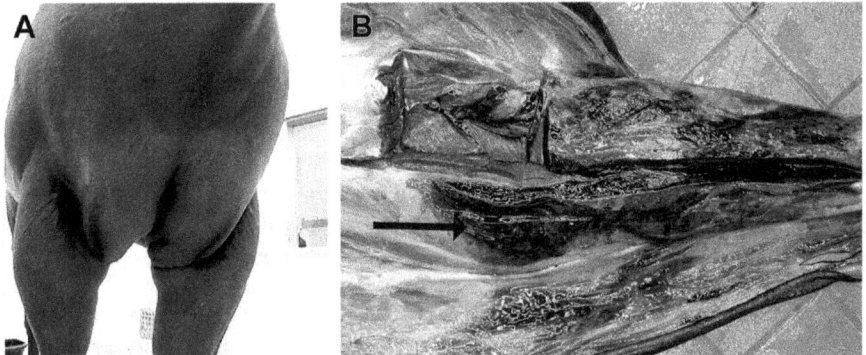

Fig. 4. (*A*) Horse with infarctive purpura hemorrhagica showing firm swelling of pectoral muscles. (*B*) Postmortem evaluation of forelimb muscles showing multiple regions of muscle infarction (*horizontal arrow*). ([*B*] *Courtesy of* Prof. Carrie J Finno.)

Diagnosis

Marked elevations in muscle enzymes, evidence of focal muscle necrosis on ultrasound, and regions of coagulative necrosis in affected muscle biopsies are indicative of IPH (**Fig. 4**A, B, **Table 1**).[1,2,12,40,41,43,44] Additionally, horses typically have a leukocytoclastic vasculitis in skin biopsies from edematous regions and high *Streptococcus equi* M (SeM) protein antibody titers (>1:1,600).[43,45]

Pathophysiology

Most horses have a history of *S. equi equi* infection or vaccination within a month of developing clinical signs.[12,46] A type III hypersensitivity reaction is thought to cause the vasculitis, edema, and extravasation of albumin.[46,47] Horses with IPH typically have large amounts of SeM-Immunoglobulin A (IgA) immune complexes in the serum.[43,45] Deposition of complement on immune complexes in blood vessel walls leads to marked leukocytoclastic vasculitis, vascular occlusion, and tissue ischemia and infarction.[12,45,46] IPH has similarities to IgA vasculitis, previously known as Henoch–Schönlein purpura in children, including having leukocytoclastic vasculitis, a recent history of an infection, especially with streptococcal species, and high levels of circulating IgA immune complexes.[48] Children with IgA vasculitis rarely develop skeletal muscle infarction but have skin rashes, nephritis, arthritis, and gastrointestinal hemorrhage.[48,49] It is thought that horses develop skeletal muscle infarction due to compression and occlusion of inflamed vessels in the muscles that are compressed during recumbency.[1]

Risk factors associated with having high SeM titers (>1:1,600) include Quarter Horses compared to Thoroughbreds and Warmbloods (odds ratio: 4.1), intranasal Strangles vaccination within the last 3 years (odds ratio: 4.7), clinical signs of Strangles within the last year (odds ratio: 7.9), and older horses (odds ratio: 1.1, for each year of increased age).[44] This suggests that it is important to test SeM titers in horses with one or more of these risk factors prior to vaccinating against *S. equi*. Horses with SeM titers greater than 1:3,200 should not be vaccinated against Strangles.[44,50]

Treatment, Prognosis, and Prevention

Without early diagnosis and treatment, the fatality rate for IPH is high.[12,41,51] High and prolonged doses of corticosteroids are required.[12] Early reduction in the corticosteroid dose based on a decrease in muscle swelling and serum CK activity should be avoided as it has led to a fatal outcome.[12] A successful regime was 0.1 mg/kg/day dexamethasone reduced by 5 mg total every other day for 5 days, then 0.6 mg/kg/day for 7 days, followed by 0.5 mg/kg/day for 7 days.[12] This horse was then switched to 2 mg/kg/day of prednisolone for 2 weeks tapered by 100 mg/week providing that serum CK activity continued declining.[12] Horses with infarction of the gastrointestinal tract rarely survive.[12] Appropriate antimicrobials, typically penicillin, should be administered if there is suspicion of concurrent *S. equi* infection.[41,46]

UNCHARACTERIZED IMMUNE-MEDIATED MUSCLE DISORDERS
Non-myosin Heavy Chain Myopathy Immune-Mediated Myositis

Notably, 9 of 71 horses diagnosed with IMM by muscle biopsy in the study that identified the MYHM variant did not carry the *MYH1* variant.[6] Two horses had moderate to severe myofiber lymphocyte infiltration and the remaining 7 had milder myofiber lymphocyte infiltration.[6] It is possible that they had a non-MYHM inflammatory myositis.[6] Such phenocopies occur because histologic differentiation between immune-mediated myopathies and inflammatory myopathies secondary to an infectious agent is difficult.[7,52,53]

Table 1
Clinical and diagnostic features of purpura hemorrhagica and infarctive purpura hemorrhagica

Diagnostic Test	PH	IPH
Hematology	Leukocytosis, neutrophilia with a left shift and toxic changes.	
Biochemistry	Mild CK elevations (CK <3,000 U/L), hyperglobulinemia and hypoalbuminemia	Marked elevations CK (>35,000 U/L) and AST (>960 U/L), hyperglobulinemia and hypoalbuminemia
SeM antibody titer	Marked elevations: >1:6,400. Frequently values are >1:12,800	
Muscle ultrasound	Normal	Areas of necrosis characterized by focal hypoechoic lesions within the muscle tissue
Ultrasound-guided muscle biopsy	Normal	Marked vasculitis, degeneration and necrosis of myofibers and in more chronic cases, connective tissue replacement of myofibers
Upper respiratory tract examination	Enlarged and/or abscessed submandibular and/or retropharyngeal lymph nodes, some horses have guttural pouch empyema	
Skin biopsy	Leukocytoclastic vasculitis	
Necropsy	Petechiae and ecchymosis of the oral and gastrointestinal mucosa, leukocytoclastic vasculitis of multiple internal organs	Petechiae and ecchymosis, leukocytoclastic vasculitis and infarction of muscles. Inflammatory cells include degenerate neutrophils, lymphocytes, plasma cells, and macrophages

Inflammatory myositis or IMM has been reported in other breeds. A 16 year old pony developed symmetric cervical muscle atrophy and weakness over 3 months with multifocal lymphocyte and plasma cell infiltration in muscle perivascular regions.[53] This pony had normal CK and AST activities and *Sarcocystis* species were not identified on muscle biopsy. The atrophy resolved with dexamethasone treatment.[53] There is also a brief report of a horse with multifocal muscle atrophy and muscle biopsy findings similar to horses with MYHM IMM.[54] Dr Valberg's database has some non-Quarter Horse breeds with inflammatory or IMM with varying degrees of lymphocyte infiltration and lymphocytic vasculitis, including 2 Thoroughbreds, and an Anglo-Arabian, a pony, a Percheron, and a Warmblood.[2] Two horses had severe acute muscle atrophy, while the atrophy was more gradual in the other horses.[2] Epaxial and gluteal muscles were affected in all horses, with 2 horses having atrophy of additional muscle groups.[2] Frequently there is concurrent infection or recent vaccination.[17,24,55] The cause of IMM is not known in these cases.[14,18]

Other Infectious Inflammatory Myopathies

Sarcocystis fayeri, Sarcocystis bertrami, and *Sarcocystis equicanis* are the most common protozoa identified in horse muscle (**Fig. 5**).[56] Sarcocysts in the muscle are usually incidental findings;[2] however, some horses develop clinical signs.[55,57] Risk factors include exposure to large numbers of sporozoan parasites in canine feces, concurrent disease, immunosuppression, and a suspected genetic predisposition.[57] Clinical signs include gluteal, epaxial, and quadriceps muscle atrophy and nonspecific signs include malaise, muscle fasciculations, anorexia, and weakness.[57] Some cases have systemic eosinophilia.[57] Diagnosis is based on muscle biopsy of affected muscles and identification of sarcocysts with concurrent infiltration of lymphocytes, macrophages, and in some cases eosinophils.[55,57] Successful treatment has included trimethoprim-sulfa and pyrimethamine, ponazuril, and/or sulfadiazine/pyrimethamine.[55,57] However, another case did not respond to aggressive treatment with sulfamethoxazole, trimethoprim, and anti-inflammatory treatment for 7 months.[57] At necropsy, this horse had disseminated nodules throughout the striated musculature, especially of the esophagus, diaphragm, large shoulder and thigh muscles, and intercostal muscles.[57] These nodules contained eosinophils with central areas of necrosis.[57]

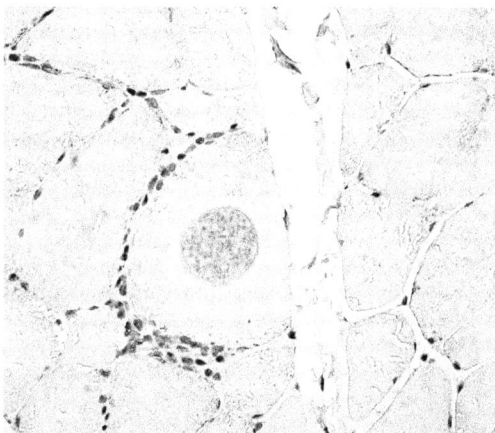

Fig. 5. A myofiber containing a sarcocyst and surrounded by leukocytes in the sacrocaudalis dorsalis medialis muscle. Succinate dehydrogenase A immunostaining 40X.

Piroplasmosis due to *Theileria equi* and *Babesia caballi* is predominantly transmitted by *Ixodes* ticks.[58,59] Horses with chronic piroplasmosis may develop mild-to-severe muscle atrophy without sex or age predilection, although all reported horses were aged 3 years or older.[58] *T. equi* and/or *B. caballi* was identified in the blood of affected horses.[58] Mild elevations in CK and AST were present.[58] Overall, 94% of muscle biopsies contained lymphocytes and lymphocyte perivascular cuffing and mild major histocompatibility class I and/or II staining.[58]

SUMMARY

Several types of inflammatory myopathy have evidence of an immune-mediated component in the horse. MYHM is caused by an E321G missense variant in *MYH1* located in a highly conserved region of the myosin heavy chain.[6] Quarter Horses with 1 or 2 copies of the MYHM variant can develop nonexertional rhabdomyolysis, IMM, and calciphylaxis.[6,10,13,15] Nonexertional rhabdomyolysis is frequently rapidly fatal and likely includes the previously named *S. equi equi* myopathy.[11,13] IPH causes infarction of skeletal muscle that can progress to infarction of other organs and, like calciphylaxis, has high fatality.[1,8,10,12,15] There are also horses with clinical signs similar to MYHM immune-mediated myopathy that do not carry the MYHM variant.[2,6,53,54] The underlying cause of muscle disease in these horses is not well understood.

CLINICS CARE POINTS

- Diagnosis of the immune mediated myositis, calciphylaxis, and nonexertional rhabdomyolysis forms of MYHM is based on clinical signs and identification of one or two copies of the MYHM variant in Quarter Horses and related breeds.

- Early diagnosis and appropriate treatment can reduce the severity of MYHM immune mediated myositis atrophy, and is essential for successful treatment of MYHM calciphylaxis and nonexertional rhabdomyolysis that have a poor prognosis.

- Prevention of MYHM related clinical signs includes minimizing exposure to infectious agents, avoiding immunostimulants, and avoiding vaccination against Strangles.

- High dose corticosteroid therapy is necessary to treat infarctive purpura hemorrhagica and corticosteroid therapy should be continued for several weeks.

DISCLOSURES

Dr S.A. Durward-Akhurst receives salary support from a K12 grant supported through the National Institutes of Health's National Center for Advancing Translational Sciences, grants UL1TR002494 and K12TR002492. S.J. Valberg directs the Valberg Neuromuscular Disease Laboratory (ValbergNMDL.com) and receives remuneration for analyzing muscle biopsies. Her website is sponsored by Kentucky Equine Research, and she receives royalties from the Polysaccharide Storage Myopathy type 1 genetic test and the feed products Re-leve and MFM pellet developed in association with Kentucky Equine Research.

REFERENCES

1. Durward-Akhurst SA, Valberg SJ. Immune-mediated muscle diseases of the horse. Vet Pathol 2018;55(1):68–75.

2. Durward-Akhurst SA, Valberg SJJ, Felippe JB. Inflammatory and immune-mediated muscle disorders, vol. 1. Wiley-Blackwell; 2016. p. 98.
3. Aleman M. Inflammatory and immune-mediated myopathies, what do we know? Vet Clin North Am Equine Pract 2024;40(2):207–18.
4. Valberg SJ, Mickelson JR, Gallant EM, et al. Exertional rhabdomyolysis in quarter horses and thoroughbreds: one syndrome, multiple aetiologies. Equine Veterinary Journalsupplement 1999;30:533–8.
5. Valberg SJ. Diseases of muscles. In: Smith BP, editor. Large animal internal medicine. Fifth: Elsevier Mosby; 2015.
6. Finno CJ, Gianino G, Perumbakkam S, et al. A missense mutation in MYH1 is associated with susceptibility to immune-mediated myositis in Quarter Horses. Skelet Muscle 2018;8(1):7.
7. Lewis SS, Valberg SJ, Nielsen IL. Suspected immune-mediated myositis in horses. J Vet Intern Med 2007;21(3):495–503.
8. Tan JY, Valberg SJ, Sebastian MM, et al. Suspected systemic calcinosis and calciphylaxis in 5 horses. Can Vet J 2010;51(9):993–9.
9. Durward-Akhurst SA, Finno CJ, Barnes N, et al. Major histocompatibility complex I and II expression and lymphocytic subtypes in muscle of horses with immune-mediated myositis. J Vet Intern Med 2016;30(4). https://doi.org/10.1111/jvim.14371.
10. Sponseller BT, Wong DM, Ruby R, et al. Systemic calcinosis in a Quarter Horse gelding homozygous for a myosin heavy chain 1 mutation. J Vet Intern Med 2022;36(4):1543–9.
11. Sponseller BT, Valberg SJ, Tennent-Brown BS, et al. Severe acute rhabdomyolysis associated with Streptococcus equi infection in four horses. J Am Vet Med Assoc 2005;227(11):1753–4, 1800-1807.
12. Kaese HJ, Valberg SJ, Hayden DW, et al. Infarctive purpura hemorrhagica in five horses. J Am Vet Med Assoc 2005;226(11):1845, 1893-1898.
13. Valberg SJ, Henry ML, Perumbakkam S, et al. An E321G MYH1 mutation is strongly associated with nonexertional rhabdomyolysis in Quarter Horses. J Vet Intern Med 2018. https://doi.org/10.1111/jvim.15299.
14. Hunyadi L, Sundman EA, Kass PH, et al. Clinical implications and hospital outcome of immune-mediated myositis in horses. J Vet Intern Med 2017. https://doi.org/10.1111/jvim.14637.
15. Faccin M, Landsgaard KA, Milliron SM, et al. Myosin heavy-chain myopathy in 2 American quarter horses. Vet Pathol 2024;61(3):462–7.
16. Hepworth-Warren KL, Young KAS, Armwood A, et al. Concurrent Streptococcus equi subsp. equi infection, purpura haemorrhagica and immune-mediated myositis in a Quarter Horse filly. Equine Vet Educ 2024;36(8):e196–202.
17. Aleman M, Scalco R, Malvick J, et al. Prevalence of genetic mutations in horses with muscle disease from a neuromuscular disease laboratory. J Equine Vet Sci 2022;118:104129.
18. Valberg SJ, Schultz AE, Finno CJ, et al. Prevalence of clinical signs and factors impacting expression of myosin heavy chain myopathy in Quarter Horse-related breeds with the MYH1E321G mutation. J Vet Intern Med 2022;36(3):1152–9.
19. Durward-Akhurst SA, Marlowe JL, Schaefer RJ, et al. Predicted genetic burden and frequency of phenotype-associated variants in the horse. Sci Rep 2024;14(1):8396.
20. Valberg SJ. Genetics of equine muscle disease. Vet Clin North Am Equine Pract 2020;36(2):353–78.

21. Sperandio LMS, Lago GR, Albertino LG, et al. Allele frequency of muscular ge-netic disorders in bull-catching (vaquejada) quarter horses. J Equine Vet Sci 2024;136:105052.
22. de Albuquerque AL, Zanzarini Delfiol DJ, Andrade DGA, et al. Prevalence of the E321G MYH1 variant in Brazilian quarter horses. Equine Vet J 2022;54(5):952–7.
23. Gianino GM, Valberg SJ, Perumbakkam S, et al. Prevalence of the E321G MYH1 variant for immune-mediated myositis and nonexertional rhabdomyolysis in per-formance subgroups of American Quarter Horses. J Vet Intern Med 2019. https://doi.org/10.1111/jvim.15393.
24. Aleman M, Vedavally U, Pusterla N, et al. Common and atypical presentations of Anaplasma phagocytophilum infection in equids with emphasis on neurologic and muscle disease. J Vet Intern Med 2023;38(1):440–8.
25. Shelton GD. From dog to man: the broad spectrum of inflammatory myopathies. Neuromuscul Disord: NMD 2007;17(9–10):663–70.
26. Jain A, Sharma MC, Sarkar C, et al. Major histocompatibility complex class I and II detection as a diagnostic tool in idiopathic inflammatory myopathies. Arch Pathol Lab Med 2007;131(7):1070.
27. Wiendl H, Hohlfeld R, Kieseier BC. Immunobiology of muscle: advances in under-standing an immunological microenvironment. Trends Immunol 2005;26(7):373–80.
28. Root-Bernstein R, Fairweather D. Unresolved issues in theories of autoimmune disease using myocarditis as a framework. J Theor Biol 2015;375:101–23.
29. Zhang P, Cox CJ, Alvarez KM, et al. Cutting edge: cardiac myosin activates innate immune responses through toll-like receptors. J Immunol 2009;183(1):27–31.
30. Quinn A, Ward K, Fischetti VA, et al. Immunological relationship between the class I epitope of streptococcal M protein and myosin. Infect Immun 1998; 66(9):4418–24.
31. Fales-Williams A, Sponseller B, Flaherty H. Idiopathic arterial medial calcification of the thoracic arteries in an adult horse. J Vet Diagn Invest 2008;20(5):692–7.
32. Quist EM, Dougherty JJ, Chaffin MK, et al. Equine rhabdomyolysis. Vet Pathol 2011;48(6):E52–8.
33. Lam J, Takeshita S, Barker JE, et al. TNF-alpha induces osteoclastogenesis by direct stimulation of macrophages exposed to permissive levels of RANK ligand. J Clin Investig 2000;106(12):1481–8.
34. Schott 2nd HC, Schott 2nd HC. Chronic renal failure in horses. Vet Clin N Am Equine Pract 2007;23(3):593–612, vi.
35. Huang L, Xu J, Kumta SM, et al. Gene expression of glucocorticoid receptor alpha and beta in giant cell tumour of bone: evidence of glucocorticoid-stimulated osteoclastogenesis by stromal-like tumour cells. Mol Cell Endocrinol 2001;181(1–2):199–206.
36. Ochala J, Finno CJ, Valberg SJ. Myofibre hyper-contractility in horses expressing the myosin heavy chain myopathy mutation, MYH1E321G. Cells 2021;10(12): 3428.
37. Brown EJ. The molecular basis of streptococcal toxic shock syndrome. N Engl J Med 2004;350(20):2093–4.
38. Aleman M. A review of equine muscle disorders. Neuromuscul Disord : NMD 2008;18(4):277–87.
39. Timoney JF. The pathogenic equine streptococci. Vet Res 2004;35(4):397–409.
40. Valberg S. Myopathies associated with Streptococcus equi equi infection. Equine Vet Educ 2024;36(8):400–2.
41. Pusterla N, Watson JL, Affolter VK, et al. Purpura haemorrhagica in 53 horses. Vet Rec 2003;153(4):118–21.

42. Trimble AC, Delph KM, Beard LA, et al. Staphyloccocus aureus-associated infarctive purpura haemorrhagica, immune-mediated haemolytic anaemia and myocarditis in a Quarter Horse mare. Equine Vet Educ 2019;31(5):230–5.

43. Sweeney CR, Timoney JF, Newton JR, et al. Streptococcus equi infections in horses: guidelines for treatment, control, and prevention of strangles. J Vet Intern Med 2005;19(1):123–34.

44. Boyle AG, Sweeney CR, Kristula M, et al. Factors associated with likelihood of horses having a high serum Streptococcus equi SeM-specific antibody titer. J Am Vet Med Assoc 2009;235(8):973–7.

45. Galan JE, Timoney JF. Immune complexes in purpura hemorrhagica of the horse contain IgA and M antigen of Streptococcus equi. J Immunol 1985;135(5):3134–7.

46. Mallicote M. Update on Streptococcus equi subsp equi infections. Vet Clin N Am Equine Pract 2015;31(1):27–41.

47. Whelchel DD, Chaffin MK. Sequelae and complications of Streptococcus equi subspecies equi infections in the horse. Equine Vet Educ 2009;21(3):135–41.

48. Saulsbury FT. Henoch-Scholein purpura. Curr Opin Rheumatol 2010;22(5):598–602.

49. Somekh E, Fried D, Hanukoglu A. Muscle involvement in Scholein-Henoch syndrome. Arch Dis Child 1983;58(11):929–30.

50. Boyle AG, Timoney JF, Newton JR, et al. Streptococcus equi infections in horses: guidelines for treatment, control, and prevention of strangles-revised consensus statement. J Vet Intern Med 2018;32(2):633–47.

51. Gunson DE, Rooney JR. Anaphylactoid purpura in a horse. Vet Pathol 1977;14(4):325–31.

52. Evans J, Levesque D, Shelton GD. Canine inflammatory myopathies: a clinicopathologic review of 200 cases. J Vet Intern Med 2004;18(5):679–91.

53. Barrott MJ, Brooks HW, McGowan CM. Suspected immune-mediated myositis in a pony. Equine Vet Educ 2004;16(2):58–61.

54. Beech J. Equine muscle disorders 2. Equine Vet Educ 2000;12(4):208–13.

55. Aleman M, Shapiro K, Siso S, et al. Sarcocystis fayeri in skeletal muscle of horses with neuromuscular disease. Neuromuscul Disord : NMD 2016;26(1):85–93.

56. Tinling SP, Cardinet GH, Blythe LL, et al. A light and electron microscopic study of sarcoysts in a horse. J Parasitol 1980;66(3):458–65.

57. Herd HR, Sula MM, Starkey LA, et al. Sarcocystis fayeri-induced granulomatous and eosinophilic myositis in 2 related horses. Vet Pathol 2015;52(6):1191–4.

58. Pasolini MP, Pagano TB, Costagliola A, et al. Inflammatory myopathy in horses with chronic piroplasmosis. Vet Pathol 2018;55(1):133–43.

59. Wise LN, Pelzel-McCluskey AM, Mealey RH, et al. Equine piroplasmosis. Vet Clin N Am Equine Pract 2014;30(3):677–93.

Vitamin E and Selenium-Related Manifestations of Muscle Disease

Carrie J. Finno, DVM, PhD[a], Erica C. McKenzie, BSc, BVMS, PhD[b],*

KEYWORDS

- Rhabdomyolysis • Nutritional myodegeneration • Alpha-tocopherol • Genetic
- Horse • Inherited • Neurodegenerative • Neuromuscular

KEY POINTS

- Nutritional deficiency of vitamin E is common in horses that are kept in a manner preventing consumption of green pasture and not provided additional directed supplementation.
- Nutritional deficiency of selenium is common in horses in regions where the soil and subsequently forage are deficient, when horses are not provided additional directed supplementation.
- Sustained deficiency of vitamin E results in neuromuscular diseases which can include equine motor neuron disease, equine neuroaxonal dystrophy/equine degenerative myeloencephalopathy, and vitamin E responsive myopathy.
- Sustained deficiency of selenium commonly causes non-exertional rhabdomyolysis and/ or muscle atrophy, with additional clinical signs possible due to degeneration of masseter muscles, pharyngeal and tongue muscles, cardiac musculature, or the developing fetus.
- Prevention of vitamin E and selenium deficiencies involves an optimal nutritional program that addresses individual physiologic needs and accounts for utilized feed sources and specific geographic and management factors.

INTRODUCTION

Vitamin E and selenium deficiencies arise from specific factors of management. Vitamin E deficiency develops in horses consuming grass hay rations and that do not receive additional supplementation. Selenium deficiency occurs in horses that consume either dried forage or green grass diets when either forage source is produced in regions where soil is deficient in selenium or vegetation uptake of selenium

[a] Department of Veterinary Population Health & Reproduction, School of Veterinary Medicine, University of California Davis, Room 4206 Vet Med 3A One Shields Avenue, Davis, CA 95616, USA; [b] Department of Clinical Sciences, Carlson College of Veterinary Medicine, Oregon State University, 227 Magruder Hall, Corvallis, OR 97331, USA
* Corresponding author.
E-mail address: erica.mckenzie@oregonstate.edu

Vet Clin Equine 41 (2025) 77–93
https://doi.org/10.1016/j.cveq.2024.11.001   vetequine.theclinics.com

is impeded.[1-4] Individual animal factors can increase the need for antioxidant protection which may exacerbate dietary deficiencies.[5-7] Clinical signs arising from these deficiencies can be very severe and challenging to completely resolve; hence, prevention of these deficiencies is critical in equine nutritional management. Vitamin E and selenium deficiencies can lead to distinct clinical disorders and both nutrients should be assessed and managed independently.

VITAMIN E REQUIREMENTS

Vitamin E is an essential fat-soluble vitamin that is required for healthy neuromuscular function. Vitamin E was originally a general term used to describe a family of 8 naturally occurring closely related compounds (**Table 1**). Alpha-tocopherol, specifically the natural RRR stereoisomer, is the most bioavailable and bioactive form in animal tissues due to preferential uptake by the liver.[8] Since α-tocopherol is also the most potent antioxidant and the only isoform that, when deficient, leads to disease in humans, a recent proposal suggests renaming vitamin E to include only alpha-tocopherol.[9] Thus, the terms α-tocopherol and vitamin E should be used interchangeably.

The major dietary source of vitamin E for horses is fresh pasture, optimally providing approximately 30 to 100 international units (IU)/kg dry matter (DM) of vitamin E.[5] With forage consumption for a healthy, mature horse estimated at 2% body weight (BW) per day, this equates to 300 to 1000 IU of vitamin E consumed by a 500 kg horse per day. The Nutritional Research Council (NRC) lists maintenance requirements of vitamin E for mature horses as 1 IU/kg BW (ie, 500 IU for a 500 kg horse), which is easily met when horses are grazing on fresh pasture multiple hours per day, but green pasture may not be available year round.[4,5] Storing of forage leads to degradation of vitamin E, with losses approaching 50% in alfalfa hay stored for 1 month.[10] Commercial feeds usually provide vitamin E in the form of synthetic vitamin E, containing a mixture of 8 isomers (dl-α-tocopherol, also called all-rac-α-tocopherol), of which only 1 is identical to the natural isomer. This form of vitamin E is a less bioavailable formulation than natural vitamin E. Thus, horses maintained on hay and grain receive far less than the recommended daily requirement of vitamin E.[5]

VITAMIN E ASSESSMENT

Whole-body deficiency of vitamin E is typically assessed by measuring serum concentrations, with normal equine serum concentrations considered to be >2 μg/mL. However, based on studies of horses maintained on pasture, target serum vitamin E concentrations between 3 and 6 μg/mL are recommended.[11] For the assessment of blood vitamin E concentrations, either serum or plasma can be sampled and concentrations are linearly correlated.[12] However, for longitudinal assessment within 1 horse, either serum or plasma should be used each time to avoid the slight variability that can

Table 1 Components of vitamin E	
Tocopherols	**Tocotrienols**
α-tocopherol 8 stereoisomers (*RRR*, SRR, RRS, RSS, RSR, SSR, RSS, SSS)	α-tocotrienol
β-tocopherol	β-tocotrienol
γ-tocopherol	γ-tocotrienol
δ-tocopherol	δ-tocotrienol

occur between sample types. Vitamin E concentration in serum is slightly higher than in plasma.[13,14]

Deficient horses may have larger fluctuations in serum vitamin E (mean coefficient of variation 41%) than nondeficient horses (mean coefficient of variation 14%) within a 24-hour period.[14] Despite these fluctuations, horses with normal vitamin E concentrations tend to maintain values within normal reference intervals based on multiple samplings over time.[15] Deficient horses (using <3 μg/mL as the lower reference point) tend to stay deficient throughout a 24-hour period (Finno CJ, unpublished data). Thus, a single sample is typically sufficient to assess serum/plasma vitamin E status. When evaluating serum/plasma vitamin E concentrations, hemolysis should be avoided since it can decrease vitamin E concentrations by up to 33%.[13] Blood tubes should be stored upright to prevent contact with the rubber stopper and should be stored refrigerated to prevent artificial decreases in vitamin E concentration.[13]

In humans, serum/plasma vitamin E concentrations are only 1% of total body stores and blood concentrations may not reflect tissue concentrations.[16] Thus, in some cases, tissue vitamin E concentrations could be a better marker of whole-body vitamin E status than serum/plasma concentrations. In healthy horses, plasma and adipose tissue concentrations[17] and plasma and hepatic and muscle concentrations[18] are linearly correlated. However, this is not the case in vitamin E responsive myopathy (VEM, see later).

VITAMIN E DEFICIENCY

Across species, clinical vitamin E deficiencies primarily target neuromuscular tissues. Although "white muscle disease" (nutritional myodegeneration) has been associated with vitamin E deficiency, the primary cause is actually selenium deficiency.[19] There are currently 3 diseases recognized as associated with vitamin E deficiency in horses: equine neuroaxonal dystrophy/degenerative myeloencephalopathy (eNAD/EDM), equine motor neuron disease (EMND), and vitamin E responsive myopathy (VEM).

When assessing myopathies associated with vitamin E deficiency, a biopsy of the sacrocaudalis dorsalis medialis muscle is required, since it contains a high proportion of the oxidative type I fibers that are affected by long-term vitamin E deficiency. Gluteal muscle biopsies are unlikely to demonstrate any pathology.[20] In the sacrocaudalis dorsalis medialis muscle, characteristic histopathologic changes are identified with EMND and VEM in type I myofibers consistent with vitamin E deficiency.[20,21] With EMND, older horses are often vitamin E deficient for 18 months or more, with clinical signs of weakness and neurogenic muscle atrophy.[22] Adult horses with VEM can present with muscle atrophy, weakness, and low muscle vitamin E concentrations, but these horses have mitochondrial alterations in muscle fibers and a preponderance of anguloid atrophied fibers that have concavity more on 1 side, rather than neurogenic atrophy, which is characterized by angular atrophied fibers that are compressed into triangular shapes (**Figs. 1** and **2**).[23] With VEM, vitamin E deficiency may be associated with poor performance. In affected horses, serum concentrations of vitamin E may be within the normal range, yet the horse will clinically respond to supplementation.[21] It is hypothesized that these horses may not be able to transport vitamin E into muscle tissue normally, and therefore maintain a normal to high serum vitamin E concentration with deficient muscle concentrations.

With "classic" eNAD/EDM, young horses do not have any pathologic changes of peripheral nerves or skeletal muscle.[23] In older horses with eNAD/EDM, long-term vitamin E deficiency can lead to mitochondrial alterations in type I myofibers. In a series of 43 older horses with postmortem lesions compatible with eNAD/EDM, >40% of

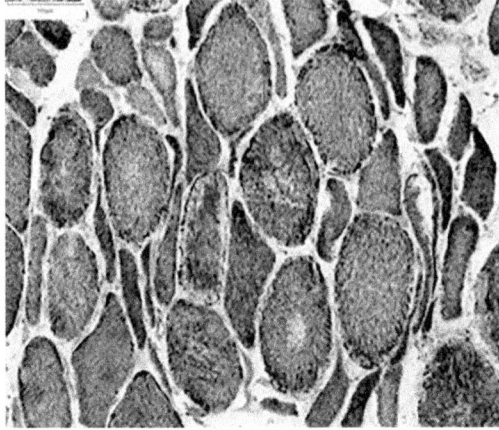

Fig. 1. Neurogenic atrophy in a cross section of the sacrocaudalis dorsalis medialis muscle in a horse with equine motor neuron disease. Note the angular atrophy of both oxidative (smaller, darker fibers) and nonoxidative muscle fibers and central pallor in large myofibers. Nicotinamide adenine dinucleotide tetrazolium reductase stain (NADH-TR; 20X).

horses had mitochondrial alterations identified on sacrocaudalis dorsalis medialis muscle biopsy.[24] However, there was no age-matched control group included, and therefore a direct association could not be concluded. Historical vitamin E deficiency can also be identified from retinal lipofuscin deposits.[25] Therefore, mitochondrial alterations in a muscle biopsy, in addition to retinal lipofuscin deposits, may provide support for historical vitamin E deficiency, but both appear to be age dependent.

VITAMIN E SUPPLEMENTATION

To correctly supplement vitamin E in the horse, the type and formulation of vitamin E supplements need to be considered.

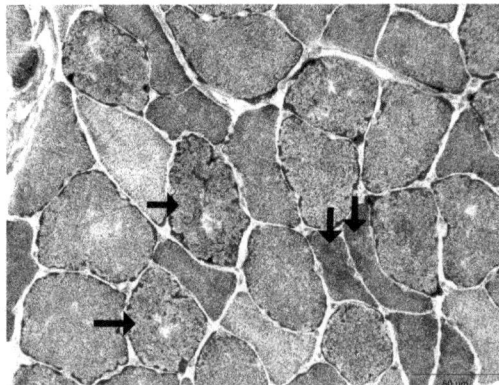

Fig. 2. A cross section of the sacrocaudalis dorsalis medialis muscle in a horse with vitamin E responsive myopathy (NADH-TR;20X). Note the anguloid atrophy (*vertical arrows*) that is typical of myogenic atrophy. There are also numerous fibers (*horizontal arrows*) with subsarcolemmal aggregates of mitochondria (*dark blue*) and these fibers also have a moth-eaten staining appearance in the myoplasm.

Formulations

Natural vitamin E, RRR-α-tocopherol, is more bioavailable than synthetic vitamin E and therefore many equine supplements now strongly market the "natural" (ie, RRR) form.[11] The natural formulation is available as an esterified form (α-tocopherol acetate) to prolong shelf life (ie, powder or pellet) or as a water dispersible (ie, liquid) formulation with higher biopotency (**Table 2**).

Dose

Most studies of vitamin E supplementation have used healthy horses and assessed serum vitamin E rather than neuromuscular tissue concentrations. The absorption and metabolism of vitamin E in healthy horses may differ from that of horses with diseases associated with vitamin E deficiency.[11,12] As a result, it is essential to measure serum vitamin E concentrations, monitor vitamin E concentrations, and adjust the dose in response to changes occurring with supplementation.

The most rapid rise in serum vitamin E concentrations is obtained by providing natural-source liquid forms of α-tocopherol at 10 IU/kg BW. The liquid formulation is 5 to 6 times more bioavailable than synthetic α-tocopherol acetate, and a 5000-IU dose/horse more than doubles serum vitamin E concentrations within 12 hours.[26] Evaluation of healthy horses with marginal or deficient serum vitamin E concentrations found that 14 days of water dispersible natural α-tocopherol supplementation at 10,000 IU/horse/day significantly increased cerebrospinal fluid (CSF) α-tocopherol concentration.[27] However, there is rarely the need to administer more than 5,000 IU/horse/day of water dispersible α-tocopherol, since more recent evidence has demonstrated an increase in CSF α-tocopherol at this dose.[28]

Many owners are reluctant to maintain horses on liquid supplementation long-term and therefore, changing to a powdered or pelleted supplement is often desired. However, veterinarians should be aware that when horses are switched from the same dose of natural water-dispersible vitamin E to the powdered acetate formulation, a precipitous drop in serum vitamin E can occur.[28] The most effective and economical approach to supplementing deficient horses over time is therefore to overlap treatment with the liquid and powder/pellet formulations, and gradually withdraw the liquid vitamin E, leading to a more stable steady state of serum vitamin E and higher tissue vitamin E concentrations with continued supplementation.[28]

If horses are deficient in vitamin E without signs of neuromuscular disease and owners find water-dispersible formulations of vitamin E cost-prohibitive, supplementation can be started with 5,000 IU/day of pelleted or powdered natural α-tocopherol

Table 2 Available forms of vitamin E supplementation			
Type of Supplement	Form of Vitamin E in Supplement	Bioavailability	Cost
Natural vitamin E (liquid)	RRR-α-tocopherol	High	High
Natural vitamin E (powder or pellet)	RRR-α-tocopheryl acetate	Intermediate	Intermediate
Synthetic vitamin E (powder or pellet)	All-rac α-tocopheryl acetate (all stereoisomers) OR dl-α-tocopheryl acetate (RRR and SRR-stereoisomers)	Low	Low

acetate. However, serum vitamin E concentrations are not expected to increase for at least 8 to 10 weeks using this protocol.[28]

Approximately 40% of EMND cases may demonstrate some improvement within 6 weeks of appropriate supplementation, and some can appear normal within 3 months.[22] In cases of eNAD/EDM, vitamin E supplementation does not improve clinical signs but may stabilize the disease process.[29] However, vitamin E supplementation of genetically susceptible foals throughout the first year of life can decrease the overall incidence of signs of eNAD/EDM.[29–31] Horses with VEM respond well to appropriate vitamin E supplementation and can regain strength and muscle mass within 3 months.[21] It is noteworthy, however, that in clinically normal vitamin E-deficient horses with mitochondrial alterations in the sacrocaudalis dorsalis medialis muscle, vitamin E supplementation does not change the percentage of fibers with mitochondrial alterations or anguloid atrophy.[20]

OTHER CONSIDERATIONS

This author (CF) has performed over 10 vitamin E supplementation trials using various formulations in healthy vitamin E-insufficient horses and in horses with specific neuromuscular diseases. Repeatable success has been demonstrated when using an RRR-α-tocopherol liquid formulation for supplementation at the doses recommended in this article.[12,20,28,31–35] There are, however, a subset of horses that fail to respond to correctly supplemented α-tocopherol. These horses may have malabsorption due to inflammation from parasitic infections or other causes of gastrointestinal inflammation.[36] There is no approved injectable vitamin E product for horses that will effectively raise serum vitamin E concentrations. Attempts to use an injectable bovine product to increase vitamin E concentrations in a study were associated with marked tissue reactions in all treated horses.[35] The only currently available U.S. Food and Drug Administration (FDA)-approved product for horses, E-SE®, will increase selenium concentrations but does not provide enough bioavailable α-tocopherol to affect serum α-tocopherol concentrations.[32]

While many nutrition companies tout their products as containing "natural vitamin E," most have not been assessed in clinical trials. For that reason, careful consideration of both product type and dose must be given when targeting vitamin E supplementation in deficient horses. For large herds, the most cost-effective means of supplementing horses is to provide fresh pasture for at least 6 months of the year.[11] Where this is not an option, targeted supplementation as recommended is advised. Assessing serum vitamin E concentrations in individuals is paramount since vitamin E metabolism differs widely from horse to horse.[28]

While vitamin E supplementation is generally considered safe, there are potential risks of over supplementation. Supplementation with vitamin E may alter drug metabolism and disposition since, in humans, the same cytochrome isoforms that metabolize vitamin E metabolize >50% of therapeutic drugs.[37] The NRC has set the upper safe dietary concentration for vitamin E at 20 IU/kg BW based on biopotency of synthetic α-tocopherol (10,000 IU/500 kg horse).[5] Above this level, coagulopathy and impaired bone mineralization have been reported.[5] Therefore, regular assessment of serum vitamin E concentrations is highly recommended in supplemented horses.

SELENIUM REQUIREMENTS

Selenium is considered an essential trace mineral, and a rare and non-renewable global resource, critical to human and animal health and utilized extensively in a range of global industrial processes.[38] Selenium has critical antioxidant functions mediated through multiple selenium-dependent peroxidase enzymes, and selenoproteins are also integral in immune function, reproductive success, and muscle and thyroid function.[6,39,40] Inadequate dietary intake of selenium is the cause of selenium deficiency in humans and animals.[38] Low soil selenium content is a major factor contributing to the production of selenium-poor forages, exacerbated by factors interfering with selenium uptake by plants, including the application of phosphate or sulfate-containing fertilizers.[6,41] Selenium-deficient soils are found in large regions of the world including much of the United States, as well as regions of Canada, Australia, New Zealand, and Europe.[1–3,38] Furthermore, consumption of sulfur, copper, and other elements can impede gastrointestinal absorption of selenium by animals, and animals under physiologic stress, such as during pregnancy, lactation, heavy exercise, or growth periods, may have increased anti-oxidant requirements including higher selenium needs.[5,6]

Due to concerns for human and animal toxicity risks, selenium content of animal feed products in the United States is controlled under the Code of Federal Regulations (CFR), which limits the addition of selenium in the forms of sodium selenite or selenate, selenium yeast (*Saccharomyces cerevisiae*), and selenomethionine hydroxy analog.[42,43] Selenium supplementation for horses is not formally recognized in the CFR, however, equine nutritional products now often align with CFR recommendations made for beef cattle. According to the relevant portion of the CFR, any of the listed selenium forms can be added to complete feeds at levels not exceeding 0.3 parts per million (ppm) DM (equivalent to 0.3 mg per kg of DM); to feed supplements for limit feeding not exceeding 3 mg total per head per day for beef cattle; or to salt-mineral mixtures up to 120 parts per million (equivalent to 120 mg/kg DM) for free-choice feeding at a rate not exceeding an intake of 3 mg per head per day for beef cattle.[42]

Clinical evidence supports a minimum total intake of 1 mg per day of selenium for a 500 kg horse, compatible with the NRC recommendations of 0.1 mg/kg DM for mature sedentary horses.[5,44] This amount will apparently maintain whole blood selenium concentrations within reference intervals for mature horses (160–275 ng/mL or ug/L) even in deficient regions.[4] However, depletion and repletion studies suggest that 0.1 mg/kg DM is close to the minimum requirement for idle mature horses, and may not be adequate to optimize blood concentrations, performance, or production. Providing selenium at 0.3 ppm DM (triple the NRC recommendations, and equivalent to approximately 2.5–3 mg total Se/day for a 500 kg horse) increases selenium status to a plateau significantly above that of horses fed at NRC recommendation.[44] All contributions of selenium to the ration should be considered during dietary evaluation to avoid the potential for toxicity, which can result in hoof and haircoat abnormalities. A maximum tolerance of between 2 and 5 mg/kg DM selenium has been suggested.[1,5,45]

Selenium sources that require voluntary intake, such as selenium-containing salt blocks, can be highly unreliable and therefore directed feeding of minimum daily requirements is recommended to prevent deficiency in equids.[4] All forms of selenium listed in the CFR are well-absorbed and suitable for prevention of deficiency in horses, with perhaps slight superiority of selenomethionine yeast.[46–48] In utero, foals derive selenium across the placenta, and hence deficient mares, and occasionally mares with adequate blood selenium concentrations can produce foals with subclinical or clinical selenium deficiency.[2,3,49] Deficiency in either mare or foal should be considered evidence of likely deficiency in the other as well as in herd mates. Selenium and vitamin E interact as antioxidants, and there is evidence to suggest that adequate status in one nutrient can confer some protective effect when the other is deficient.[6,7,40] However, severe clinical selenium deficiency including cardiac damage can occur in neonatal and mature equids even in spite of adequate vitamin E status, and ideally both nutrients should be assessed when clinical signs and management factors suggest deficiency of either nutrient.[3,50–53]

SELENIUM DEFICIENCY

Mature horses likely sustain suboptimal blood and liver selenium concentrations for months before the onset of overt clinical signs of deficiency and some individuals can be clinically asymptomatic in spite of very low blood selenium concentrations.[44,54] However, it is likely that deficient horses go through a period of subclinical disease. During this time, they potentially have suboptimal immune responses and suboptimal reproductive function, with pregnant mares also at risk of dystocia, abortion, or producing foals with clinical deficiency.[6,55,56] Clinical signs of deficiency are reported with the greatest frequency in foals, and usually relate to the presence of severe rhabdomyolysis, referred to as nutritional myodegeneration or white muscle disease.[3,19,49,53,57] Affected foals may be born with clinical signs or develop them days to months after birth.[3,19,57,58] Foals may be recumbent or weak, and may display low head carriage related to weakness and necrosis of cervical musculature. Visible myoglobinuria may be evident when large amounts of muscle tissue are compromised and secondary renal damage can occur.[57] Cardiac arrythmias may be evident related to accompanying myocardial necrosis or severe electrolyte disturbances associated with massive rhabdomyolysis.[57–59] Signs related to disturbed oropharyngeal function including milk from the nostrils and aspiration pneumonia often occur, related to compromise to the musculature of the tongue and/or pharynx (**Fig. 3**).[51,57] In Europe, severe panniculitis or steatitis ("yellow fat disease") is also reported to occur in foals and young horses, potentially related to combined deficiencies of selenium and vitamin E.[60]

Though foals have been suggested to be much more susceptible to nutritional myodegeneration, there are multiple reports describing severe clinical disease and death in mature equids as a result of selenium deficiency.[51,52,56,60–66] The clinical presentation of severe and prolonged selenium deficiency in mature horses can be highly variable, often contributing to misdiagnosis and delayed recognition and treatment. The

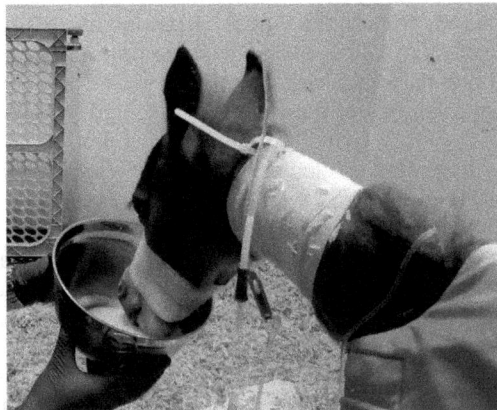

Fig. 3. Weak foals born with rhabdomyolysis and dysphagia related to selenium deficiency may require enteral and pan feeding to provide adequate nutrition while minimizing aspiration.

list of tissues that may be affected in selenium deficiency and the associated clinical signs that can be encountered as a result are included in **Table 3**, and combinations of potentially any of these signs can arise in an individual. Clinical signs can present acutely, despite the chronic nature of the underlying disease, or subtle anomalies including diffuse muscle atrophy and abnormal prehension can develop over weeks to months, sometimes preceding an acute crisis of non-exertional rhabdomyolysis with or without accompanying indications of cardiac muscle damage.[51,62] External stressors, such as moving environments, can precipitate the onset of overt clinical signs in chronically deficient horses.[62] Clinical presentations of confirmed severe selenium deficiency in mature equids (horses, donkeys, mules, zebras) that have been reported in the literature and anecdotally observed include and are not limited to acute non-exertional rhabdomyolysis, diffuse severe chronic muscle atrophy and weakness, abnormal prehension with quidding of feed and trismus (**Fig. 4**), oropharyngeal dysphagia, signs of left-sided (pulmonary edema) and right-sided (ventral edema, cavitary effusions, distended peripheral vasculature, diarrhea) congestive heart failure with accompanying rhabdomyolysis, spontaneous ventricular tachycardia, respiratory failure related to diaphragmatic necrosis, and panniculitis.[51,52,56,60–66] Multiple deaths can occur in groups of mature equids as a result of severe sustained selenium deficiency particularly when the underlying cause is not identified promptly.[65]

DIAGNOSIS OF SELENIUM DEFICIENCY

In clinically diseased horses, the diagnosis of selenium deficiency is usually supported by compatible dietary history and clinical signs, (variably) elevated serum creatine kinase (CK) and aspartate transaminase (AST) activities, and measurement of whole blood selenium or other blood-based indicators of selenium status. Additional diagnostics are typically focused on evaluating the presence and severity of the primary and secondary consequences of this deficiency.

Subclinical selenium deficiency is very common in some regions, and confirmation requires blood testing.[2–4,53] Suspicion for deficiency can be readily established by

Table 3
Tissues and systems that can be affected in severe selenium deficiency in foals and horses, and associated clinical signs and consequences

Tissue or System Affected	Consequences
Tongue	Ptyalism, tongue swelling and protrusion, oropharyngeal dysphagia
Pharynx	Oropharyngeal dysphagia, aspiration pneumonia (more common in foals)
Masseter	Trismus, dysfunctional prehension, masseter swelling or atrophy
Cardiac muscle	Tachycardia, arrythmias, peripheral edema, respiratory distress (pulmonary edema), and other signs of congestive heart failure
Diaphragm	Respiratory difficulty
Skeletal muscle	Weakness, diffuse muscle atrophy, low head carriage, fasciculations, recumbency, myoglobinuria. Signs accompanied by variable elevation of CK and AST, and variable electrolyte disturbances
Reproductive tract	Reproductive failure (males and females), dystocia, retained placenta, weak or dead foals
Adipose	Subcutaneous edema, swelling of supraorbital fat, pain on palpation
Immune system	Compromised immunity including reduced vaccine response

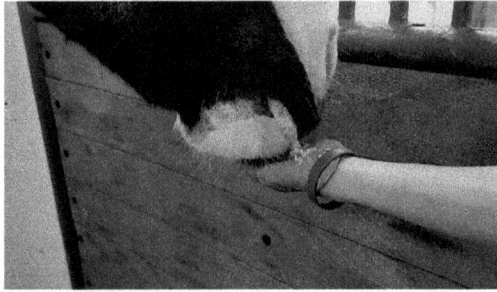

Fig. 4. A 22-year-old Mustang gelding showing trismus, abnormal prehension, quidding, and ptyalism. Blood selenium was critically low at 13 ng/mL (reference: 160–275 ng/mL or ug/L), CK moderately elevated at 10,241 U/L (reference: 145–633 U/L), and AST severely elevated at 13,393 U/L (reference: 212–453 U/L). The horse was euthanized after 3 weeks of intensive treatment when it continued to be unable to eat even a modified diet due to ongoing anomalies of prehension and swallowing.

ration review, where the amount of each component fed and its reported or estimated selenium content are collated to determine if minimum requirements for the individual are likely being met.[4,5] Generally, in deficient regions, forage whether green or dried should be considered a negligible selenium source due to low intrinsic selenium content, as should salt blocks since highly variable and unreliable daily consumption patterns occur.[4] Confirmation of suboptimal selenium status can be determined by measurement of several variables, including plasma or serum selenium, whole blood glutathione peroxidase activity (a selenium-dependent enzyme), or whole blood selenium concentration. Extensive literature exists for all of these measures in horses, and measurement of whole blood selenium concentration is the preferred methodology to detect deficiency due to greater reliability of results and capacity to more accurately differentiate deficient from adequate status.[6,47,53] Though serum or plasma selenium concentration more accurately reflects recent supplementation status, measurement of whole blood selenium is a good indicator of chronic supplementation status, and both are convenient in foals, where ration review has less utility. Mare and foal selenium status is moderately to highly correlated and horse and donkey foals typically have lower plasma and blood selenium values than their dams, even when blood glutathione peroxidase does not differ.[2,45,67,68] Nonetheless, mares with apparently adequate selenium status on blood testing can still produce clinically selenium-deficient foals, but do so much less frequently than mares with inadequate status.[2,3,49] It is also possible to observe features suggestive of nutritional myodegeneration, particularly in the masseter muscles, in horses with apparently normal blood selenium status suggesting complex etiology in some cases.[51,69] Liver tissue can also be collected by biopsy or postmortem sampling for measurement of selenium concentration as an accurate indicator of whole body selenium status.

Elevation of serum CK and AST activities are encountered in most cases of clinical selenium deficiency of foals and mature horses and can vary widely from hundreds to hundreds of thousands, though values are rarely completely normal.[3,49,51,59] Very high CK values (>30,000 U/L) and myoglobinuria indicate the presence of severe rhabdomyolysis involving a large amount of muscle tissue. Modest elevations can occur in chronically diseased animals that also have severe dysfunction, and anecdotally, there appears to be poor correlation between how high serum CK activities are and prognosis for survival. In cases with acute, profound rhabdomyolysis, additional biochemical disturbances can be encountered, including azotemia, hypoalbuminemia, hyperkalemia, hyperphosphatemia, and reductions in serum sodium, chloride, and calcium. In foals, this necessitates the exclusion of urinary tract disruption as a cause of azotemia and electrolyte disturbances by abdominal ultrasound and potentially peritoneal fluid analysis.[57] Urine of equids with rhabdomyolysis should be evaluated for the presence of visible or occult pigmenturia, and specific gravity recorded prior to fluid therapy if possible.

Measurement of blood cardiac troponin I, in addition to ECG monitoring and echo-cardiography can help establish the presence and severity of cardiac involvement in selenium deficiency cases which has implications potentially for survival and future performance (**Figs. 5** and **6**).[52,59] Non-exertional rhabdomyolysis with cardiac involvement may necessitate additional diagnostic steps to exclude toxic etiologies including ionophores and hypoglycin A.[64,70] For horses with masseter involvement, other causes of trismus and masseter myodegeneration might require consideration, including hypocalcemia, hyperkalemic periodic paralysis, tetanus, and jaw trauma. Imaging via radiography and ultrasound should be considered.[66,69] Dysphagic foals and horses may require endoscopy and other diagnostics for upper gastrointestinal and respiratory tract assessment. Ultrasonography has been used to confirm steatitis in horses with nutritional deficiencies reflected by abnormally increased echogenicity of adipose tissue, including in the peri-renal, coronary, pericardial, and ventral extra-peritoneal regions, confirmed by adipose biopsy.[60]

Histopathology of skeletal muscle tissue can be used to identify patchy monophasic (acute) or polyphasic (chronic) necrosis and dystrophic calcification suggestive of nutritional myodegeneration, and to exclude other causes of atrophy and/or non-exertional rhabdomyolysis, including vitamin E deficiency disorders and hypoglycin A toxicity.[51,71,72] Where relevant, specific genetic testing can be used to exclude glycogen branching enzyme deficiency (foals), myosin heavy chain myopathy, and

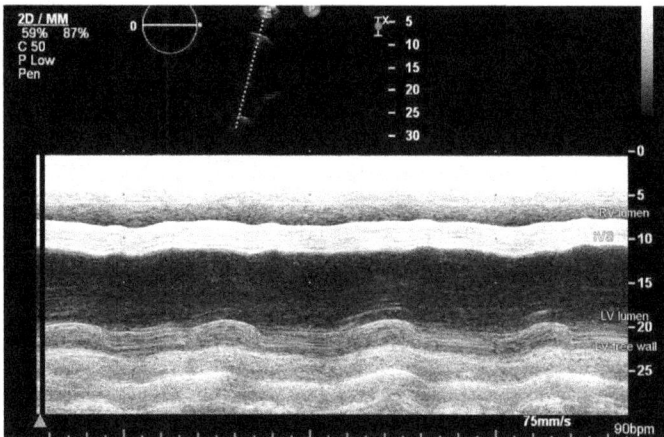

Fig. 5. M-mode of the cardiac ventricles from a 12-year-old mare presenting with acute respiratory distress related to cardiogenic pulmonary edema from selenium deficiency. Systolic function is severely impaired (fractional shortening 13%) and cardiac troponin I very high at 103 ng/mL (reference <0.2 ng/mL). Serum CK of the mare was moderately elevated 8,992 (reference 145–633 U/L) and serum AST proportionally much more elevated at 3,372 (212–453 U/L) consistent with non-exertional rhabdomyolysis. Whole blood selenium was critically low at 23 ng/mL (reference: 160–275 ng/mL). (*Image courtesy of* Dr. Kate Scollan.)

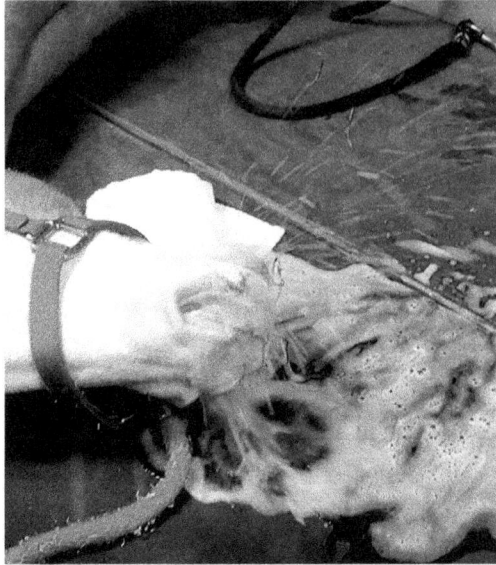

Fig. 6. Edema fluid erupting from the nostrils of the mare in **Fig. 5** immediately after euthanasia, reflecting severe pulmonary edema.

type 1 polysaccharide storage myopathy which can also all be associated with non-exertional rhabdomyolysis.[61,72,73]

Treatment of Selenium Deficiency

Rectifying the absolute deficiency is usually readily achieved by injecting affected equids intramuscularly with inorganic selenium at a dose of 0.055 mg/kg. This can be repeated in 7 to 10 days if very low blood concentrations (<60 ng/mL) are observed.[74] Repeat evaluation of whole blood selenium 4 weeks after treatment commences is recommended. Where there is a high index of suspicion for deficiency, horses should be provided injectable selenium prior to return of results related to measurement of selenium status, to optimize the chance of successful outcome. Due to the constellation of involved tissues in many cases, and the severity of clinical signs that can occur, it is not uncommon for affected foals and adults to require prolonged and extensive treatment sometimes stretching over multiple weeks. Complete recovery can take months, and permanent fibrosis and atrophy of damaged musculature can occur. Treatment and monitoring of clinical deficiency cases should subscribe to the following tenets as necessary.

1. Prevent progressive rhabdomyolysis—provide injectable selenium, oral dantrolene sodium, appropriate bedding and sling support if necessary. Monitor serum CK and AST for response to treatment.
2. Prevent recumbency-related complications—remove shoes, wrap limbs, protect head and eyes.
3. Provide analgesia—caution with non-steroidal drugs if renal challenges are present.
4. Prevent renal damage from vasomotor phenomena and pigmenturia—fluid therapy, judicious use of nephrotoxic agents, and alkalinization if acid urine pH is present concurrently with myoglobinuria.

5. Correct severe electrolyte disturbances.
6. Provide nutritional support in animals with dysphagia, trismus, or anorexia. Parenteral and enteral nutrition may be necessary, or modified (mash) diets, along with protein and amino acid supplementation. Miniature horses, ponies, and donkeys in particular require careful management to prevent secondary hepatic lipidosis.
7. Antioxidant treatment—high-dose vitamin E (5000 IU natural alpha-tocopherol), 0.3 to 0.5 ppm DM selenium in total ration, and consider vitamin C supplementation.
8. Control head position to prevent additional swelling of the head and tongue; muscle relaxants (methocarbamol, dantrolene) may aid relaxation of trismus.
9. Control cardiac arrhythmias—ventricular tachycardia may require first-line therapy with lidocaine or magnesium sulfate; repeat echocardiography to monitor circulating volume and cardiac function.
10. Antibiotic coverage—usually only indicated in high-risk patients (neonates) and those with aspiration secondary to oropharyngeal dysphagia.

Prevention of Selenium Deficiency

Deficiency is readily prevented by daily dietary supplementation which induces peak plasma and blood concentrations within 28 to 112 days after supplementation commences, even with minimal change in plasma glutathione peroxidase.[45,47,75] Supplementation of pregnant mares is recommended throughout gestation to optimize selenium status of the developing foal. It has been demonstrated to reliably increase muscle and plasma selenium concentrations in mares and the foals they produce, as well as increasing colostrum selenium concentrations.[45] Reference values for whole blood selenium concentration in mature horses may vary somewhat between laboratories, but a range between 160 and 275 ng/mL (equivalent to ug/L) is consistent with values that have been applied in the last 3 decades and likely promote optimal function.[4,76] The origin of reference values for whole blood selenium values in foals is less clear, with a large study employing relatively disparate values of >0.76 μm/L (60 ng/mL) in foals under 10 days of age, and $\geq$2.15 μm/L (170 ng/mL) for horses over 10 days of age.[53] Foals from supplemented mares in a longitudinal trial had plasma selenium values of 0.149 and 0.158 ug/mL (149–158 ng/mL) when mares were receiving 0.5 to 0.65 mg/kg DM in the ration during gestation.[45]

CLINICS CARE POINTS

- Subclinical and clinical nutritional deficiencies of vitamin E and selenium are prevalent which relate to modern systems of equine management and geographic features. Both can result in severe disease that can be difficult to resolve, and prevention is paramount.

- Vitamin E deficiency disorders tend to present with gait abnormalities, weakness, and muscle atrophy with or without evidence of rhabdomyolysis on clinical pathology screening.

- Selenium deficiency has a more variable clinical presentation, and non-exertional rhabdomyolysis, symmetric masseter swelling or atrophy, dysphagia, and cardiac disease are common clinical signs in mature equids, and weakness and dysphagia in foals.

- Both deficiencies can be readily prevented through appropriate daily dietary supplementation of vitamin E at a minimum 1 IU/kg BW and selenium at 0.1 to 0.3 ppm DM of the ration (or a minimum of 1 mg/horse/day).

- Vitamin E status can be assessed through measurement of serum or plasma concentrations (values preferably over >3 μg/mL) and selenium status preferably on whole blood (values preferably between 160 and 275 ng/mL).

- Selenium supplementation is particularly crucial throughout gestation to reduce the chance of a clinically deficient foal.

DISCLOSURES

The authors have nothing to disclose.

REFERENCES

1. Edmonson AJ, Norman BB, Suther D. Survey of state veterinarians and state veterinary diagnostic laboratories for selenium deficiency and toxicosis in animals. J Am Vet Med Assoc 1993;202(6):865–72.
2. Muirhead TL, Wichtel JJ, Stryhn H, et al. The selenium and vitamin E status of horses in Prince Edward Island. Can Vet J 2010;51(9):979–85.
3. Delesalle C, de Bruijn M, Wilmink S, et al. White muscle disease in foals: focus on selenium soil content. A case series. BMC Vet Res 2017;13(1):121.
4. Pitel MO, McKenzie EC, Johns JL, et al. Influence of specific management practices on blood selenium, vitamin E, and beta-carotene concentrations in horses and risk of nutritional deficiency. J Vet Intern Med 2020;34(5):2132–41.
5. National Research Council (NRC). Minerals. In: National Research Council, editor. Nutrient requirements of horses. 6th edition. Washington, DC: National Academies Press; 2007. p. 17–8.
6. Hosnedlova B, Kepinska M, Skalickova S, et al. A summary of New findings on the biological effects of selenium in selected animal species-A critical review. Int J Mol Sci 2017;18(10):2209.
7. Owen RN, Semanchik PL, Latham CM, et al. Elevated dietary selenium rescues mitochondrial capacity impairment induced by decreased vitamin E intake in young exercising horses. J Anim Sci 2022;100(8):172.
8. Leonard SW, Terasawa Y, Farese RV Jr, et al. Incorporation of deuterated RRR- or all-rac-alpha-tocopherol in plasma and tissues of alpha-tocopherol transfer protein-null mice. Am J Clin Nutr 2002;75:555–60.
9. Azzi A, Atkinson J, Ozer NK, et al. Vitamin E discussion forum position paper on the revision of the nomenclature of vitamin E. Free Radic Biol Med 2023;207: 178–80.
10. McDowell LR. Vitamin E. In: McDowell LR, editor. Vitamins in animal nutrition. San Diego, CA: Academic Press, Inc.; 1989. p. 93–131.
11. Finno CJ, Valberg SJ. A comparative review of vitamin E and associated equine disorders. J Vet Intern Med 2012;26:1251–66.
12. Hales EN, Habib H, Favro G, et al. Increased alpha-tocopherol metabolism in horses with equine neuroaxonal dystrophy. J Vet Intern Med 2021;35:2473–85.
13. Craig AM, Blythe LL, Rowe KE, et al. Variability of alpha-tocopherol values associated with procurement, storage, and freezing of equine serum and plasma samples. Am J Vet Res 1992;53:2228–34.
14. Vanschandevijl K, Nollet H, Deprez P, et al. Variation in deficient serum vitamin E levels and impact on assessment of the vitamin E status in horses. Vlaams Diergeneeskunidig Tijdschrift 2009;78:28–33.
15. Lindholm A, Asheim A. Vitamin E and certain muscular enzymes in the blood serum of horses. Acta Agric Scand Suppl 1973;19:40–2.
16. Traber MG. Vitamin E inadequacy in humans: causes and consequences. Adv Nutr 2014;5:503–14.

17. Steiss JE, Traber MG, Williams MA, et al. Alpha tocopherol concentrations in clinically normal adult horses. Equine Vet J 1994;26:417–9.
18. Roneus BO, Hakkarainen RV, Lindholm CA, et al. Vitamin E requirements of adult Standardbred horses evaluated by tissue depletion and repletion. Equine Vet J 1986;18:50–8.
19. Lofstedt J. White muscle disease of foals. Vet Clin N Am Equine Pract 1997;13: 169–85.
20. Bookbinder L, Finno CJ, Firshman AM, et al. Impact of alpha-tocopherol deficiency and supplementation on sacrocaudalis and gluteal muscle fiber histopathology and morphology in horses. J Vet Intern Med 2019;33:2770–9.
21. Bedford HE, Valberg SJ, Firshman AM, et al. Histopathologic findings in the sacrocaudalis dorsalis medialis muscle of horses with vitamin E-responsive muscle atrophy and weakness. J Am Vet Med Assoc 2013;242:1127–37.
22. Divers TJ, De Lahunta A, Hintz HF, et al. Equine motor neuron disease. Equine Vet Educ 2001;13:63–7.
23. Finno CJ, Higgins RJ, Aleman M, et al. Equine degenerative myeloencephalopathy in Lusitano horses. J Vet Intern Med 2011;25:1439–46.
24. Colmer SF, Valberg SJ, Bender SJ, et al. Association of vitamin E-responsive myopathy and equine neuroaxonal dystrophy/equine degenerative myeloencephalopathy. American Association of Equine Practitioners 2023;454–5.
25. Riis RC, Jackson C, Rebhun W, et al. Ocular manifestations of equine motor neuron disease. Equine Vet J 1999;31:99–110.
26. Pagan JD, Lennox M, Perry L, et al. Form of α-tocopherol affects vitamin E bioavailability in Thoroughbred horses. Nordic Feed Science 2010;112–5.
27. Higgins JK, Puschner B, Kass PH, et al. Assessment of vitamin E concentrations in serum and cerebrospinal fluid of horses following oral administration of vitamin E. Am J Vet Res 2008;69:785–90.
28. Brown JC, Valberg SJ, Hogg M, et al. Effects of feeding two RRR-alpha-tocopherol formulations on serum, cerebrospinal fluid and muscle alpha-tocopherol concentrations in horses with subclinical vitamin E deficiency. Equine Vet J 2017;49:753–8.
29. Burns EN, Finno CJ. Equine degenerative myeloencephalopathy: prevalence, impact, and management. Vet Med (Auckl) 2018;9:63–7.
30. Mayhew IG, Brown CM, Stowe HD, et al. Equine degenerative myeloencephalopathy: a vitamin E deficiency that may be familial. J Vet Intern Med 1987;1:45–50.
31. Aleman M, Finno CJ, Higgins RJ, et al. Evaluation of epidemiological, clinical, and pathological features of neuroaxonal dystrophy in Quarter Horses. J Am Vet Med Assoc 2011;239:823–33.
32. Finno CJ, Estell KE, Katzman S, et al. Blood and cerebrospinal fluid alpha-tocopherol and selenium concentrations in neonatal foals with neuroaxonal dystrophy. J Vet Intern Med 2015;29:1667–75.
33. Powers A, Peek SF, Reed S, et al. Equine neuroaxonal dystrophy/degenerative myeloencephalopathy in Gypsy Vanner horses. J Vet Intern Med 2024;38:1792–8.
34. Donnelly CG, Finno CJ. Vitamin E depletion is associated with subclinical axonal degeneration in juvenile horses. Equine Vet J 2023;55(5):884–90.
35. Donnelly CG, Burns E, Easton-Jones CA, et al. Safety and efficacy of subcutaneous alpha-tocopherol in healthy adult horses. Equine Vet Educ 2021;33:215–9.
36. Diez de Castro E, Zafra R, Acevedo LM, et al. Eosinophilic enteritis in horses with motor neuron disease. J Vet Intern Med 2016;30:873–9.
37. Kluth D, Landes N, Pfluger P, et al. Modulation of Cyp3a11 mRNA expression by alpha-tocopherol but not gamma-tocotrienol in mice. Free Radic Biol Med 2005; 38:507–14.

38. Haug A, Graham RD, Christophersen OA, et al. How to use the world's scarce selenium resources efficiently to increase the selenium concentration in food. Microb Ecol Health Dis 2007;19(4):209–28.

39. Arthur JR, McKenzie RC, Beckett GJ. Selenium in the immune system. J Nutr 2003;133(5 Suppl 1):1457S–9S.

40. Rederstorff M, Krol A, Lescure A. Understanding the importance of selenium and selenoproteins in muscle function. Cell Mol Life Sci 2006;63(1):52–9.

41. Gupta M, Gupta S. An overview of selenium uptake, metabolism, and toxicity in plants. Front Plant Sci 2017;7:2074.

42. Code of federal Regulations. Available at: https://www.ecfr.gov/current/title-21/chapter-I/subchapter-E/part-573.

43. Ullrey DE. Basis for regulation of selenium supplements in animal diets. J Anim Sci 1992;70(12):3922–7.

44. Brummer M, Hayes S, Dawson KA, et al. Measures of antioxidant status of the horse in response to selenium depletion and repletion. J Anim Sci 2013;91(5):2158–68.

45. Karren BJ, Thorson JF, Cavinder CA, et al. Effect of selenium supplementation and plane of nutrition on mares and their foals: selenium concentrations and glutathione peroxidase. J Anim Sci 2010;88(3):991–7.

46. Podoll KL, Bernard JB, Ullrey DE, et al. Dietary selenate versus selenite for cattle, sheep, and horses. J Anim Sci 1992;70(6):1965–70.

47. Richardson SM, Siciliano PD, Engle TE, et al. Effect of selenium supplementation and source on the selenium status of horses. J Anim Sci 2006;84(7):1742–8.

48. Calamari L, Ferrari A, Bertin G. Effect of selenium source and dose on selenium status of mature horses. J Anim Sci 2009;87(1):167–78.

49. Katz L, O'Dwyer S, Pollock P. Nutritional muscular dystrophy in a four-day-old Connemara foal. Ir Vet J 2009;62(2):119–24.

50. Owen R, Moore JN, Hopkins JB, et al. Dystrophic myodegeneration in adult horses. J Am Vet Med Assoc 1977;171:343–9.

51. Pearson EG, Snyder SP, Saulez MN. Masseter myodegeneration as a cause of trismus or dysphagia in adult horses. Vet Rec 2005;156(20):642–6.

52. Schefer KD, Hagen R, Ringer SK, et al. Laboratory, electrocardiographic, and echocardiographic detection of myocardial damage and dysfunction in an Arabian mare with nutritional masseter myodegeneration. J Vet Intern Med 2011;25(5):1171–80.

53. Streeter RM, Divers TJ, Mittel L, et al. Selenium deficiency associations with gender, breed, serum vitamin E and creatine kinase, clinical signs and diagnoses in horses of different age groups: a retrospective examination 1996-2011. Equine Vet J Suppl 2012;43:31–5.

54. Ronéus B. Glutathione peroxidase and selenium in the blood of healthy horses and foals affected by muscular dystrophy. Nord Vet Med 1982;34(10):350–3.

55. Brummer M, Hayes S, Adams AA, et al. The effect of selenium supplementation on vaccination response and immune function in adult horses. J Anim Sci 2013;91(8):3702–15.

56. Busse NI, Uberti B. Uterine inertia due to severe selenium deficiency in a parturient mare. J Equine Vet Sci 2020;85:102845.

57. Perkins G, Valberg SJ, Madigan JM, et al. Electrolyte disturbances in foals with severe rhabdomyolysis. J Vet Intern Med 1998;12(3):173–7.

58. MacQuarrie J. Congenital nutritional myodegeneration in a neonatal foal. Can Vet J 2016;57(7):781–4.

59. Conze TM, Falkenau A, Goehring LS, et al. Complete AV block in a neonatal foal suffering from nutritional myodegeneration. Equine Vet Educ 2022;34:e282–8.
60. Paulussen E, Lefère L, Bauwens C, et al. Yellow fat disease (steatitis) in 20 equids: description of clinical and ultrasonographic findings. Equine Vet Educ 2019;31:321–7.
61. Valentine BA, Hammock PD, Lemiski D, et al. Severe diaphragmatic necrosis in 4 horses with degenerative myopathy. Can Vet J 2002;43(8):614–6.
62. Ludvikova E, Jahn P, Lukas Z. Nutritional myodegeneration as a cause of dysphagia in adult horses: three case reports. Vet Med 2007;52(6):267–72.
63. Conwell R. Hyperlipaemia in a pregnant mare with suspected masseter myodegeneration. Vet Rec 2010;166(4):116–7.
64. Gomez DE, Valberg SJ, Magdesian KG, et al. Acquired multiple acyl-CoA dehydrogenase deficiency and marked selenium deficiency causing severe rhabdomyolysis in a horse. Can Vet J 2015;56(11):1166–71.
65. Chen F, Gao J, Wu D, et al. Clinical and pathologic features of a suspected selenium deficiency in captive plains zebras. Biol Trace Elem Res 2017;176:114–9.
66. Aleman M. Brief review of masseter muscle disorders. Equine Vet Educ 2023; 35(6):305–10.
67. Quaresma M, Marín C, Bacellar D, et al. Selenium and vitamin E concentrations in miranda jennies and foals (*Equus asinus*) in Northeast Portugal. Animals (Basel) 2021;11(6):1772.
68. Bazzano M, McLean A, Tesei B, et al. Selenium and vitamin E concentrations in a healthy donkey population in Central Italy. J Equine Vet Sci 2019;78:112–6.
69. Wilson A, Talbot A, Crosby-Durrani H, et al. Masseter myodegeneration in the horse: suggested approach to diagnosis and treatment. Equine Vet Educ 2023; 35:300–4.
70. Gy C, Leclere M, Bélanger MC, et al. Acute, subacute and chronic sequelae of horses accidently exposed to monensin-contaminated feed. Equine Vet J 2020; 52(6):848–56.
71. Valberg SJ. Muscle conditions affecting sport horses. Vet Clin N Am Equine Pract 2018;34(2):253–76.
72. Aleman M. A review of equine muscle disorders. Neuromuscul Disord 2008;18(4): 277–87.
73. Valberg SJ. Genetics of equine muscle disease. Vet Clin N Am Equine Pract 2020;36(2):353–78.
74. Urschel KL, McKenzie EC. Nutritional influences on skeletal muscle and muscular disease. Vet Clin N Am Equine Pract 2021;37(1):139.
75. Shellow JS, Jackson SG, Baker JP, et al. The influence of dietary selenium levels on blood levels of selenium and glutathione peroxidase activity in the horse. J Anim Sci 1985;61(3):590–4.
76. Stowe HD. Selenium supplementation for horse feed. In: Pagan JD, editor. Advances in equine nutrition. Nottingham, UK: Nottingham Univ. Press; 1998. p. 97–103.

Nonexertional Rhabdomyolysis

Stephanie J. Valberg, DVM, PhD[1]

KEYWORDS

- Tying up • Muscle disease • Myopathy • Myoglobinuria • Myositis

KEY POINTS

- Serum creatine kinase (CK) activity reflects the extent of muscle damage and serial dilutions should be performed to ascertain the maximal CK value rather than relying on a nonspecific reading of "above the limit of detection."
- Early diagnosis and treatment are key to ensuring a horse's survival from nonexertional rhabdomyolysis (nonER).
- The Quarter Horse breed is particularly susceptible to several genetic causes of nonER.
- Other causes include toxic, inflammatory/infectious, nutritional, and traumatic disorders.
- Obtaining a specific diagnosis helps to prevent the development of further cases in a group when there are genetic, toxic, or nutritional origins to disease.

INTRODUCTION

Rhabdomyolysis literally means the dissolution of striated muscle and clinically it is defined by increased serum creatine kinase (CK) and aspartate transaminase (AST) activities. The degree of elevation of serum CK, when blood is obtained at least 4 to 6 hours after onset of rhabdomyolysis, is a good indicator of the extent of muscle damage. Benchtop analyzers may report serum CK activities as "above the limit of detection"; in such cases, serial dilutions or submission to an outside laboratory is critical to establish an approximate maximum value, which helps determine the extent of muscle damage and the best treatment regime. Values can be serially monitored to determine whether the treatment is successfully diminishing rhabdomyolysis. There are numerous forms of nonexertional rhabdomyolysis (nonER). Their etiologies can be broadly categorized as toxic, genetic, inflammatory/infectious, nutritional, and traumatic (**Box 1**) and the list of differential diagnoses narrowed by careful evaluation of signalment and history (**Fig. 1**). This study discusses causes of nonER, applicable diagnostic tests, and treatments that are specific to each etiology. General treatment

College of Veterinary Medicine, Michigan State University, East Lansing, MI, USA
[1] Present address: Director Valberg Neuromuscular Diagnostic Laboratory, 833 Blacksmith Trail, Williamston, MI 48895.
E-mail address: valbergs@msu.edu

Vet Clin Equine 41 (2025) 95–110
https://doi.org/10.1016/j.cveq.2024.11.002
0749-0739/25/© 2024 Elsevier Inc. All rights reserved, including those for text and data mining, AI training, and similar technologies.

> **Box 1**
> **Causes of nonexertional rhabdomyolysis**
>
> 1. Metabolic myopathy
>   - Glycogen branching enzyme deficiency
>   - Type 1 polysaccharide storage myopathy
>   - Type 2 polysaccharide storage myopathy (Quarter Horses)
>   - Malignant hyperthermia
>
> 2. Myosin heavy chain myopathy
>   - Immune-mediated myositis
>   - Nonexertional rhabdomyolysis
>   - Systemic calcinosis
>
> 3. Inflammatory myopathies
>   - Immune mediated
>   - Infarctive hemorrhagic purpura
>
> 4. Infectious
>   - Clostridial myositis
>   - Viral myositis
>   - Sarcocystis myositis
>
> 5. Nutritional myopathy
>   - Vitamin E deficiency
>   - Selenium deficiency
>   - Myofibrillar myopathy-ER (oxidative stress)
>
> 6. Toxic myopathy
>   - Ionophore toxicity
>   - Hypoglycin A myopathy
>   Seasonal pasture myopathy
>   Atypical myopathy
>   - Rayless golden rod/white snakeroot
>   - Cassia occidentalis
>
> 7. Traumatic myopathy
>   - Compressive anesthetic myopathy
>   - Trauma

of acute rhabdomyolysis is covered in detail in Stephanie J. Valberg's article, "Sporadic and Recurrent Exertional Rhabdomyolysis," in this issue.[1]

TOXIC CAUSES OF NONEXERTIONAL RHABDOMYOLYSIS
Hypoglycin A Myopathy

Hypoglycin A myopathy, also known as seasonal pasture myopathy or atypical myopathy, has a particular geographic and seasonal occurrence with cases occurring in the early Spring or Autumn after cool, wet windy weather. Horses housed on wooded pastures for greater than 12 hours a day without additional feed provided are most susceptible.[2–4] The occurrence of disease overlaps with the distribution of box elder (*Acer negundo*) trees in North America (**Fig. 2**) and European sycamore maple trees (*Acer pseudoplatanus*) in northern and central Europe (**Fig. 2**), the United Kingdom, and New Zealand.[5–7]

Pathogenesis

Hypoglycin A myopathy is caused by the toxin hypoglycin A, which is a nonproteogenic amino acid found in seeds from box elder and sycamore maple trees.[5,6,8] It is quickly metabolized in the liver to methylene cyclopropyl acetic acid (MCPA) that

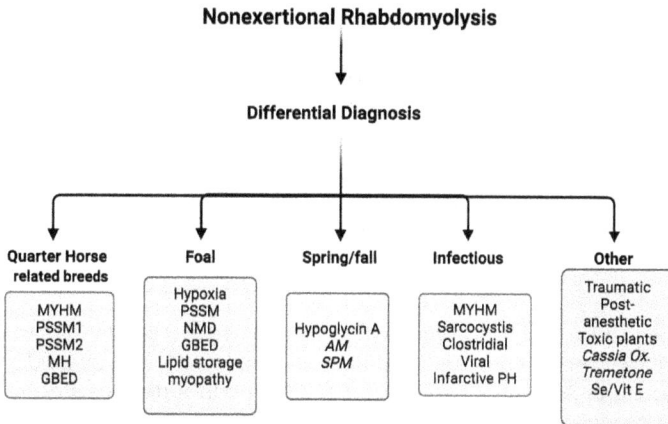

Fig. 1. Differential diagnosis for nonexertional rhabdomyolysis organized by signalment, environment, and infectious disease exposure.

irreversibly binds to multiple acyl coenzyme A (CoA) dehydrogenases in the mitochondria. This impairs metabolism of short and medium-chain fatty acids and branched-chain amino acids.[9,10] The resulting accumulation of fat esters damages muscle cell membranes and impairs mitochondrial respiratory capacity leading to weakness and muscle degeneration.[11] Ingestion of about 20 g of seeds, 50 seedlings, or 2 L of water that has been in contact with seedlings is proposed to be the maximum tolerated dose before disease develops.[12] Horses aged less than 3 years, horses new to

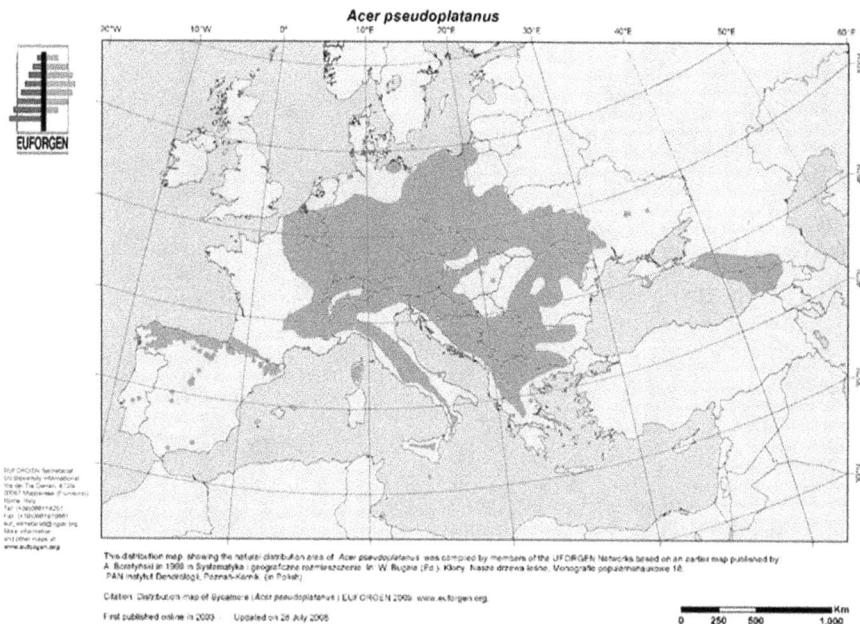

Fig. 2. The distribution of European sycamore maple trees (*Acer pseudoplantanus*) in Europe. Blue is the native continuous range. (*EUFORGEN European forest genetic resources programme.* www.euforgen.org. https://www.euforgen.org/).

affected pastures, and selenium-deficient horses (due to increased vulnerability to oxidative damage) are most likely to develop clinical disease.[13]

Within 3 to 5 days of ingesting enough seeds or young shoots, horses develop muscular weakness, sweating, fasciculations, stiffness, and potentially tachycardia, tachypnea, recumbency, and esophageal obstruction. When urine is observed, myoglobinuria is evident. A rapid rise in respiratory rate is usually followed by collapse and death from respiratory or cardiac failure. Pasture mates can be subclinically affected as evidenced by the presence of low serum hypoglycin A concentrations or mild elevations in serum CK activity.[14]

Diagnosis

The index of suspicion of hypoglycin A myopathy is raised if serum CK and AST activities are markedly elevated (>10,000 U/L), and urine is dark with an acidic pH during the early Spring or Autumn. The fastest way to support a diagnosis of hypoglycin A myopathy is to inspect pastures for box elder (**Fig. 3**A) or European sycamore maple trees (**Fig. 3**B,C) that are laden with seeds on or near the pastures. Typical alterations in serum biochemistry profiles include markedly increased serum CK and AST activities, hyperglycemia, hypocalcemia, lacticacidemia, and in some cases elevated serum troponin I concentrations.[4,15]

A definitive diagnosis can be made by identifying a specific pattern of accumulation of serum acylcarnitines and urine organic acids and glycine conjugates typical of a multiple acyl CoA dehydrogenase deficiency as well as isolation of the conjugated toxic metabolite MCPA or hypoglycin A in blood or urine.[9,10,16] All acylcarnitines

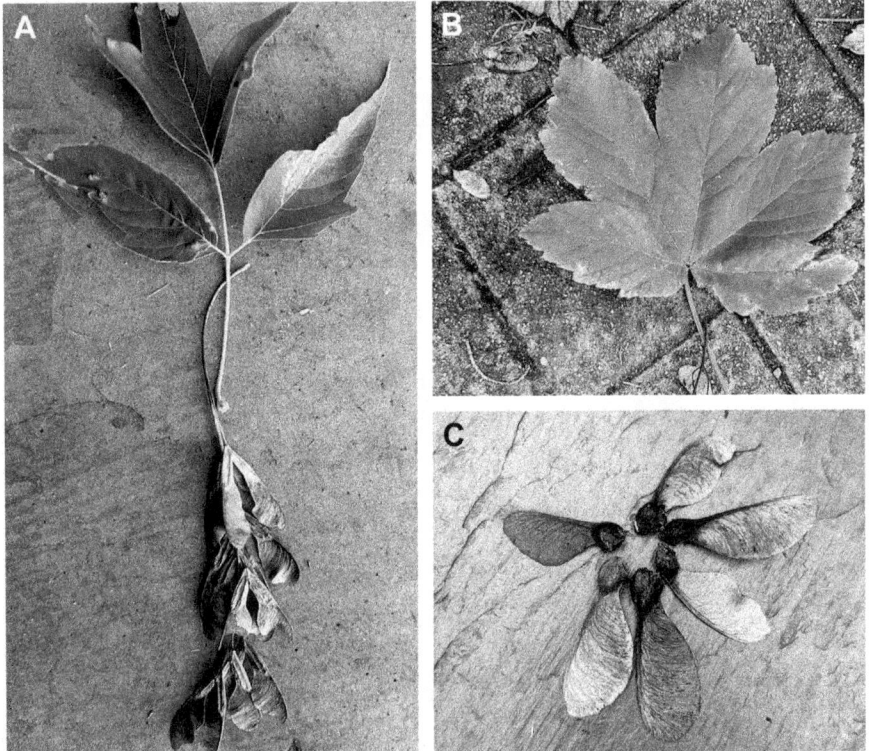

Fig. 3. (A) The leaves and seeds (samaras) of the box elder tree. (B) A leaf from the European sycamore maple. (C) Seeds (samaras) from the European sycamore maple.

(C2–C16) are elevated in diseased horses with the exception of long chain C18.[14] C5 acylcarnitine is reported to have the best diagnostic and prognostic value.[14]

Postmortem findings include extensive necrosis in deep postural and respiratory muscles and in 50% or more of cases, the myocardium. Frozen sections of myocardium, intercostal, diaphragm, or deep postural muscles show marked intracellular lipid accumulation in oxidative fibers (oil red O stain).[4,17]

Treatment and prognosis

The affected horse and co-grazing horses should be removed from the source of seeds immediately. For clinically affected horses, early treatment is imperative and includes aggressive fluid therapy, antioxidants, and anti-inflammatories that can include dimethylsulfoxide, vitamin E, vitamin C, nonsteroidal antiinflammatory drugs (NSAIDs), and potentially riboflavin (**Table 1**).[4,18] Activated charcoal given enterally may decrease toxin absorption.[19] The mortality rate for horses with overt clinical signs is high at 75%; however, early recognition may improve the prognosis.[3]

Prevention

All horses, but if not possible, particularly young horses or horses new to the property should not be pastured with box elder or European sycamore maple trees in the Autumn or early Spring. The incidence of disease can be minimized by providing feed on pasture or reducing grazing time during these periods of the year. Current recommendations are to mow pastures to reduce seedlings in the Spring, followed by hand collection of sycamore seedlings in contaminated pastures.[20] Pastures contaminated with sycamore material should not be used to produce processed hay or silage as both seedlings and seeds present in the bales still pose a risk of intoxication.[20]

Table 1
Treatment of horses with hypoglycin A myopathy (seasonal pasture myopathy, atypical myoglobinuria)

Treatment	Route	Dose	Comment
Activated charcoal	Oral/enteral	250 g/foal, 750 g/adult	Decrease toxin absorption
Keep head up, deep bedding, warm, minimize exertion			Prevent nasal edema and further rhabdomyolysis
Nasal oxygen			If low Pao_2 or increased respiratory rate
Fluids (myoglobinuria, hyperkalemia)	IV	Until urine yellow	Monitor electrolytes, empty bladder
NSAIDs Flunixin meglumine	IV	1 mg/kg	For pain
Acepromazine	IM	0.03–0.1 mg/kg	To decrease anxiety, muscle relaxation
B vitamins	IV or oral	44 µg/kg Riboflavin/day	Cofactor in fat metabolism
Vitamin C	Oral	5 g/day	Antioxidant
Vitamin E	Oral	5000–10,000 IU/day	Antioxidant, ideally d-alpha-tocopherol (natural form)
Carnitine	IV	18–22 mg/kg	Fat metabolism

Adapted from Fabius and Westerman 2017.[18]

OTHER PLANTS CAUSING NONEXERTIONAL RHABDOMYOLYSIS

Malva parviflora (marsh mallow) in Australia can cause clinical signs and biochemical profile findings similar to hypoglycin A myopathy. A component of this plant is believed to interfere with β oxidation of fatty acids causing similar plasma carnitine profiles to hypoglycin A myopathy.[21]

Blister beetle toxicosis can cause elevations in serum CK in some horses. *Cassia obtusifolia* (sicklepod) is prevalent in the southeastern United States and ingestion of seeds can cause degenerative myopathy and cardiomyopathy with evidence of myofiber atrophy, segmental necrosis, and mitochondrial disruption.[22] Additionally, tremetone-containing plants can cause fatal cardiomyopathy and severe skeletal muscle degeneration in horses when ingested at 0.5% to 2% of body weight.[23] Both white snakeroot *(Eupatorium rugosum)*, which grows in shaded areas of the eastern and central United States, and rayless goldenrod *(Isocoma wrightii)*, which is common in the southwest United States on open pastures, contain tremetone. Tremetone remains active in hay, and in the stalks of the dead plants on pasture, so both the fresh and the dried form of the plants should be kept from horses.[24] Microsomal activation of the toxin in the liver may be necessary for toxic effects.[25]

CHEMICAL CAUSES OF NONEXERTIONAL RHABDOMYOLYSIS

Ionophores can be introduced into equine feed products if they are mixed in a feed mill that did not properly clean machinery after producing cattle feeds or other feed products containing ionophores. Most ionophore toxicities in horses cause cardiomyopathy and/or neurologic disease rather than overt rhabdomyolysis. Tetrachlorvinphos, an oral fly control agent, has been reported to cause nonER in miniature horses being fed a complete feed containing this agent.[26] Affected horses showed signs of lethargy, dysphagia, fasciculations, tachypnea, and tachycardia. Cases had evidence of chronic myonecrosis of the masseters, tongue, neck, respiratory and postural muscles, and occasionally cardiac muscle.[26] Myonecrosis was attributed to acetylcholine accumulation at muscarinic and nicotinic sites producing oxidant stress. Low selenium status may contribute to this toxicosis.

METABOLIC CAUSES OF NONEXERTIONAL RHABDOMYOLYSIS
Polysaccharide Storage Myopathy

Both type 1 polysaccharide storage myopathy (PSSM1) and type 2 PSSM (PSSM2) can cause nonER and are covered in detail in Anna M. Firshman and Stephanie J. Valberg's article, "Polysaccharide Storage Myopathy," in this issue.[27] PSSM1 is caused by an autosomal dominant mutation in glycogen synthase (*GYS1*) and PSSM2 in Quarter Horse-related breeds is also a glycogen storage disorder; however, the metabolic defect causing PSSM2 is unknown. Horses with PSSM1 and PSSM2-ER usually have a history of exertional rhabdomyolysis but may also develop nonER after turnout, particularly if they have been stall rested for 2 or more days. In foals, PSSM1 can cause nonER following turnout or with concurrent respiratory or intestinal infection.[28,29] Clinical signs are typical of nonER with muscle pain, stiffness, sweating, reluctance to move, and potentially pawing and recumbency accompanied by marked elevation in serum CK and AST. A diagnosis of PSSM1 is based on genetic testing and, for PSSM2-ER, a biopsy of the gluteal or semimembranosus muscles. Hallmark features are dark staining for glycogen and the presence of abnormal polysaccharide. The general treatment of acute rhabdomyolysis is described in the Stephanie J. Valberg's article, "Sporadic and Recurrent Exertional Rhabdomyolysis," in this issue.[27] Serum

CK activity declines slowly during treatment of acute rhabdomyolysis in PSSM1 horses (**Fig. 4**).

Glycogen Branching Enzyme Deficiency

Glycogen branching enzyme deficiency (GBED) in Quarter Horse-related breeds is a fatal disease of foals, caused by an autosomal recessive mutation in the glycogen branching enzyme (*GBE1*) gene.[30] The prevalence of carriers is particularly high in pleasure horses of these breeds, affecting 26%.[31] Clinical signs include abortion in second or third trimesters, stillbirth, hypothermia at birth, mild flexural deformities, intermittent seizures, skeletal and respiratory muscle weakness, and sudden death.[30,32,33] Persistent leukopenia, intermittent hypoglycemia, and moderately high serum CK (1000–15,000 U/L), AST, and γ-glutamyl transferase activities are usually present in affected foals. Although foals initially respond to treatment in neonatal intensive care, all foals with GBED have died, often suddenly, by the age of 18 weeks. A diagnosis is established through genetic testing. Muscle biopsy reveals typical periodic acid-positive (PAS) inclusions and negligible normal glycogen staining (**Fig. 5**). Gross necropsy changes are minimal and routine hematoxylin and eosin stains of tissues may be normal or show basophilic inclusions in skeletal muscle and cardiac tissues. Periodic acid Schiff's (PAS) stains of skeletal and cardiac muscle, brain, and liver are required to reveal the distinctive abnormal polysaccharide inclusions with lack of normal background glycogen staining.

Lipid Storage Myopathy

There is a report of a 12-h-old Paint Filly with a lipid storage myopathy suspected to be due to multiple acyl-CoA dehydrogenase deficiency (MADD).[34] The foal presented with weakness and dull mentation after birth. Despite intravenous (IV) administered dextrose, the foal remained persistently hypoglycemic (12 mg/dL) with increases in serum activity of CK (4476 U/L), AST (638 U/L), mildly increased gamma-glutamyl transferase activity, and hyper lactatemia. Muscle biopsy of the semimembranosus muscle identified

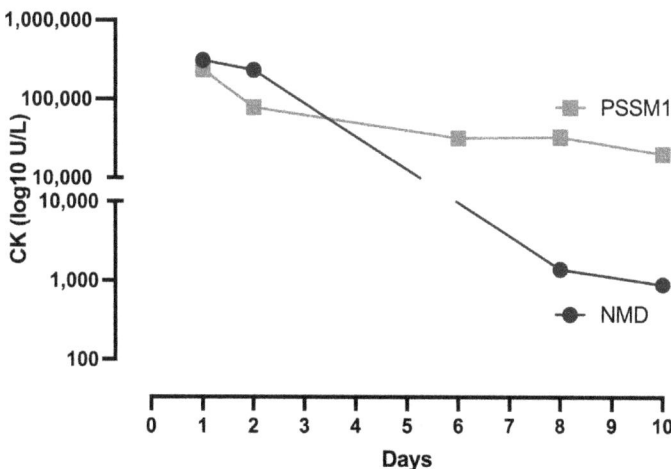

Fig. 4. Serum creatine kinase (CK) activity in 2 foals with nonER. The foal with nutritional myodegeneration (NMD) due to selenium deficiency shows a rapid decline in CK activity with treatment. The foal with PSSM1 shows a slow decline in CK with treatment because of an innate error in metabolism.

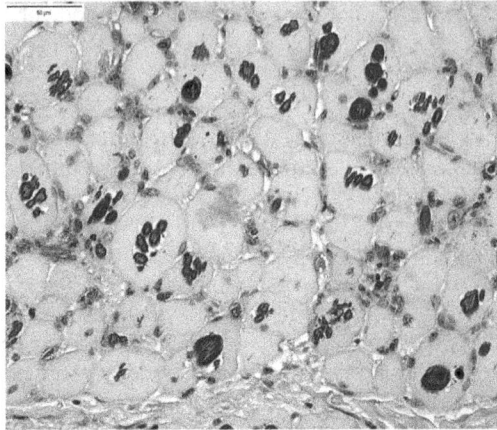

Fig. 5. Accumulation of abnormal polysaccharide and a lack of normal background staining in semimembranosus muscle from a foal with glycogen branching enzyme deficiency.

marked storage of large lipid droplets in myofibers without evidence of myofiber degeneration.[34] Elevated urine organic acids, including ethylmalonic, methylsuccinic, glutaric, butyrylglycine, isovalerylglycine, 2-hydroxyglutaric, and hexanoylglycine, were consistent with MADD. Serum-free acylcarnitines and C2-C18 acylcarnitines were elevated consistent with MADD. Following publication of this case report, stored serum was found and hypoglycin A measurement was normal ruling out hypoglycin A myopathy (personal communication Dr Toby Pinn). Lipid storage myopathies should be included as a differential diagnosis in foals with persistent weakness and hypoglycemia.

Malignant Hyperthermia

Quarter Horses with a mutation in the ryanodine receptor 1 (*RYR1*) gene that causes malignant hyperthermia (MH) can develop clinical signs of nonER as well as exertional rhabdomyolysis.[35,36]

Episodes of rhabdomyolysis are often severe, accompanied by elevated rectal temperatures, and can culminate in sudden death. A definitive diagnosis is established through genetic testing. Treatment with dantrolene at 2 mg/kg three times a day (TID) until serum CK is steadily declining is warranted in MH horses because dantrolene will slow release of calcium through the skeletal muscle ryanodine receptor, RYR1.[37] If hyperthermia is severe, attempts to cool the animal with alcohol or cold water baths are indicated.

INFLAMMATORY CAUSES OF NONEXERTIONAL RHABDOMYOLYSIS

Infarctive Hemorrhagic Purpura

Infarctive purpura hemorrhagica (IHP) is a severe form of purpura with a high fatality rate and is discussed in detail in Sian A. Durward-Akhurst and Stephanie J. Valberg's article, "Myosin Heavy Chain Myopathy and Immune-Mediated Muscle Disorders," in this issue.[38] Infarctions in these cases usually occur in skeletal muscles that are compressed during recumbency and progress to involve multiple organs including mucous membranes and the gastrointestinal tract.[39] Deposition of complement near immune complexes in vessel walls may result in cell membrane destruction, cell death, and vascular occlusion. Horses present with acute painful lameness with limb swelling, muscle stiffness, and/or colic.[39] Petechiae, well-demarcated limb edema and focal firm intramuscular swellings in abdominal, pectoral, adductor, and tarsocrural muscles, are evident on physical examination. Leukocytosis, hyperproteinemia from hyperglobulinemia, hypoalbuminemia, and marked elevations in CK (47,000–280,000 U/L) and AST (960–7000 U/L) activities are evident.[39] Serum titers for strepotococcal M protein on enzyme-linked immunosorbent assay are usually markedly elevated. Ultrasonographic examination of swollen muscle reveals focal hypoechoic lesions within muscle tissue that represent infarcted regions of acute coagulative necrosis. Infarctions in numerous organs are evident at necropsy and *Streptococcus equi* abscessation of a lymph node is usually present.[39]

Early recognition of clinical signs and aggressive antibiotic and corticosteroid treatment are essential to combat the high fatality rate from IHP. Penicillin, NSAIDs, and 3 weeks of dexamethasone (0.1 mg/kg, tapering to 0.07 mg/kg) followed by a 10 week tapering course of oral prednisolone (2 mg/kg dose initially) have been successful treatments.

Sarcocystosis

It is not uncommon in equine muscle to see one or 2 dormant cysts of the sporozoan parasite *Sarcocystis fayeri*, for which the dog is the definitive host.[40] Large numbers of *S fayeri*, however, can cause fever, malaise, chronic muscle atrophy, stiffness, weakness, and muscle fasciculations.[40–43] Chronic weight loss, muscle pain, recurrent esophageal dysphagia, granulomatous masses, and marked persistent eosinophilia have also been reported with sarcocystosis.[44] Sarcocystosis and vitamin E responsive myopathy can occur concurrently.[41] Clinicopathology is typified by normochromic normocytic anemia, mild hypoalbuminemia, hyperglobulinemia, and elevations in CK and AST activities.[42,45] Diagnosis of sarcocystosis requires history, clinical signs, laboratory and serologic evaluation, and the demonstration of numerous immature cysts in muscle biopsies ideally in conjunction with inflammatory infiltrates.

Successful treatment of sarcocystosis is reported using phenylbutazone, and prolonged treatment with trimethoprim-sulfamethoxazole, and pyrimethamine.[41,42] Current antiparasitic medications such as diclazuril should also be effective. Control involves preventing gross contamination of equine feeds with carnivore feces.

Viral Nonexertional Rhabdomyolysis

Skeletal muscle degeneration and stiffness are rarely reported in association with equine influenza A2 and equine herpes virus 1 infection, with concurrent clinical signs typical of these viral diseases.[46,47]

Clostridial Myonecrosis

Infection with a variety of clostridial bacteria, most commonly *Clostridium perfringens*, can cause severe systemic toxicosis with moderate elevations in serum CK and AST activities. Most reports of clostridial myonecrosis in horses follow intramuscular injections and less often puncture wounds.[48–50] When local tissue is devitalized, and conditions become appropriate, spores germinate releasing powerful exotoxins that act locally and systemically to create widespread organ dysfunction. *Clostridium septicum*, *Clostridium chauvoei*, *Clostridium sporogenes*, and mixed infections are associated with a high fatality rate, whereas *C perfringens* type A has a mortality rate of 20% with early and aggressive treatment.[49] Swelling and crepitus at the wound/injection site is accompanied by depression, fever, toxemia, and tachypnea. Clostridial infection can migrate along fascial planes to affect additional sites in the body which often results in the spread of crepitus. Tremors, ataxia, dyspnea, recumbency, coma, and death can occur within 12 to 24 hour depending on the type of clostridial infection.

Myocardial damage occurs in some horses. Wound fenestration and aggressive surgical debridement over the entire affected area are required for successful treatment.[49] Additional treatment includes high doses of IV potassium penicillin every 2 to 4 hours until the animal is stable (1–5 days) combined with or followed by oral metronidazole along with supportive fluid therapy and NSAIDs.

Myosin Heavy Chain Myopathy

Myosin heavy chain myopathy (MYHM) comprises 3 clinical presentations, nonER, immune-mediated myositis, and calciphylaxis, covered in detail in Sian A. Durward-Akhurst and Stephanie J. Valberg's article, "Myosin Heavy Chain Myopathy and Immune-Mediated Muscle Disorders," in this issue.[38] It occurs in horses with Quarter Horse-related bloodlines, including American Paints, Appaloosas, and their crosses, with the highest frequency in reining and working cow horses.[51] Disease has a bimodal age distribution with young horses most impacted by the disease.

MYHM is caused by a codominant E321G mutation in *MYH1* encoding myosin heavy chain 2X that is found in type 2X fibers, the predominant fiber type in equine locomotor muscles.[52] Seven percent of Quarter Horses have the mutation, with the highest prevalence in reining (24%), working cow (17%), and halter (16%) horse bloodlines.[53,54] Clinical signs occur in about 20% of heterozygotes and in most homozygous horses. Homozygotes have more severe and more recurrent clinical signs than heterozygotes.[55]

The trigger for nonER may not be apparent in many cases or can be recent vaccination for *Streptococcus equi equi* or influenza/rhinopneumonitis (3–4 weeks before signs) or concurrent infections with *S equi, Anaplasma phagocytophilum,* or *Corynebacterium pseudotuberculosis.*[51,56–59] It is not clear whether autoimmunity is the driver of rhabdomyolysis because lymphocytic infiltrates are rare in the affected muscles unlike horses with the immune-meditated myositis form of MYHM. A molecular and cellular hyper-contractile phenotype has been identified in *MYH1* homozygous horses that could contribute to the development of nonER.[60]

Typical clinical signs of the nonER presentation of MYHM include stiffness, and markedly firm, painful epaxial and gluteal muscles that rapidly progresses to recumbency (**Fig. 6**A).[51,61] Atrophy may or may not follow nonER. Affected horses may have evidence of a concurrent infection such as submandibular lymphadenopathy,

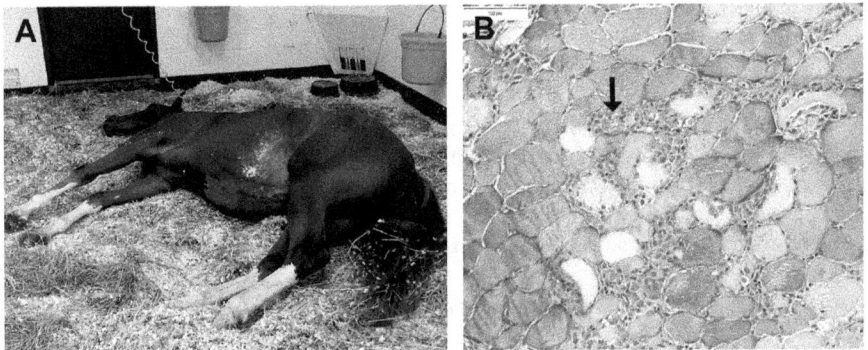

Fig. 6. (*A*) A horse with nonER due to myosin heavy chain myopathy (MYHM) with firm hard painful muscles, and inability to rise resulting in involuntary recumbency. (*B*) Gluteal muscle from an MYHM horse with nonER showing 40% of fibers that are either acutely necrotic (pale staining) or degenerating with macrophage infiltration (*arrow*). Periodic acid Schiff's stain 20X.

pneumonia, or guttural pouch empyema.[57] Marked elevations in serum CK (115,000–1,000,000 U/L) and AST activities are evident in biochemistry profiles, and in very severe cases, hyperkalemia, hyperphosphatemia, hyponatremia, hypochloremia, and hypocalcemia occur because of loss of the distinction between extracellular and intracellular compartments arising from massive tissue necrosis.[62] If horses have concurrent infections, leukocytosis, or leukopenia, neutrophilia and elevated fibrinogen may be present.

Diagnosis
A definitive diagnosis of MYHM is achieved through genetic testing for the E321G *MYH1* mutation.[52] If a biopsy is performed, the gluteal muscle should be sampled as this muscle shows acute necrosis, extensive macrophage infiltration of degenerating myocytes, and glycogen depletion in large muscle fibers with MYHM (**Fig. 6**B).

Treatment
Hydration status should be assessed before addressing muscle pain using NSAIDs. In severe cases, constant-rate infusions of butorphanol or detomidine can be used. In the author's experience, early institution of dantrolene administered TID at 2 to 4 mg/kg orally until CK is close to the normal range is the most effective means of halting rhabdomyolysis. Dexamethasone (0.07–0.08 mg/kg IV) for 3 days, followed by prednisolone (1 mg/kg per os [PO]) for 7 to 10 days tapered by 100 mg per week over 1 month, is recommended.[51] Their dose and use are tempered by the presence of any underlying infections. Horses should be placed in a deeply bedded stall and rotated from side to side every 4 hours if they are unable to rise. Some horses may benefit from a sling if they will bear weight on their hind limbs when assisted to stand.

Without early treatment, horses may be euthanized due to recumbency, myoglobinuric renal failure, or the severity of rhabdomyolysis. If horses are homozygous for the mutation, a discussion with the owner about the high likelihood that clinical signs of nonER or immune-mediated myositis will recur should ensue.

NUTRITIONAL CAUSES
Nutritional Myodegeneration

In-depth coverage of myopathies associated with selenium and vitamin E deficiencies can be found in the chapter by Carrie J. Finno and Erica C. McKenzie "Vitamin E and Selenium-Related Manifestions of Muscle Disease" in this issue.[63] Brief information on foals with nutritional myodegeneration (NMD) can be found here. Foals with NMD present with signs of weakness, trembling, stiffness, and inability to stand for more than short periods and aspiration pneumonia. Affected muscle groups might be firm and painful to palpation. Some foals present with a cardiorespiratory syndrome characterized by dyspnea, a rapid irregular heartbeat, profound weakness, recumbency, and sudden death.[62,64] NMD is caused by a dietary deficiency of selenium and/or vitamin E (alpha-tocopherol) in young rapidly growing foals born to dams that consumed selenium-deficient diets during gestation.[64,65] Selenium and vitamin E appear to be synergistic in preventing NMD; however, selenium deficiency appears to be the most important contributor to oxidant damage of muscle cell membranes.

A diagnosis involves demonstration of increased serum CK and AST activities and low selenium in whole blood samples with or without low serum vitamin E (reference ranges: whole blood selenium 160–275 ng/mL, alpha-tocopherol 2–4 μg/mL). Foals may have slightly lower normal values.[63] With severe rhabdomyolysis, hyperkalemia, hyperphosphatemia, hyponatremia, hypochloremia, and hypocalcemia can occur because of loss of the distinction between extracellular and intracellular compartments arising from massive tissue necrosis.[62]

Treatment

Treatment with intramuscular (IM) selenium at a dose of 0.055–0.067 mg/kg (2.5–3 mg/ 45 kg) body weight often results in a rapid decline in serum CK and clinical improvement after a few days of rest barring other complications (see **Fig. 4**). Injectable selenium products contain a minimal amount of alpha-tocopherol (68 IU per ml) and additional oral supplementation with water-dispersible RRR-alpha-tocopherol is recommended (10 IU/kg body weight). When dysphagia is present, feeding via nasogastric tube, provision of adequate energy intake and attention to fluid and electrolyte balance are of critical importance if recovery is to be successful. Hyperkalemia can be life-threatening and mineralocorticoids, alkalinizing fluids, dextrose, and insulin are used to reduce circulating potassium concentrations.[62] Note that pseudohyperkalemia occurs when serum CK is high and electrolytes assessed on an Abaxis VetScan2 analyzer.[66] The prognosis for foals with the skeletal muscle form of NMD is good, whereas the cardiorespiratory form has a guarded prognosis, and foals with severe dysphagia may require extended management.

In summary, there are numerous causes of nonER. A detailed history, physical examination, evaluations of serum muscle enzymes and selection of appropriate hematological, serologic, or genetic tests, or muscle biopsy will lead to a specific diagnosis and optimal treatment.

DISCLOSURES

S.J. Valberg directs the Valberg Neuromuscular Disease Laboratory (ValbergNMDL. com) and receives remuneration for analyzing muscle biopsies. Her Web site is sponsored by Kentucky Equine Research, and she receives royalties from the PSSM1 genetic test and the feed products Re-leve and MFM pellet developed in association with Kentucky Equine Research.

CLINICS CARE POINTS

- Serial dilution of serum CK will indicate the extent of muscle damage and response to treatment.
- High serum CK can cause pseudohyperkalemia when using the Abaxis VetScan2 analyzer.
- Determining the specific basis for nonER will aid in establishing a prognosis and selecting targeted treatment.

REFERENCES

1. Valberg SJ. Sporadic and recurrent exertional rhabdomyolysis. In: McKenzie EC, Valberg SJ, editors. Muscle disorders of horses: Veterinary Clinics of North America: equine practice. 2025. p. 111–24.
2. van Galen G, Marcillaud PC, Saegerman C, et al. European outbreaks of atypical myopathy in grazing equids (2006-2009): spatiotemporal distribution, history and clinical features. Equine Vet J 2012;44:614–20.
3. van Galen G, Saegerman C, Marcillaud PC, et al. European outbreaks of atypical myopathy in grazing horses (2006-2009): determination of indicators for risk and prognostic factors. Equine Vet J 2012;44:621–5.

4. Finno CJ, Valberg SJ, Wünschmann A, et al. Seasonal pasture myopathy in horses in the midwestern United States: 14 cases (1998-2005). J Am Vet Med Assoc 2006;229:1134–41.

5. Unger L, Nicholson A, Jewitt EM, et al. Hypoglycin A concentrations in seeds of Acer pseudoplatanus trees growing on atypical myopathy-affected and control pastures. J Vet Intern Med 2014;28:1289–93.

6. Valberg SJ, Sponseller BT, Hegeman AD, et al. Seasonal pasture myopathy/atypical myopathy in North America associated with ingestion of hypoglycin A within seeds of the box elder tree. Equine Vet J 2013;45:419–26.

7. Votion DM, Van Galen G, Sweetman L, et al. Identification of methylenecyclopropyl acetic acid in serum of E uropean horses with atypical myopathy. Equine Vet J 2014;46:146–9.

8. Baise E, Habyarimana J, Amory H, et al. Samaras and seedlings of Acer pseudoplatanus are potential sources of hypoglycin A intoxication in atypical myopathy without necessarily inducing clinical signs. Equine Vet J 2016;48:414–7.

9. Westermann CM, Dorland L, Votion DM, et al. Acquired multiple Acyl-CoA dehydrogenase deficiency in 10 horses with atypical myopathy. Neuromuscul Disord 2008;18:355–64.

10. Sponseller BT, Valberg SJ, Schultz NE, et al. Equine multiple acyl-CoA dehydrogenase deficiency (MADD) associated with seasonal pasture myopathy in the midwestern United States. J Vet Intern Med 2012;26:1012–8.

11. Lemieux H, Boemer F, Van Galen G, et al. Mitochondrial function is altered in horse atypical myopathy. Mitochondrion 2016;30:35–41.

12. Votion DM, Habyarimana JA, Scippo ML, et al. Potential new sources of hypoglycin A poisoning for equids kept at pasture in spring: a field pilot study. Vet Rec 2019;184:740.

13. Gomez DE, Valberg SJ, Magdesian KG, et al. Acquired multiple acyl-CoA dehydrogenase deficiency and marked selenium deficiency causing severe rhabdomyolysis in a horse. Can Vet J 2015;56:1166–71.

14. Renaud B, Kruse C-J, François A-C, et al. Large-scale study of blood markers in equine atypical myopathy reveals subclinical poisoning and advances in diagnostic and prognostic criteria. Environ Toxicol Pharmacol 2024;110:104515.

15. van Galen G, Cerri S, Porter S, et al. Traditional and quantitative assessment of acid-base and shock variables in horses with atypical myopathy. J Vet Intern Med 2012;27(1):186–93.

16. Bochnia M, Ziegler J, Sander J, et al. Hypoglycin A content in blood and urine discriminates horses with atypical myopathy from clinically normal horses grazing on the same pasture. PLoS One 2015;10:e0136785.

17. Cassart D, Baise E, Cherel Y, et al. Morphological alterations in oxidative muscles and mitochondrial structure associated with equine atypical myopathy. Equine Vet J 2007;39:26–32.

18. Fabius L, Westermann C. Evidence-based therapy for atypical myopathy in horses. Equine Vet Educ 2018;30:616–22.

19. Krägeloh T, Cavalleri J, Ziegler J, et al. Identification of hypoglycin A binding adsorbents as potential preventive measures in co-grazers of atypical myopathy affected horses. Equine Vet J 2018;50:220–7.

20. González-Medina S, Montesso F, Chang YM, et al. Atypical myopathy-associated hypoglycin A toxin remains in sycamore seedlings despite mowing, herbicidal spraying or storage in hay and silage. Equine Vet J 2019;51:701–4.

21. Bauquier J, Stent A, Gibney J, et al. Evidence for marsh mallow (Malva parviflora) toxicosis causing myocardial disease and myopathy in four horses. Equine Vet J 2017;49:307-13.

22. Putnam MR, Boosinger T, Spano J, et al. Evaluation of Cassia obtusifolia (sicklepod) seed consumption in Holstein calves. Vet Hum Toxicol 1988;30:316-8.

23. Beier RC, Norman JO. The toxic factor in white snakeroot: identity, analysis and prevention. Vet Hum Toxicol 1990;32(Suppl):81-8.

24. Thompson LJ. Depression and choke in a horse: probable white snakeroot toxicosis. Vet Hum Toxicol 1989;31:321-2.

25. Beier RC, Norman JO, Irvin TR, et al. Microsomal activation of constituents of white snakeroot (Eupatorium rugosum Houtt) to form toxic products. Am J Vet Res 1987;48:583-5.

26. Myers CJ, Aleman M, Heidmann R, et al. Myopathy in American miniature horses. Equine Vet J 2006;38:272-6.

27. Firshman AC, Valberg SJ. Polysaccharide Storage Myopathy. In: McKenzie EC, Valberg SJ, editors. Muscle Disorders of Horses: An Issue of Veterinary Clinics of North America: Equine Practice. 2025. p. 125-37.

28. De La Corte FD, Valberg SJ, MacLeay JM, et al. Developmental onset of polysaccharide storage myopathy in 4 Quarter Horse foals. J Vet Intern Med 2002;16: 581-7.

29. Byrne E, Cohen N, Jones SL, et al. Rhabdomyolysis in two foals with polysaccharide storage myopathy. Comp Cont Educ 2000;22:503-7.

30. Ward TL, Valberg SJ, Adelson DL, et al. Glycogen branching enzyme (GBE1) mutation causing equine glycogen storage disease IV. Mamm Genome 2004;15:570-7.

31. Tryon RC, Penedo MC, McCue ME, et al. Evaluation of allele frequencies of inherited disease genes in subgroups of American Quarter Horses. J Am Vet Med Assoc 2009;234:120-5.

32. Wagner ML, Valberg SJ, Ames EG, et al. Allele frequency and likely impact of the glycogen branching enzyme deficiency gene in Quarter Horse and Paint Horse populations. J Vet Intern Med 2006;20:1207-11.

33. Valberg SJ, Ward TL, Rush B, et al. Glycogen branching enzyme deficiency in quarter horse foals. J Vet Intern Med 2001;15:572-80.

34. Pinn TL, Divers TJ, Southard T, et al. Persistent hypoglycemia associated with lipid storage myopathy in a paint foal. J Vet Intern Med 2018;32:1442-6.

35. Aleman M, Brosnan RJ, Williams DC, et al. Malignant hyperthermia in a horse anesthetized with halothane. J Vet Intern Med 2005;19:363-6.

36. Aleman M, Riehl J, Aldridge BM, et al. Association of a mutation in the ryanodine receptor 1 gene with equine malignant hyperthermia. Muscle Nerve 2004;30: 356-65.

37. Zhao F, Li P, Chen SW, et al. Dantrolene inhibition of ryanodine receptor Ca2+ release channels: molecular mechanism and isoform selectivity. J Biol Chem 2001;276:13810-6.

38. Durward-Akhurst SA. Myosin heavy chain myopathy and immune mediated muscle disorders. In: McKenzie EC, Valberg SJ, editors. Muscle disorders of horses: Veterinary Clinics of North America: equine practice. 2025. p. 61-75.

39. Kaese HJ, Valberg SJ, Hayden DW, et al. Infarctive purpura hemorrhagica in five horses. J Am Vet Med Assoc 2005;226:1893-8.

40. Aleman M, Shapiro K, Sisó S, et al. Sarcocystis fayeri in skeletal muscle of horses with neuromuscular disease. Neuromuscul Disord 2016;26:85-93.

41. Trimble A, Delph K, Perry E, et al. Sarcocystis myositis and vitamin E deficiency in a Gypsy Vanner stallion suspected of having equine motor neuron disease. Equine Vet Educ 2020;32:e235–9.

42. Traub-Dargatz JL, Schlipf JW Jr, Granstrom DE, et al. Multifocal myositis associated with Sarcocystis sp in a horse. J Am Vet Med Assoc 1994;205: 1574–6.

43. Coultous RM, Raftery AG, Shiels BR, et al. Molecular confirmation of Sarcocystis fayeri in a donkey. Vet Parasitol 2017;240:30–3.

44. Herd H, Sula M, Starkey L, et al. Sarcocystis fayeri–induced granulomatous and eosinophilic myositis in 2 related horses. Vet Pathol 2015;52:1191–4.

45. Fayer R, Dubey JP. Development of Sarcocystis fayeri in the equine. J Parasitol 1982;68:856–60.

46. Harris PA. An outbreak of the equine rhabdomyolysis syndrome in a racing yard. Vet Rec 1990;127:468–70.

47. Freestone JF, Carlson GR. Muscle disorders in the horse: a retrospective study. Equine Vet J 1991;23:86–90.

48. Rebhun WC, Shin SJ, King JM, et al. Malignant edema in horses. J Am Vet Med Assoc 1985;187:732–6.

49. Peek SF, Semrad SD, Perkins GA. Clostridial myonecrosis in horses (37 cases 1985-2000). Equine Vet J 2003;35:86–92.

50. Valberg SJ, McKinnon AO. Clostridial cellulitis in the horse: a report of five cases. Can Vet J 1984;25:67–71.

51. Lewis SS, Valberg SJ, Nielsen IL. Suspected immune-mediated myositis in horses. J Vet Intern Med 2007;21:495–503.

52. Finno CJ, Gianino G, Perumbakkam S, et al. A missense mutation in MYH1 is associated with susceptibility to immune-mediated myositis in Quarter Horses. Skelet Muscle 2018;8:7.

53. Gianino GM, Valberg SJ, Perumbakkam S, et al. Prevalence of the E321G MYH1 variant for immune-mediated myositis and nonexertional rhabdomyolysis in performance subgroups of American Quarter Horses. J Vet Intern Med 2019;33: 897–901.

54. Albuquerque ALH, Delfiol DJZ, Andrade DGA, et al. Prevalence of the E321G MYH1 variant in Brazilian quarter horses. Equine Vet J 2021;54(5):952–7.

55. Valberg SJ, Schultz AE, Finno CJ, et al. Prevalence of clinical signs and factors impacting expression of myosin heavy chain myopathy in Quarter Horse-related breeds with the MYH1 E321G mutation. J Vet Intern Med 2022;36: 1152–9.

56. Hunyadi L, Sundman E, Kass P, et al. Clinical implications and hospital outcome of immune-mediated myositis in horses. J Vet Intern Med 2017;31:170–5.

57. Sponseller BT, Valberg SJ, Tennent-Brown BS, et al. Severe acute rhabdomyolysis associated with Streptococcus equi infection in four horses. J Am Vet Med Assoc 2005;227:1800–4.

58. Hilton H, Madigan JE, Aleman M. Rhabdomyolysis associated with Anaplasma phagocytophilum infection in a horse. J Vet Intern Med 2008;22:1061–4.

59. Valberg SJ, Henry ML, Perumbakkam S, et al. An E321G MYH1 mutation is strongly associated with nonexertional rhabdomyolysis in Quarter Horses. J Vet Intern Med 2018;32:1718–25.

60. Ochala J, Finno CJ, Valberg SJ. Myofibre hyper-contractility in horses expressing the myosin heavy chain myopathy mutation, MYH1E321G. Cells 2021;10:3428.

61. Hunyadi L, Sundman EA, Kass PH, et al. Clinical implications and hospital outcome of immune-mediated myositis in horses. J Vet Intern Med 2017;31: 170–5.
62. Perkins G, Valberg SJ, Madigan JM, et al. Electrolyte disturbances in foals with severe rhabdomyolysis. J Vet Intern Med 1998;12:173–7.
63. McKenzie EC, Finno CJ. Vitamin E and selenium related manifestations of muscle disease. In: Muscle disorders of the horses. Veterinary Clinics of North America: Equine Practice. 2025. p. 77–93.
64. Dill SG, Rebhun WC. White muscle disease in foals. Comp Cont Educ Pract Vet 1985;7:S627–36.
65. Maylin GA, Rubin DS, Lein DH. Selenium and vitamin E in horses. Cornell Vet 1980;70:272–89.
66. Valberg SJ, Clancey NP, Salinger A, et al. Pseudohyperkalemia in horses with rhabdomyolysis reported by an enzymatic chemistry analyzer. J Am Vet Med Assoc 2024;262:1–5.

Sporadic and Recurrent Exertional Rhabdomyolysis

Stephanie J. Valberg, DVM, PhD

KEYWORDS

- Skeletal muscle • Tying up • Rhabdomyolysis • Myopathy

KEY POINTS

- Horses have key adaptations in genes and proteins relating to intracellular calcium flux that may make them particularly susceptible to exertional rhabdomyolysis (ER).
- The final common pathway for rhabdomyolysis across species is usually an excessive rise in myoplasmic calcium concentrations.
- Changes in diet, training, or environment can trigger a sporadic episode of ER.
- Recurrent ER, a chronic form of ER, occurs in fit horses when trained in stress-inducing environments.
- Minimizing stress, altering the diet and providing medications that reduce calcium release from the sarcoplasmic reticulum reduce clinical episodes of recurrent ER.

INTRODUCTION

Skeletal muscle has remarkable ability to respond to electrical stimuli, contracting and relaxing within milliseconds (**Fig. 1**). Muscle contraction requires the following components (see **Fig. 1**):

1. Initiation and propagation of a plasma membrane action potential throughout the transverse tubule system (T-tubule)
2. Dihydropyridine receptors that detect changes in plasma membrane potential
3. Interaction between these receptors and the sarcoplasmic reticulum (SR) calcium release channel also known as the ryanodine receptor (ryanodine receptor 1 [RYR1])
4. Release of calcium from the SR via RYR1 producing a transient increase of myoplasmic calcium concentration
5. Activation of the contractile apparatus through calcium binding to troponin facilitating actin–myosin crossbridge formation

Michigan State University, Large Animal Clinical Sciences, College of Veterinary Medicine, East Lansing, MI, USA
E-mail address: sjvalberg@gmail.com

Vet Clin Equine 41 (2025) 111–124
https://doi.org/10.1016/j.cveq.2024.11.003
0749-0739/25/© 2024 Elsevier Inc. All rights are reserved, including those for text and data mining, AI training, and similar technologies.

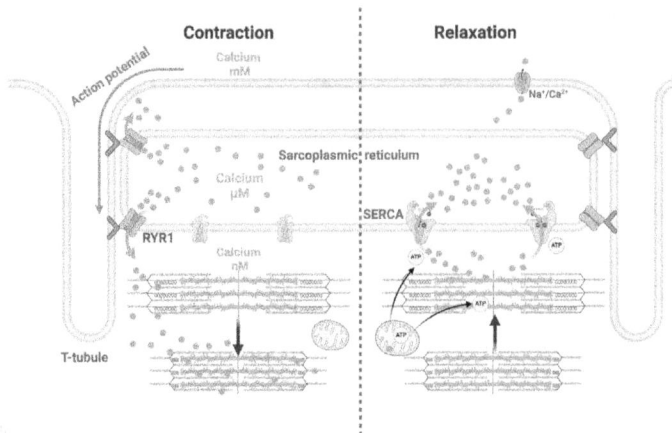

Fig. 1. The process of muscle contraction and relaxation requires tight regulation of intramuscular calcium concentrations. Contraction begins with (1) initiation and propagation of a plasma membrane action potential throughout the transverse tubule system (T-tubules), (2) dihydropyridine receptors (*brown arrow head*) that detect changes in membrane potential, (3) allosteric interaction between these receptors and sarcoplasmic reticulum (SR) calcium release channel also known as the ryanodine receptor (RYR1), (4) release of Ca^{2+} from the SR via RYR1 producing a transient increase of myoplasmic calcium concentration, (5) activation of the contractile apparatus. Relaxation of contraction is an energy-dependent process requiring adenosine triphosphate (ATP) dependent release of myosin from actin-binding sites and ATP dependent calcium reuptake into the SR through the SR Ca^{2+} adenosine triphosphatase (SERCA). (*Created in* Bio-Render. Valberg, S. (2025) https://BioRender.com/h33a961.)

6. Relaxation of contraction through calcium reuptake into the SR through the SR calcium adenosine triphosphatase (sarcoplasmic reticulum calcium atpase [SERCA]), and potentially into mitochondria.[1]

ATP from aerobic or anaerobic metabolism is required to fuel relaxation of contractile filaments, SERCA, and sarcolemmal pumps. Although a diverse spectrum of inherited and acquired disorders can cause exertional rhabdomyolysis (ER), the final common pathophysiological mechanism initiating cellular damage is usually an uncontrolled rise in free cytoplasmic calcium that activates calcium-dependent proteases leading to myofibrillar lysis and lysosomal digestion of muscle fiber contents.[2] Macrophages arrive after several hours to remove debris, followed by regeneration of the damaged muscle segment by activated satellite cells that form myotubes. With ER, complete repair of fibers usually takes approximately 4 weeks (**Fig. 2**).

CLINICAL SIGNS OF EXERTIONAL RHABDOMYOLYSIS

Horses with ER can have a range of clinical signs depending on the severity. With mild cases, stiffness during exercise and a decrease in willingness to work may be noted. As severity increases, bilaterally symmetric signs will include

- A short stride
- Shifting lameness
- Stiffness
- Sweating
- Reluctance to go forward
- Firm muscles particularly in the hindquarters
- Inappropriately rapid respiratory and heart rates

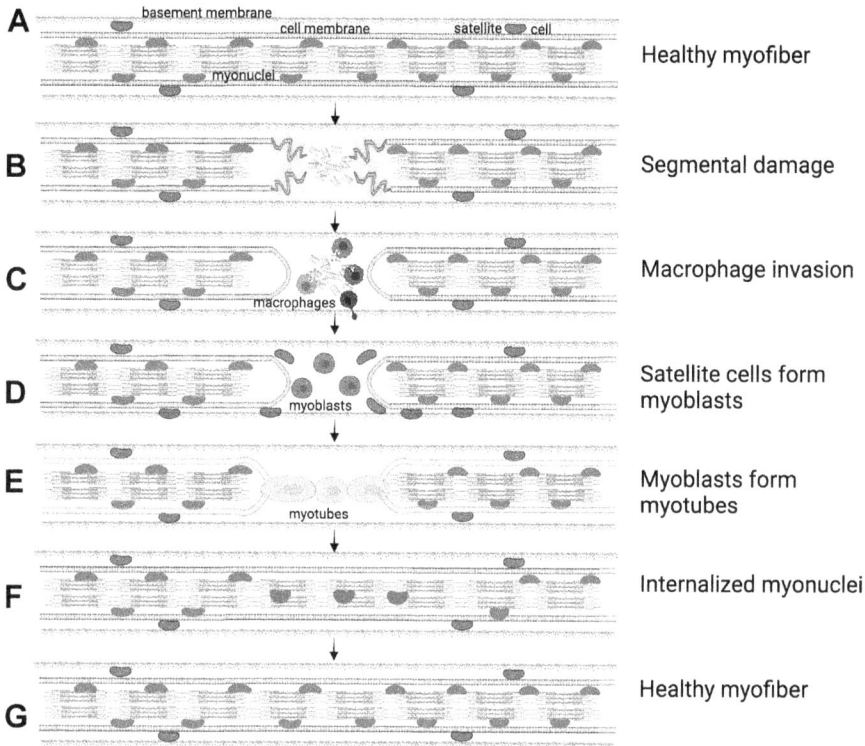

Fig. 2. The sequence of events that occur with myofiber degeneration and regeneration. (*A*) A longitudinal view of a healthy myofiber containing an outer layer of connective tissue (epimysium) and a cell membrane with satellite cells lying in between. An orderly array of myofilaments is present and myonuclei lie just under the cell membrane. (*B*) Exertional rhabdomyolysis damages a segment of a muscle fiber. (*C*) Within hours, the ends of the myofiber are sealed, and within 12–24 h, macrophages migrate into the damaged segment and phagocytize the degenerating organelles. (*D*) Within days, satellite cells are activated and migrate into the damaged segment to form myoblasts. (*E*) Myoblasts fuse to form myotubes which then regenerate myofilaments and organelles. (*F*) For 2–3 weeks after the fiber is damaged, the myonuclei in the damaged segment remain in a central position. (*G*) Within 4 weeks, the myonuclei migrate to a position under the cell membrane and the myofiber has fully regenerated. (*Created in* BioRender. Valberg, S. (2025) https://BioRender.com/w28j649.)

- Pawing
- Severe cases can be recumbent and unwilling to rise

Diagnosis of ER: Damage to the cell membrane leads to release of muscle components such as creatine kinase (CK), aspartate aminotransferase (AST), and lactate dehydrogenase into the serum, and thus, increases in the activity of these enzymes in serum are the cornerstone for diagnosing rhabdomyolysis.[3] Serum CK activity increases within hours of a muscle insult, peaks within 4 to 6 hours after injury, and usually declines to the normal range within 48 hours of an insult if there is no ongoing muscle damage (longer if peak activity exceeded 100,000 U/L). Serum AST activity is not specific for skeletal and cardiac muscle damage because it is also present in liver, red blood cells, and other tissues. However, assessing AST in muscle disease is useful for assessing chronicity because it persists in serum for 2 to 3 weeks following muscle damage, and evaluation of other serum variables can be used to determine muscle origin of AST.

TREATMENT OF ACUTE RHABDOMYOLYSIS

Hand walking horses with acute rhabdomyolysis is contraindicated as it exacerbates muscle damage. During a competition, it is best to treat rhabdomyolysis on site and avoid long-distance transport for at least 24 to 48 hours. Dehydration should be assessed before beginning treatment because myoglobinuria, dehydration, and nonsteroidal anti-inflammatory drugs (NSAIDs) can all be nephrotoxic. Tranquilizers provide immediate relief from pain and anxiety. An alpha-adrenergic antagonist such as acepromazine is a good choice if the pain is moderate and the horse well hydrated and can be repeated if needed after 2 hours (**Table 1**). Alternatively, xylazine or, in more painful horses, detomidine combined with butorphanol provides excellent sedation and analgesia. NSAIDs can be given to hydrated horses to provide additional pain relief. Analgesic treatment is continued to effect, but most horses are relatively pain free within 18 to 24 hours. For horses with extreme pain and distress, a constant rate infusion of detomidine or lidocaine or butorphanol can make the difference between adequate time for recovery and euthanasia (see **Table 1**). Muscle relaxants such as methocarbamol may be of some benefit. Dantrolene is both a muscle relaxant and has the beneficial effect of reducing ongoing rhabdomyolysis by decreasing release of calcium from the SR.[4] Dantrolene can be given orally three times a day (TID) to four times a day (QID) at 2 mg/kg until serum CK is dropping substantially. Caution is advised when administering dantrolene to horses with hyperkalemic periodic paralysis (HYPP) as it can elevate serum potassium concentrations and

Table 1			
Medications that can be used to treat rhabdomyolysis along with their dose, route, and frequency of use			
Drug	**Dose**	**Route**	**Frequency**
Anxiety relief (choose one)			
Acepromazine	0.04–0.07 mg/kg	IM or IV	Once to q 8 h
Xylazine	0.2–0.5 mg/kg	IV	Once
Detomidine	0.02–0.04 mg/kg	IM or IV	Once
Butorphanol	0.1 mg/kg	IV	Once
Pain relief once hydrated (choose one)			
Ketoprofen	2.2 mg/kg	IV	q 12 h
Phenylbutazone	2.2–4.4 mg/kg	Oral	q 12 h
Flunixin meglumine	1.1 mg/kg	Oral	q 12 h
Severe pain constant rate infusions (choose one)			
Detomidine loading dose	0.01 mg/kg	IV	
Detomidine CRI	0.01 mg/kg/h	IV	
Lidocaine loading dose	1.3 mg/kg	IV over 15 min	
Lidocaine CRI	0.05 mg/kg/min	IV	
Butorphanol CRI	13 mcg/kg/hour	IV	
Muscle relaxation			
Methocarbamol	5–22 mg/kg	IV slowly or orally	q 12 h
Prevent further rhabdomyolysis			
Dantrolene	2–4 mg/kg	Oral—ensure recent feed intake (within 4 h)	q 8–12 h

Abbreviations: CRI, constant rate infusion; IV, intravenous; mcg, micrograms.

precipitate an episode.[5] It should be administered in recent proximity to feeding to aid absorption.

Well-hydrated horses should have access to fresh water and a second bucket of electrolyte solution. For mildly dehydrated horses, fluids can be administered via nasogastric tube. For horses with moderate dehydration and horses with myoglobinuria, intravenously administered fluids are optimal. Ideally, serum electrolytes should be evaluated because marked hyponatremia, hypochloremia, hypocalcemia, hyperkalemia, and hyperphosphatemia can occur with severe rhabdomyolysis.[6] Balanced polyionic electrolyte solutions are usually best, with specific supplementation as needed. If severe rhabdomyolysis is present, then isotonic saline or 2.5% dextrose in 0.45% saline may be beneficial. If hypocalcemia is present, supplementing IV fluids with 100 to 200 mL of 23% calcium borogluconate in 5 L of fluids is recommended, but serum calcium should be monitored and should not exceed a low normal range. Horses with ER are usually alkalotic, making bicarbonate therapy inappropriate unless metabolic acidosis and myoglobinuria are concurrently present.

Sporadic Exertional Rhabdomyolysis

Horses have a much higher prevalence of ER than other species. For example, ER occurs in 2% to 3% of horses across breeds compared to an annual incidence of ER in human military recruits of 0.04%.[7,8] This low threshold for developing ER in equine muscle may be due to evolutionary adaptations for speed. Equine muscle has

1. Large amounts of a high affinity binding protein, calsequestrin, in the SR allowing more calcium to be stored and released down a concentration gradient with each contraction.[9]
2. A truncated sarcolipin gene resulting in undetectable skeletal muscle sarcolipin, a key inhibitory regulator of SERCA activity, resulting in continual high SERCA activity.[9,10]
3. A robust fight or flight response resulting in epinephrine release that enhances calcium release via RYR1.[11]

These adaptations should enhance muscle contraction and relaxation rates; however, while they provide the benefit of enhanced muscle performance on one side, they may also enhance the risk of exceeding tolerable cytoplasmic calcium concentrations that will trigger rhabdomyolysis. Causes of sporadic ER include exercise performed beyond training adaptation or to the point of exhaustion, dietary imbalances of electrolytes, antioxidants, or nonstructural carbohydrates (NSCs) or exercising in the face of underlying respiratory viral disease.

Overexertion: Horses that have not received an adequate base of conditioning prior to more strenuous exercise may develop ER from overexertion. For example, 81% of cases of ER in Polo horses are attributed to overexertion, with 30% of cases occurring after a day of rest.[12] Exhaustion occurs most commonly in endurance horses or racehorses exercising in hot, humid weather. Signs of heat exhaustion include rectal temperatures of 40.5°C to 42.2°C (105–108°F), weakness, ataxia, rapid breathing, muscle fasciculations, sweating, and in severe cases collapse. With overexertion, muscles are firm and horses stiff, and with heat exhaustion, muscles are frequently not firm on palpation, although serum CK activity can be markedly elevated and myoglobinuria may be noted in both cases.[13]

Dietary imbalances: Diets with a high NSC content and low forage content,[14,15] deficient in electrolytes, or inadequate in selenium and vitamin E may precipitate episodes of ER. Whole blood selenium concentrations measured in ethylenediaminetetraacetic acid (EDTA), or serum should be assessed when horses are in geographic areas with selenium-deficient soil. Vitamin E concentration should be measured in serum or plasma samples kept chilled and protected from light. To ensure the diet is balanced to prevent further episodes, a nutrition consultation is advised.

Management of sporadic ER: Following treatment of acute ER, rest with regular access to a paddock once stiffness resides and weekly monitoring of serum CK activity is recommended. Allowing horses to calmly determine their own exercise through turnout is preferable to hand walking, which should be limited to no more than a few minutes at a time initially. The diet is assessed to ensure that the ration is fed in an amount recommended by the manufacturer for the corresponding level of exercise. Good-quality grass or grass-legume mixed hay (55%–65% neutral detergent fiber [NDF], 10%–12% crude protein [CP], 10%–17% NSC by weight) and concentrates providing moderate levels of soluble carbohydrate (20%–30% NSC by weight in the concentrate), fat (4%–8%), and fiber (20%–30% NDF) are appropriate. Horses with sporadic ER do not necessarily benefit from increased dietary fat, so addition of fat should depend upon caloric needs. A salt block or 30 to 50 g (1–3 tablespoons) of salt per day will provide the necessary amount of sodium chloride, with the amount required depending on the heat, humidity, and intensity and duration of exercise. Once serum CK returns to normal and muscle fibers have regenerated, usually within 2 to 3 weeks, training can be resumed gradually. A regular exercise schedule, beginning with 20 min or less of exercise per day, is gradually increased to eventually match the expected amount of daily exercise to the underlying state of conditioning.

Some horses when put back into exercise will have chronic episodes of muscle pain despite reasonable management. The management plan for these horses differs from sporadic ER. An intrinsic abnormality in muscle function is believed to cause their repeated episodes of rhabdomyolysis and several specific causes have been identified and are described in this and subsequent articles (**Fig. 3**). For horses with chronic

Exertional Rhabdomyolysis

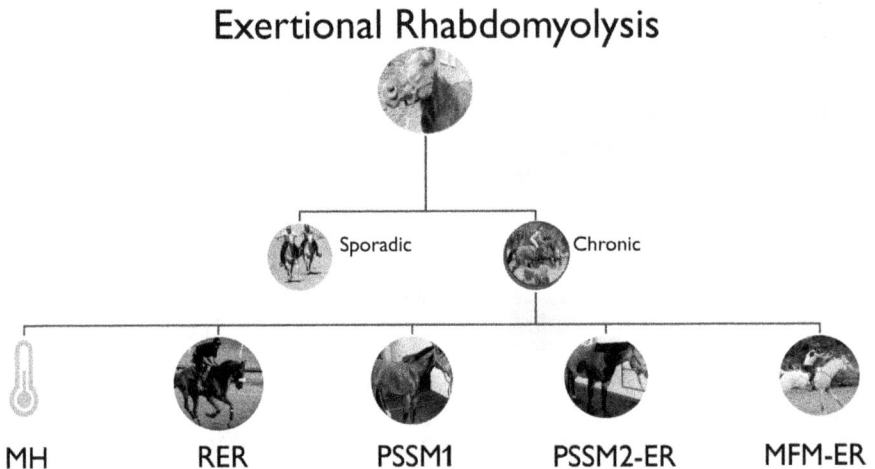

Fig. 3. A diagnosis of exertional rhabdomyolysis (ER) requires establishing that serum creatine kinase (CK) activity is elevated in association with clinical signs of muscle pain and stiffness. ER has several different causes. Sporadic ER occurs from extrinsic factors. Chronic ER occurs from intrinsic abnormalities that cause muscle dysfunction. Causes of chronic ER include malignant hyperthermia (MH), recurrent exertional rhabdomyolysis (RER), type 1 polysaccharide storage myopathy (PSSM1), type 2 polysaccharide storage myopathy-ER (PSSM2-ER), and myofibrillar myopathy in Arabian horses (MFM-ER).

ER, this prolonged period of rest is not recommended, and horses are gradually put back into work as soon as they are pain free and moving normally.

Chronic Exertional Rhabdomyolysis

Causes of chronic ER include malignant hyperthermia (MH) and recurrent exertional rhabdomyolysis (RER) that are included in this article (see **Fig. 3**). Other causes such as type 1 polysaccharide storage myopathy (PSSM1) and type 2 polysaccharide storage myopathy-ER (PSSM2-ER) can be found in the article Polysaccharide Storage Myopathy by Firshman and Valberg[16] in this issue and Myofibrillar Myopathy in Arabian horses (MFM-ER) can be found in the article Myofibrillar Myopathy by Williams and Valberg (see **Fig. 3**).[17]

Recurrent Exertional Rhabdomyolysis

RER is one form of chronic ER that affects 5% to 7% of Thoroughbreds and 6% of Standardbreds across the globe.[7,18–21] Based on overlapping histories, clinical signs, muscle biopsy findings, and response to management, RER likely also occurs in Arabians, Warmbloods, racing Quarter Horses, and other breeds.[22] Young mares develop RER more often than geldings although episodes or rhabdomyolysis are not correlated with stages of the estrus cycle.[18,23] A nervous/excitable temperament is associated with RER, and in Thoroughbreds, young fillies are most likely to have this temperament as well as a high prevalence of RER.[18,20,21] High grain diets and, in some studies, lameness can potentiate rhabdomyolysis in RER-susceptible horses.[18,24]

Clinical signs: Horses with a history of RER can be clinically normal when unfit or exercising in low-stress environments. However, when fit and in a race training environment or when training for, or competing at horse shows or 3 day events, horses intermittently develop classic signs of muscle pain and stiffness typical of those described earlier for ER. These signs are usually apparent within 30 min or less of commencing exercise but may not be apparent until after exercise ceases. A day or more of rest before exercise increases the incidence of rhabdomyolysis.[25] In Standardbreds, ER commonly occurs while jogging and in Thoroughbreds, 3 day event horses and Arabians, signs usually occur when horses are held back by the rider.[18,20,26] ER rarely occurs when horses are allowed to achieve maximal exercise speeds such as racing.

Pathogenesis: RER is characterized by a sharp rise in serum myoglobin concentrations and serum CK activity.[27] The trigger for episodes is often excitement in a horse that already has an underlying nervous temperament or is often fighting with the rider to go faster.[18,19] With an acute episode of RER, gluteus medius muscle biopsies show segmental necrosis in fewer than 5% of fast-twitch type 2A and 2X myofibers. Physiologic studies of muscle contraction in response to agents that trigger SR calcium release in intact muscle fiber bundles and muscle cultures indicate that RER is due to an abnormality in the regulation of intracellular calcium flux from or into the SR that is intermittently triggered in skeletal muscle.[28–30] Transcriptomic and proteomic studies of gluteal muscle from RER susceptible Thoroughbreds between episodes of rhabdomyolysis show that RER horses have higher RYR1 (the calcium release channel) content, increased calsequestrin (a high affinity calcium-binding protein in the SR), enhanced pathways for beta-adrenergic stimulation of RYR1, and indicators of mitochondrial apoptosis compared to controls.[31] This led to the hypothesis that episodes of rhabdomyolysis in RER horses are easily triggered by excitement that causes the following phenomena (**Fig. 4**):

1. Intermittent prolonged opening of RYR1
2. Excessive release of calcium into the myoplasm

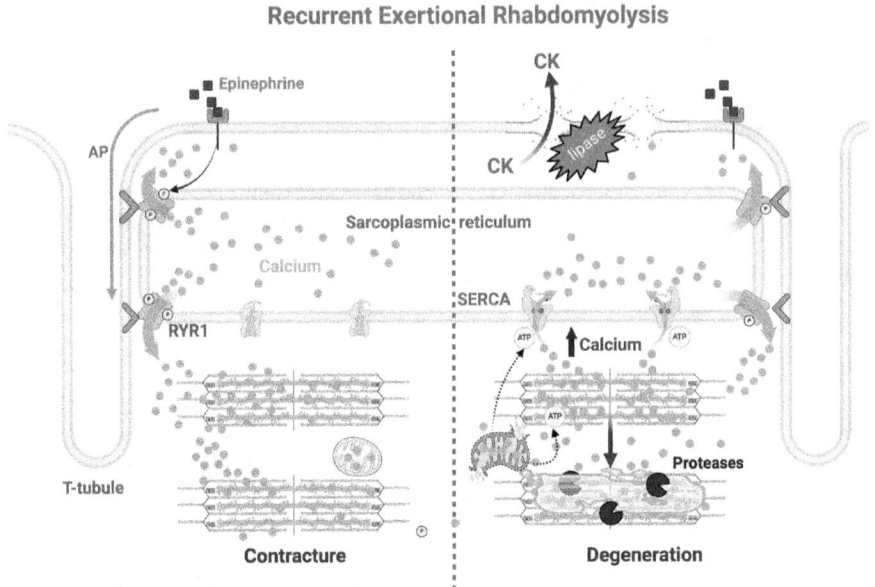

Fig. 4. A scenario for the development of rhabdomyolysis in RER-susceptible horses. A high stress environment resulting in beta-adrenergic activation of secondary messengers will phosphorylate RYR1 and increase the open probability of RYR1. This allows excessive calcium (*green circles*) to be released from the sarcoplasmic reticulum into the myoplasm. Myoplasmic calcium interacts with contractile filaments and, when not adequately pumped back into the SR, produces persistent contracture of the sarcomere (*left* portion of figure). Mitochondria attempt to buffer excessive myoplasmic calcium; however, in excess, calcium uncouples oxygen consumption from electron transport and ATP production and releases reactive oxygen species (ROS) (*right* portion of figure). Calcium activation of proteases such as calpain and lipases results in degradation of myofilaments, other cellular proteins, and cell membranes resulting in the release of creatine kinase (CK) into the bloodstream. (*Created in* BioRender. Valberg, S. (2025) https://BioRender.com/h96y301.)

3. Persistent muscle contracture
4. Excessive mitochondrial calcium uptake
5. Uncoupling of the mitochondrial electron transfer system
6. Mitochondrial degeneration
7. Activation of proteases and loss of myofiber integrity

In Standardbreds, transcriptomic and proteomic analyses of gluteal muscle suggest that pathways of calcium regulation, cellular/oxidative stress, and inflammation characterize susceptibility to RER.[31,32] Thus, it appears that intermittently there is dysregulation of SR calcium release in RER horses resulting in an excessive rise in myoplasmic calcium and muscle degeneration.

Genetic basis for RER: There is a familial tendency for RER with heritability estimated at 0.40; however, a simple Mendelian basis for RER has not been identified and no validated genetic tests are available.[33–35]

Diagnosis: A diagnosis of RER is based on clinical signs, presence of risk factors commonly associated with RER, and determination of elevations in serum CK and AST activities in association with exercise and clinical signs. Two year old fillies generally have greater fluctuations in serum CK activity during race training than 3 year old fillies or geldings.[36] Fit RER horses often show intermittent elevations in serum CK activity that can exceed 1000 U/L that return to normal relatively quickly during training. Timing of the sample with regard to the onset of ER is important with samples ideally obtained 4 to 6 hours after an episode at a time when serum CK peaks. Muscle histopathology is nonspecific in RER horses; either no abnormalities or evidence of centrally located nuclei in mature fibers and potentially waves of myofiber degeneration or regeneration is found. The value of muscle biopsy as a diagnostic tool in horses with suspected RER is largely confined to particularly recurrent unmanageable cases where a need arises to evaluate for other forms of ER.

MANAGEMENT

Prevention of rhabdomyolysis in horses susceptible to RER is complex and multiple factors need to be changed to decrease episodes. These factors include the environment, the exercise regime, and diet. In addition, medication may be needed at times to prevent further episodes of muscle damage.

Environment: Because excitement and nervousness often trigger rhabdomyolysis, stressful situations in the environment that can be modified need to be identified. This may involve a change to a smaller barn with fewer horses, fewer handlers and turnout paddocks, compatible equine companions, and a more consistent daily routine. The use of hot walkers, exercise machines, and swimming pools needs to be evaluated on an individual basis, as some horses develop rhabdomyolysis when using this type of equipment. Horses that develop RER at specific events, such as horse shows, may need to be reconditioned to decrease the stress level associated with such events or tranquilized as part of the accommodation process. Providing daily turnout with other horses seems to be very beneficial for RER horses and may decrease anxiety and thereby the likelihood of rhabdomyolysis.

Exercise: Although rest is recommended for sporadic forms of ER, it is not recommended for horses with RER because more than 2 days of rest increase serum CK activity and the likelihood of developing ER with the next exercise session.[25,37] Clinical judgment should be used, but often horses are returned to regular daily exercise when serum CK falls below about 3000 U/L. During time off, turnout is highly recommended. Horses with more severe episodes of rhabdomyolysis may require additional time off in a paddock before gradually resuming exercise. Once back in training, some form of daily exercise is recommended. Avoiding fighting to hold horses to slower speeds is important and in Standardbreds, interval training and reduction of jog miles to no more than 15 minutes per session are beneficial. Event horses may require training that incorporates calm exposure to speeds achieved during the cross-country phase and Arabian endurance horses might benefit from delaying their start until most horses have left so they can begin calmly.

Diet: A nutritionally balanced diet with appropriate caloric intake and adequate vitamin and mineral intake is the core element of managing RER. For RER Thoroughbreds and Standardbreds in training, the challenge is usually supplying enough calories in a highly palatable form to meet their daily energy demands. This is in part because they often require greater than 30 Mcal of digestible energy (DE) a day (provided by 5 kg sweet feed and 1.5% of body weight in hay), and because of their nervous temperament, they may be more discriminating in their eating habits or prone to gastric ulcers. Hay with an NSC as high as 17% can be fed to RER Thoroughbreds. Some RER horses have a higher propensity to develop episodes of ER if fed alfalfa hay. Concentrates for RER horses should contain 12% to 18% NSC and 10% to 13% fat by weight and be fed according to manufacturer instructions to provide the needed balance of vitamins and minerals. To maintain high energy densities (3.2–3.4 Mcal DE/kg), feed products should also contain sources of highly digestible fiber such as beet pulp or soy hulls. The benefit of a high-fat diet for RER does not appear to result from a change in muscle metabolism.[24] Rather, low-NSC, high-fat diets in RER horses may decrease muscle damage by assuaging anxiety and excitability, which are tightly linked to development of rhabdomyolysis in susceptible horses.[38]

Standardbreds have molecular signatures of persistent inflammation in their muscle even between episodes of ER.[39] Eicosatetraenoic acid and docosahexaenoic acid are long-chain omega-3 polyunsaturated fatty acids that can be of additional benefit when managing RER in Standardbred horses (Valberg personal observation).

Further information on nutritional support for RER horses can be found in the article the Role of Nutrition in Managing Muscle Disorders by Pagan in this issue.[40]

Medications: Dantrolene acts to decrease release of calcium from the ryanodine receptor in skeletal muscle and lowers elevated myoplasmic calcium concentrations in horses experiencing ER.[41] Treatment with 1 to 2 mg/kg dantrolene 60 minutes before exercise mitigates the differences in gene expression between horses susceptible to RER and control horses in a racing environment.[31] Controlled and field studies have also shown that dantrolene (800 mg up to 4 mg/kg PO) given orally 60 to 90 minutes before exercise can significantly decrease signs of rhabdomyolysis in RER horses.[37,42] As such, it is an ideal means to manage RER outside of drug-restricted competition. Absorption of dantrolene is superior in fed versus fasted horses.[43]

Low doses of tranquillizers, such as acepromazine, before exercise have been used in RER horses prone to excitement.[44] A dose of 7 mg IV 20 minutes before exercise is reported to make horses more relaxed and manageable. Reserpine and fluphenazine, which have a longer duration of effect, have also been used for this purpose. Horses given fluphenazine may occasionally exhibit prolonged bizarre behavior. Use of tranquilizers may only be necessary when horses are in their initial phase of training and during accommodation to a new environment (Valberg personal observation). Horses cannot compete on these medications and withdrawal times must be observed.

Some mares appear to exhibit signs of rhabdomyolysis during estrus, and it may well be of benefit in these horses to suppress estrus behavior using progesterone injections.

Adjunct therapies: Massage, myofascial release, mesotherapy, stretching, aqua-treadmills, and hot/cold therapy performed by experienced therapists may be of benefit in individual cases.[45] Their use may promote relaxation and normal muscle tension and build muscle strength.

MALIGNANT HYPERTHERMIA

MH is another cause of chronic ER that is due to an abnormality in intramuscular calcium regulation. It is caused by an autosomal dominant mutation in the skeletal muscle *RYR1*.[46,47] The mutation lowers the activation and heightens the deactivation threshold of RYR1, which intermittently can result in a drastic efflux of calcium from the SR, increasing myoplasmic calcium and producing contracture and myodegeneration.[48]

MH affects less than 1% of Quarter Horses and Paint horses and is most common in halter and pleasure horse lines. In many horses, clinical signs are completely inapparent or very intermittent in nature. Rhabdomyolysis with MH can be induced by exercise but can also occur with stress or anesthesia.[47] Some horses have both the MH mutation and the glyocgen synthase 1 gene (*GYS1*) mutation for PSSM1 which make clinical signs more severe and harder to manage.[49]

Clinical signs: Horses will intermittently exhibit classic signs of ER but additionally will have a very elevated rectal temperature during signs.

Diagnosis: Genetic testing is required to diagnose MH. Muscle biopsies are often normal or have nonspecific signs of muscle degeneration.

Treatment: Although dantrolene is designed to block the excessive leak of calcium through RYR1 that occurs with MH, the unpredictable occurrence of episodes of ER is such that it is difficult or excessively expensive to use dantrolene on a daily basis to prevent rhabdomyolysis in susceptible horses.

In summary, ER is a common occurrence in horses. It can occur sporadically due to extrinsic influences or chronically from a variety of intrinsic abnormalities in muscle function. RER is one form of chronic ER that causes intermittent episodes of ER in fit horses that often have a nervous temperament or fight the rider when being held back under saddle. Careful management of their diet, environment, and training regimes can help maintain the horse's athletic performance.

CLINICS CARE POINTS

- While sporadic cases of ER can be rested after an episode, horses with chronic exertional rhabdomyolysis require regular daily exercise.
- Horses with myoglobinuria should receive intravenous fluids to prevent renal damage.

DISCLOSURE

S.J. Valberg directs the Valberg Neuromuscular Disease Laboratory (ValbergNMDL.com) and receives remuneration for analyzing muscle biopsies. Her Web site is sponsored by Kentucky Equine Research, United States, and she receives royalties from the PSSM1 genetic test and the feed products Re-leve and MFM pellet developed in association with Kentucky Equine Research.

REFERENCES

1. Calderón JC, Bolaños P, Caputo C. The excitation-contraction coupling mechanism in skeletal muscle. Biophys Rev 2014;6:133–60.
2. Warren JD, Blumbergs PC, Thompson PD. Rhabdomyolysis: a review. Muscle Nerve 2002;25:332–47.
3. Cardinet GH, Littrell JF, Freedland RA. Comparative investigations of serum creatine phosphokinase and glutamic-oxaloacetic transaminase activities in equine paralytic myoglobinuria. Res Vet Sci 1967;8:219–26.
4. Zhao F, Li P, Chen SW, et al. Dantrolene inhibition of ryanodine receptor Ca2+ release channels: molecular mechanism and isoform selectivity. J Biol Chem 2001;276:13810–6.
5. McKenzie EC, Di Concetto S, Payton ME, et al. Effect of dantrolene premedication on various cardiovascular and biochemical variables and the recovery in healthy isoflurane-anesthetized horses. Am J. Vet Res 2015;76:293–301.
6. Perkins G, Valberg SJ, Madigan JM, et al. Electrolyte disturbances in foals with severe rhabdomyolysis. J Vet Intern Med 1998;12:173–7.
7. Cole FL, Mellor DJ, Hodgson DR, et al. Prevalence and demographic characteristics of exertional rhabdomyolysis in horses in Australia. Vet Rec 2004;155:625–30.

8. Exertional rhabdomyolysis among active component members of the U.S. Armed Forces, 2019-2023. Msmr 2024;31:9–14.

9. Autry JM, Svensson B, Carlson SF, et al. Sarcoplasmic reticulum from horse gluteal muscle is Poised for enhanced calcium transport. Vet Sci 2021;8:289.

10. Autry JM, Karim CB, Perumbakkam S, et al. Sarcolipin exhibits abundant RNA transcription and minimal protein expression in horse gluteal muscle. Vet Sci 2020;7:178.

11. Andersson DC, Betzenhauser MJ, Reiken S, et al. Stress-induced increase in skeletal muscle force requires protein kinase A phosphorylation of the ryanodine receptor. J Physiol 2012;590:6381–7.

12. McGowan CM, Posner RE, Christley RM. Incidence of exertional rhabdomyolysis in polo horses in the USA and the United Kingdom in the 1999/2000 season. Vet Rec 2002;150:535–7.

13. Muñoz A, Castejón-Riber C, Riber C, et al. Current knowledge of pathologic mechanisms and derived practical applications to prevent metabolic disturbances and exhaustion in the endurance horse. J Equine Vet Sci 2017;51:24–33.

14. Valentine BA, Van Saun RJ, Thompson KN, et al. Role of dietary carbohydrate and fat in horses with equine polysaccharide storage myopathy. J Am Vet Med Assoc 2001;219:1537–44.

15. Valentine BA, Hintz HF, Freels KM, et al. Dietary control of exertional rhabdomyolysis in horses. J Am Vet Med Assoc 1998;212:1588–93.

16. Firshman AC, Valberg SJ. Polysaccharide Storage Myopathy. In: McKenzie EC,Valberg SJ, editor. Muscle Disorders of Horses: An Issue of Veterinary Clinics of North America: Equine Practice. 2025. p. 125–37.

17. Williams ZJ, Valberg SJ. Myofibrillar Myopathy. In: McKenzie EC, Valberg SJ, editors. Muscle Disorders of Horses: An Issue of Veterinary Clinics of North America: Equine Practice. 2025. p. 139–50.

18. MacLeay JM, Sorum SA, Valberg SJ, et al. Epidemiologic analysis of factors influencing exertional rhabdomyolysis in Thoroughbreds. Am J Vet Res 1999;60:1562–6.

19. McGowan CM, Fordham T, Christley RM. Incidence and risk factors for exertional rhabdomyolysis in thoroughbred racehorses in the United Kingdom. Vet Rec 2002;151:623–6.

20. Upjohn MM, Archer RM, Christley RM, et al. Incidence and risk factors associated with exertional rhabdomyolysis syndrome in National Hunt racehorses in Great Britain. Vet Rec 2005;156:763–6.

21. Isgren CM, Upjohn MM, Fernandez-Fuente M, et al. Epidemiology of exertional rhabdomyolysis susceptibility in standardbred horses reveals associated risk factors and underlying enhanced performance. PLoS One 2010;5:e11594.

22. Hunt LM, Valberg SJ, Steffenhagen K, et al. An epidemiological study of myopathies in Warmblood horses. Equine Vet J 2008;40:171–7.

23. Frauenfelder HC, Rossdale PD, Ricketts SW, et al. Changes in serum muscle enzyme levels associated with training schedules and stage of the oestrous cycle in Thoroughbred racehorses. Equine Vet J 1986;18:371–4.

24. MacLeay JM, Valberg SJ, Pagan JD, et al. Effect of ration and exercise on plasma creatine kinase activity and lactate concentration in Thoroughbred horses with recurrent exertional rhabdomyolysis. Am J Vet Res 2000;61:1390–5.

25. McKenzie EC, Valberg SJ, Godden SM, et al. Effect of dietary starch, fat, and bicarbonate content on exercise responses and serum creatine kinase activity in equine recurrent exertional rhabdomyolysis. J Vet Intern Med 2003;17:693–701.

26. Valberg S, Jonsson L, Lindholm A, et al. Muscle histopathology and plasma aspartate aminotransferase, creatine kinase and myoglobin changes with exercise in horses with recurrent exertional rhabdomyolysis. Equine Vet J 1993; 25:11–6.

27. Valberg S, Haggendal J, Lindholm A. Blood chemistry and skeletal muscle metabolic responses to exercise in horses with recurrent exertional rhabdomyolysis. Equine Vet J 1993;25:17–22.

28. Lentz LR, Valberg SJ, Balog EM, et al. Abnormal regulation of muscle contraction in horses with recurrent exertional rhabdomyolysis. Am J Vet Res 1999;60:992–9.

29. Lentz LR, Valberg SJ, Herold LV, et al. Myoplasmic calcium regulation in myotubes from horses with recurrent exertional rhabdomyolysis. Am J Vet Res 2002;63:1724–31.

30. Beech J, Lindborg S, Fletcher JE, et al. Caffeine contractures, twitch characteristics and the threshold for Ca(2+)-induced Ca2+ release in skeletal muscle from horses with chronic intermittent rhabdomyolysis. Res Vet Sci 1993;54:110–7.

31. Aldrich K, Velez-Irizarry D, Fenger C, et al. Pathways of calcium regulation, electron transport, and mitochondrial protein translation are molecular signatures of susceptibility to recurrent exertional rhabdomyolysis in Thoroughbred racehorses. PLoS One 2021;16:e0244556.

32. Barrey E, Jayr L, Mucher E, et al. Transcriptome analysis of muscle in horses suffering from recurrent exertional rhabdomyolysis revealed energetic pathway alterations and disruption in the cytosolic calcium regulation. Anim Genet 2012; 43:271–81.

33. Dranchak PK, Valberg SJ, Onan GW, et al. Inheritance of recurrent exertional rhabdomyolysis in thoroughbreds. J Am Vet Med Assoc 2005;227:762–7.

34. MacLeay JM, Valberg SJ, Sorum SA, et al. Heritability of recurrent exertional rhabdomyolysis in Thoroughbred racehorses. Am J Vet Res 1999;60:250–6.

35. Norton EM, Mickelson JR, Binns MM, et al. Heritability of recurrent exertional rhabdomyolysis in Standardbred and Thoroughbred racehorses derived from SNP genotyping data. J Hered 2016;107:537–43.

36. Harris PA, Snow DH, Greet TR, et al. Some factors influencing plasma AST/CK activities in thoroughbred racehorses. Equine Vet J Suppl 1990;66–71.

37. McKenzie EC, Valberg SJ, Godden SM, et al. Effect of oral administration of dantrolene sodium on serum creatine kinase activity after exercise in horses with recurrent exertional rhabdomyolysis. Am J Vet Res 2004;65:74–9.

38. Finno CJ, McKenzie E, Valberg SJ, et al. Effect of fitness on glucose, insulin and cortisol responses to diets varying in starch and fat content in Thoroughbred horses with recurrent exertional rhabdomyolysis. Equine Vet J Suppl 2010;323–8.

39. Valberg SJ, Velez-Irizarry D, Williams ZJ, et al. Enriched pathways of calcium regulation, cellular/oxidative stress, inflammation, and cell proliferation characterize gluteal muscle of standardbred horses between episodes of recurrent exertional rhabdomyolysis. Genes 2022;13:1853.

40. Pagan JD, Valberg SJ. The role of nutrition in muscle disorders. In: McKenzie EC, Valberg SJ, editors. Muscle Disorders of Horses An Issue of Veterinary Clinics of North America: Equine Practice. 2025. p. 151–63.

41. Lopez JR, Linares N, Cordovez G, et al. Elevated myoplasmic calcium in exercise-induced equine rhabdomyolysis. Pflugers Arch 1995;430:293–5.

42. Edwards JG, Newtont JR, Ramzan PH, et al. The efficacy of dantrolene sodium in controlling exertional rhabdomyolysis in the Thoroughbred racehorse. Equine Vet J 2003;35:707–11.

43. Mc Kenzie E, Garrett R, Payton M, et al. Effect of feed restriction on plasma dantrolene concentrations in horses. Equine Vet J 2010;42:613–7.

44. Freestone JF, Wolfsheimer KJ, Kamerling SG, et al. Exercise induced hormonal and metabolic changes in Thoroughbred horses: effects of conditioning and acepromazine. Equine Vet J 1991;23:219–23.

45. Tiidus PM. Manual massage and recovery of muscle function following exercise: a literature review. J Orthop Sports Phys Ther 1997;25:107–12.

46. Aleman M, Riehl J, Aldridge BM, et al. Association of a mutation in the ryanodine receptor 1 gene with equine malignant hyperthermia. Muscle Nerve 2004;30: 356–65.

47. Aleman M, Nieto JE, Magdesian KG. Malignant hyperthermia associated with ryanodine receptor 1 (C7360G) mutation in Quarter Horses. J Vet Intern Med 2009;23:329–34.

48. Mickelson JR, Louis CF. Malignant hyperthermia: excitation-contraction coupling, Ca2+ release channel, and cell Ca2+ regulation defects. Physiol Rev 1996;76: 537–92.

49. McCue ME, Valberg SJ, Jackson M, et al. Polysaccharide storage myopathy phenotype in quarter horse-related breeds is modified by the presence of an RYR1 mutation. Neuromuscul Disord 2009;19:37–43.

Polysaccharide Storage Myopathy

Anna M. Firshman, BVSc, PhD[a],*, Stephanie J. Valberg, DVM, PhD[b]

KEYWORDS

- Skeletal muscle • Horse • Glycogen synthase • Glycogenosis • Glycogen

KEY POINTS

- Polysaccharide Storage Myopathy is a glycogen storage disease currently divided into Type 1 PSSM and Type 2 PSSM. Type 1 PSSM is caused by an autosomal dominant mutation in glycogen synthase 1 (*GYS1*). A specific genetic mutation has not been validated for PSSM2.
- The clinical presentation of PSSM1 varies from asymptomatic to muscle soreness, exertional rhabdomyolysis (ER) and occasionally in homozygotes, symmetric topline atrophy.
- Type 2 PSSM with ER (PSSM2-ER) is found in Quarter Horses and likely other breeds and presents as muscle stiffness and pain with high serum creatine kinase.
- Horses with PSSM1 and PSSM2-ER can be managed with a low nonstructural carbohydrate, high fat diet combined with regular exercise.
- Other subsets of PSSM2 are not glycogen storage disorders and have now been termed myofibrillar myopathy based on research; Warmblood breeds are particularly predisposed.

INTRODUCTION/HISTORY/BACKGROUND

Polysaccharide Storage Myopathy (PSSM) was first described in 1992 in 9 horses of Quarter Horse-related breeds with chronic exertional rhabdomyolysis (ER) and was characterized by 2-fold higher-than-normal muscle glycogen concentrations and the presence of periodic acid Schiff's (PAS)-positive abnormal polysaccharide inclusions that were resistant to amylase digestion within the cytoplasm of muscle cells.[1,2] In the following years, several acronyms were used for polysaccharide storage myopathy besides PSSM,[3] including EPSM and EPSSM,[4,5] which caused some debate as to whether they were all the same condition. In 2008, a mutation in the glycogen synthase 1 gene (*GYS1*) was determined to be highly associated with the presence of amylase-resistant polysaccharide in skeletal muscle in many horses with PSSM diagnosed by

[a] Department of Veterinary Population Medicine, University of Minnesota, 225k VMC, 1365 Gortner Avenue, Saint Paul, MN 55108, USA; [b] Department of Large Animal Clinical Sciences, Michigan State University, East Lansing, MI, USA
* Corresponding author.
E-mail address: firsh001@umn.edu

Vet Clin Equine 41 (2025) 125–137
https://doi.org/10.1016/j.cveq.2024.11.004
0749-0739/25/© 2024 Elsevier Inc. All rights reserved, including those for text and data mining, AI training, and similar technologies.
vetequine.theclinics.com

muscle biopsy.[6] Some cases diagnosed with PSSM by muscle biopsy did not possess the genetic mutation however, and this suggested that there were at least 2 forms of PSSM.[7,8] The form of PSSM caused by the *GYS1* mutation is now termed type 1 (PSSM1) whereas the form(s) of PSSM not associated with the *GYS1* mutation is termed type 2 (PSSM2).[7] Recent research has further subdivided PSSM2 into PSSM2-ER, myofibrillar myopathy-ER (MFM-ER), and myofibrillar myopathy in Warmblood horses (MFM-WB) that does not present with ER, but rather with exercise intolerance.[9–11] (**Fig. 1**) See the article "Myofibrillar Myopathy" by Williams and Valberg in this issue for discussion regarding forms of MFM.[12]

TYPE 1 POLYSACCHARIDE STORAGE MYOPATHY

PSSM1 is estimated to have emerged approximately 1600 years ago when the Great Horse or War Horse of the Middle Ages was being developed from European draft and light horse breeds to carry horsemen with heavy armor into battle.[6] It is likely the same disorder that was called "Azoturia" or "Monday Morning Disease" in work horses in the nineteenth and twentieth centuries. PSSM1 is now known to be caused by an autosomal dominant missense mutation in *GYS1* that results in an arginine substitution for histidine at codon 309 in glycogen synthase.[6] The effect of this amino acid substitution is a higher-than-normal activity of glycogen synthase both at basal states and when activated by glucose-6-phosphate, twice normal glycogen concentrations and the formation of amylase-resistant polysaccharide (**Figs. 2**A, B and **3**A).[6,13] Foals and yearlings with the *GYS1* mutation rarely have abnormal polysaccharide in skeletal muscle, yet they have rhabdomyolysis.[14] Thus, abnormal polysaccharide appears to be an indicator of PSSM1 but not the direct cause for rhabdomyolysis.

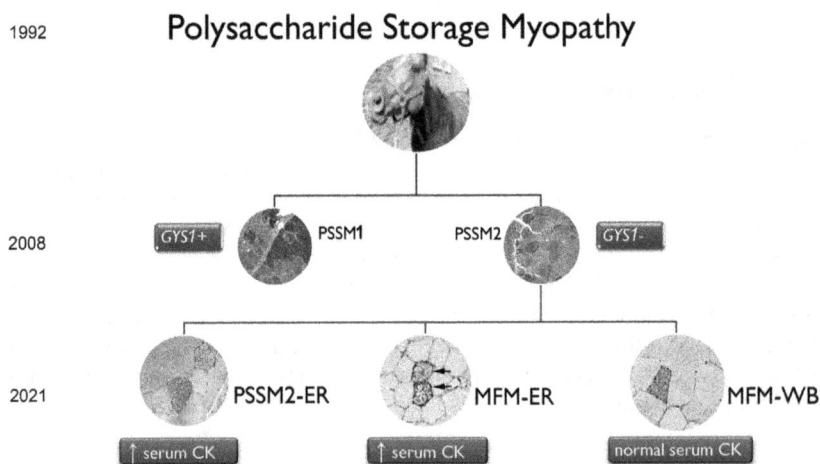

Fig. 1. PSSM was identified in 1992 based on abnormal staining for polysaccharide. In 2008, it was subdivided into PSSM1 and PSSM2 based on the presence (PSSM1) or absence (PSSM2) of the *GYS1* mutation. PSSM2 was later divided into PSSM2-ER, a glycogen storage disorder, and MFM in 2021. A diagnosis of PSSM2-ER was based on high muscle glycogen concentrations and exertional rhabdomyolysis and a diagnosis of MFM was based on normal muscle glycogen concentrations and the presence of desmin aggregation in muscle samples. MFM has now been determined to have 2 distinct forms: One characterized by ER (now termed MFM-ER) and the other by exercise intolerance in Warmbloods (now termed MFM-WB).

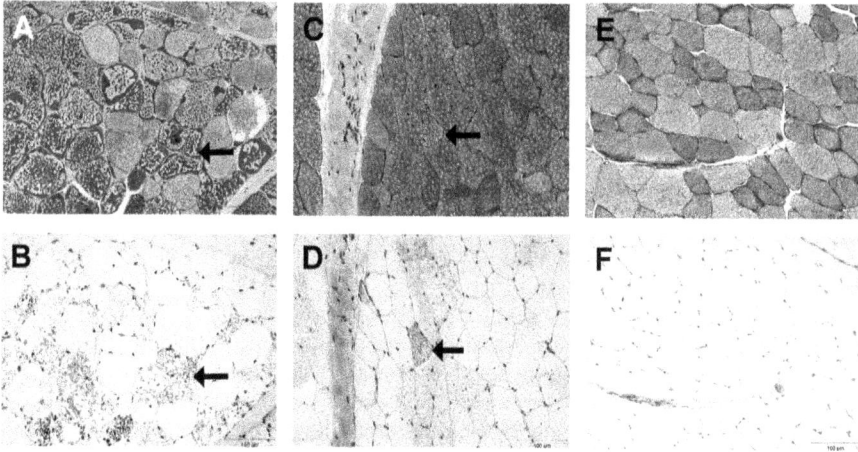

Fig. 2. Cross-sections of semimembranosus muscle biopsies from PSSM1, PSSM2-ER and control Quarter Horses 20X. (*A*) PAS of muscle from a PSSM1 horse with over 50% of muscle fibers in this fascicle containing excessive glycogen and abnormal polysaccharide inclusions (*arrow*). (*B*) Amylase-PAS stain of the same PSSM1 muscle sample in A showing that the polysaccharide (*arrow*) is resistant to amylase digestion. (*C*) PAS stain of muscle from a PSSM2-ER horse with dark staining indicating increased glycogen and a few fibers (*arrow*) with abnormal polysaccharide. (*D*) Amylase-PAS stain of the same PSSM2 muscle sample in C showing that the abnormal polysaccharide (*arrow*) is amylase-resistant. (*E*) A normal PAS stain. (*F*) A normal amylase PAS stain showing all the glycogen is digested.

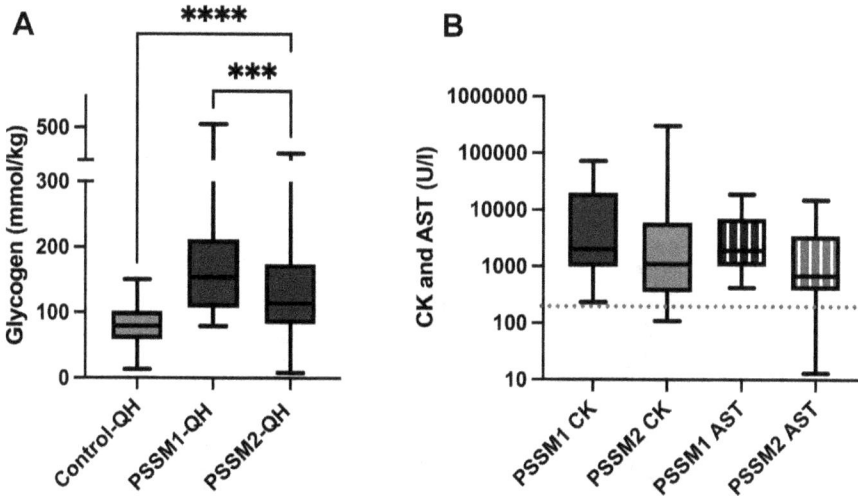

Fig. 3. (*A*) The mean and range of muscle glycogen concentrations in control horses and Quarter Horses (QH) with PSSM1 or Quarter Horses with PSSM2-ER. Glycogen concentrations in PSSM2-QH were significantly higher (**** $P<0.0001$) than controls and significantly lower (*** $P<0.001$) than PSSM1 Quarter Horses. (*B*) The mean and range of serum CK and aspartate AST activities in control horses and QH with PSSM1 or PSSM2-ER (*dotted line* indicates approximate normal range).[9]

Prevalence

- More than 20 breeds have the *GYS1* mutation responsible for PSSM1.[8,15–17]
- Continental European draft horse breeds have the highest prevalence (90% prevalence of PSSM1 in Trekpaards with 40% of tested Belgian Trekpaards homozygous).[15]
- United Kingdom-derived draft breeds such as Shires and Clydesdales, have a low prevalence but PSSM1 is present in other UK horse breeds such as Irish Drafts, Cob, and Connemara.[15,18]
- North American Belgians and Percherons have a prevalence of 36%, and 54% respectively.[16]
- Prevalence estimates of PSSM1 in Quarter Horses, American Paint, and Appaloosa horses range from 6% to 10% with the highest frequency of PSSM1 in Quarter Horses occurring in halter horses (28% affected) and the lowest frequency in racing Quarter Horses.[19]
- Arabians, Standardbreds, and Thoroughbreds have not been identified as possessing the PSSM1 mutation.[16]

Clinical Signs

The severity of clinical signs of PSSM1 varies widely from no clinical signs to muscle soreness, ER, gait abnormalities, severe weakness, and recumbency.[20] There is no evidence of impaired myocardial function in horses with PSSM1.[21]

- Individuals may first show signs of PSSM1 at an average of 5 years of age (range from 1 to 14 years of age).[19]
- Horses can have elevated serum creatine kinase (CK) and aspartate transaminase (AST) activities and in severe cases myoglobinuria can occur (**Fig. 3**B).[20]
- Acutely, signs of tucking up of the abdomen, flank fasciculations, muscle stiffness, sweating, reluctance to move forward, and firm muscle contractures lasting more than 2 hours are observed (**Fig. 4**). Some affected horses will paw and roll resembling colic or become recumbent.[20]
- Hindquarters are most often affected, but back, abdomen, and forelimb muscles may also be involved.[20]
- Gradual pronounced topline muscle atrophy can occur in homozygotes.

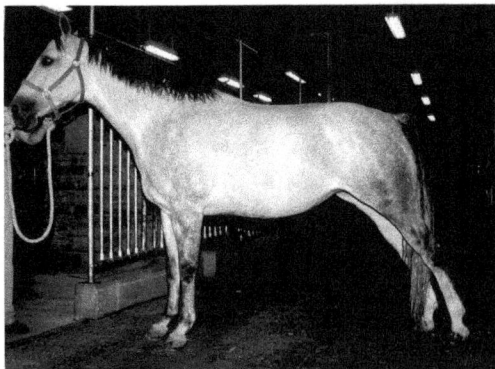

Fig. 4. 5-year-old Quarter Horse mare with PSSM1, stretching abnormally as a sign of muscle pain due to the development of rhabdomyolysis after 10 minutes of walking excercise.

Chronic clinical signs

- A lack of energy under saddle, reluctance to move, stopping and stretching out as if to urinate and a sour attitude toward exercise can develop.[20]
- Horses may have a combination of low-grade reluctance to exercise, poor performance and repeated episodes of ER.[17,22]
- Dressage horses and show jumpers can show chronic back pain, failure to round over fences and fasciculations, or pain upon palpation of lumbar muscles.[23]

Clinical signs in draft horses

- Many draft horses with PSSM are asymptomatic.[24]
- The average age of draft horses diagnosed with PSSM is approximately 8 years.[24]
- Draft horses homozygous for the GYS1 mutation have higher serum muscle enzyme activities compared to healthy or heterozygous draft horses[25]
- Signs of severe rhabdomyolysis and myoglobinuria may occur in draft horses fed high-grain diets, exercised irregularly with little turn-out, or draft horses that undergo general anesthesia.[26,27]
- Rhabdomyolysis can be so severe that it leads to recumbency and death.[26,28]
- Other signs of PSSM reported in draft horses include progressive weakness and muscle loss resulting in difficulty rising.[28]
- Pronounced weakness is more prevalent in draft horses homozygous for the GYS1 mutation.[25]
- Although the condition 'Shivers' was previously attributed to PSSM, studies have found no causal association between these 2 conditions; simply that they are both highly prevalent in specific draft breeds.[24]

Clinical signs associated with concurrent malignant hyperthermia mutation

- A small proportion of Quarter Horses and Paint Horses have both the GYS1 mutation and the ryanodine receptor (RYR1) mutation associated with malignant hyperthermia (MH).[29]
- This combination occurs most often in halter and pleasure horses and results in particularly severe signs of ER, including excessively high body temperatures and sudden death, and limited response to management changes intended to prevent episodes.

Factors Precipitating Episodes of Exertional Rhabdomyolysis

- No significant temperament, body type, or sex predilection for PSSM1 are recognized.[20]
- The variability in clinical presentation is likely because of the influence of diet, exercise, environmental factors, and other genes on the expression of the disease.[29]
- Aerobic exercise lasting below 20 min is the most common trigger for clinical signs particularly if the horse has been rested for several days before exercise or is unfit.[20]
- ER is more common if diets are high in nonstructural carbohydrate (NSC) and reluctance to exercise occurs if horses do not have sufficient dietary fat.[30]
- About 40% of owners feel there is a Spring or wet Summer associated pattern to the development of clinical signs, which some have attributed to quality of grass available at the time.[20,31]
- Quarter and Paint Horse foals and weanlings may develop rhabdomyolysis in conjunction with a systemic illness.

Diagnosis

1. Serum muscle enzymes:
   ○ Persistent elevations in serum CK and AST activities even at rest are common in symptomatic horses with PSSM1 (see **Fig. 3B**).
   ○ If serum muscle enzymes are normal at rest, an exercise test consisting of a maximum of 15 minutes lunging at a walk and trot can be performed to determine if subclinical ER is present. An elevation of CK activity, from baseline, of more than 2 to 3 fold, 4 hours after exercise is considered abnormal.[3]
2. The gold standard for diagnosis of PSSM1 is genetic testing for the *GYS1* mutation performed on hair root samples.[6]
3. A muscle biopsy is no longer required to diagnose PSSM1. The distinctive features of PSSM1 in muscle biopsy samples are numerous subsarcolemmal vacuoles and dense, crystalline PAS-positive, amylase-resistant inclusions in fast twitch fibers (see **Fig. 2A–C**).[1] Muscle biopsy abnormalities may not be present if biopsy samples are small or if horses are less than 2 years old.

Clinical judgment must be used when interpreting a positive genetic test from breeds such as draft horses of continental European origin because the very high prevalence of PSSM1 means that there is a high chance that any clinical sign they exhibit could be falsely associated with the *GYS1* mutation.[15]

TYPE 2 POLYSACCHARIDE STORAGE MYOPATHY

In the original study that identified the PSSM1 genetic mutation, 28% of the 99 Quarter Horses diagnosed with PSSM by amylase-resistant polysaccharide in muscle biopsy lacked the R309H *GYS1* genetic mutation.[6] Further, a high proportion of Warmblood horses diagnosed with PSSM by muscle biopsy lacked the PSSM1 mutation.[32] The term PSSM2 was coined to encompass this group of horses that had some form of increased glycogen or anormal polysaccharide in skeletal muscle.[7] In essence, a diagnosis of PSSM2 was based on a histopathologic description of muscle glycogen in horses with signs of muscle pain.

With further research using a breed-specific approach, PSSM2 terminology has evolved to comprise (see **Fig. 1**):

1. Horses with ER and a true glycogen storage disease—now termed PSSM2-ER.[33]
2. Arabian endurance horses with ER and distinctive desmin aggregates in skeletal muscle—termed MFM-ER.[10]
3. Warmblood horses presenting with exercise intolerance, normal serum CK and desmin aggregates in skeletal muscle—termed MFM-WB.[34]

It is imperative to ascertain whether horses potentially afflicted with PSSM2 demonstrate an abnormal increase in serum CK activity because management for PSSM2-ER, MFM-ER, and MFM-WB differ substantially. See the article "Myofibrillar Myopathy" by Williams and Valberg in this issue for details on the pathophysiology and management of MFM disorders.[12]

Type-2 Polysaccharide Storage Myopathy with Exertional Rhabdomyolysis

Key Points

- Research into PSSM2-ER has focused on Quarter Horses, but this form of ER likely occurs in other breeds.
- In Quarter Horses, PSSM2-ER occurs in barrel racing, working cow, and reining performance horses.[9]

- PSSM2-ER in Quarter Horses is a glycogen storage disease that responds well to the same dietary and exercise recommendations made for PSSM1.[9]

Pathophysiology

Quarter Horses with PSSM2-ER have muscle glycogen concentrations 60% higher than normal, establishing this as a glycogen storage disorder (see **Fig. 3**A).[9] The amount of abnormal polysaccharide and glycogen in skeletal muscle is less than in horses with PSSM1, and the electron microscopic appearance of abnormal polysaccharide is different from PSSM1.[9] PSSM2-ER has been diagnosed in other breeds based on increased amylase-sensitive glycogen in muscle biopsies, but further research into actual concentrations of muscle glycogen in these breeds has not been performed (Valberg personal observation). Horses with recurrent exertional rhabdomyolysis (RER) can also have dark PAS stains and subsarcolemmal glycogen accumulation related to an increase in skeletal muscle glycogen concentrations associated with training.[5,7,8,35] Thus, there can be some overlap in muscle histology between the 2 diseases; however, the presence of abnormal polysaccharide distinguishes PSSM2-ER from RER.

Clinical Signs

Clinical signs of PSSM2-ER in QHs are typical of ER; pain, sweating, firm hard muscles, stiffness, and reluctance to move developing after light exercise.[9] Some horses develop rhabdomyolysis on pasture. Other less common clinical signs include low-grade lameness, stiffness, and muscle fasciculations.

Diagnosis

A diagnosis of PSSM2-ER is based on documented elevations in serum CK and AST activities following exercise (see **Fig. 3**B) and on muscle biopsy evaluation, which shows a homogeneously dark glycogen stain, increased subsarcolemmal glycogen, and in many cases a small number of fibers with coarse granular PAS positive inclusions (see **Fig. 2**C–F).[9] Horses with PSSM2-ER lack aggregates of desmin, which are characteristic of MFM in immunohistochemical preparations.

Genetics

- A genetic basis for PSSM2-ER is suspected in Quarter Horses based on identification of familial relationships in affected horses.[9]
- A specific genetic mutation in genes demonstrated to cause muscle glycogenoses in other species has not been identified from analysis of whole genome sequences of PSSM2-ER horses.
- A commercial company (Equiseq.com, accessed July 2024) offers genetic testing for PSSM2 based on genetic variants (termed P2, P3, and P4) in genes that cause MFM or muscular dystrophies in humans. Scientifically reviewed studies have not found these commercial tests to be diagnostic for either PSSM2 or MFM in horses with a diagnosis established by muscle histopathology.[36–38] These genetic tests have been found to cause a false positive diagnosis of PSSM in 57% of healthy Quarter Horses with normal biopsies and a false negative diagnosis of PSSM2 in 40% of Quarter Horses that have histopathologic evidence of PSSM2.[36,37] Further, although these variants are found in genes linked to MFM in humans, none of the hundreds of Quarter Horses evaluated had evidence of MFM in immunohistochemical preparations targeting desmin aggregation in skeletal muscle.[39]
- Based on this research, the use of commercial variant tests for diagnosis of PSSM2 and MFM is not recommended.

TREATMENT AND MANAGEMENT OF PSSM
Treatment of Acute Exertional Rhabdomyolysis

- The aim of treatment of an acute episode of ER is to reduce anxiety and discomfort; correct fluid, electrolyte, and acid-base disturbances; and prevent renal compromise and additional muscle injury.
- Nephrotoxic drugs should be used judiciously.
- During an acute episode of ER minimize exercise of any kind and stall rest the patient.
- Treat dehydration, azotemia, and myoglobinuria by administering enteral and/or IV fluids, and address any electrolyte or metabolic disturbances.
- Acepromazine is anxiolytic and may benefit muscle blood flow (NB: caution in stallions and geldings because of possible link to paraphimosis).
- Other muscle relaxants that can be used include methocarbamol (15–20 mg/kg PO q24 h) or dantrolene sodium (2 mg/kg PO q8–12h, with food to ensure absorption).
- Analgesia choice (eg, Nonsteroidal Anti-Inflammatory Drug [NSAIDs], opiates, lidocaine continuous rate infusion [CRI]) depends on the severity of pain and degree of dehydration, renal compromise, and myoglobinuria.
- Possible complications of an acute ER event include renal insufficiency, recumbency, laminitis and muscle atrophy.

Management of Type 1 and Type 2 Polysaccharide Storage Myopathy Associated with Exertional Rhabdomyolysis

Key points

- PSSM horses will always have a tendency for muscle soreness and management of clinical disease should be the goal, as cure is not currently possible.
- Both PSSM1 and PSSM2-ER horses can respond well to a low NSC, high fat diet combined with regular exercise.

Diet

A low NSC, high fat diet is the standard for PSSM diets, which aims to decrease uptake of glucose into skeletal muscle cells, making less substrate available and reducing stimulation of glycogen synthesis, and to provide another source of metabolizable energy in the form of fat and protein.[30,40] A diet of hay with 12% or less NSC and a ration balancer low in NSC (<15%) with added plant-based oil (250–400 mL) is recommended in amounts that do not promote excessive weight gain.[30,41] Owners report that this type of diet improves clinical signs of muscle pain, stiffness, and exercise tolerance.[9,20] There is a great deal of variation in individual tolerance to dietary starch and horses with more severe clinical signs of PSSM appear to require the greatest restriction of starch intake. See the article "The role of nutrition in muscle disorders" by Pagan in this issue for specific details of dietary management of equine muscle disorders.[42]

Supplements

- There are no specific supplements that have been shown to benefit horses with PSSM.
- Chromium, which is reported to increase glucose absorption, may be contraindicated in PSSM horses because it can enhance insulin sensitivity.[43]
- Carnitine is a dietary supplement that may replenish muscle carnitine stores if depleted and assists transport of fat into the mitochondria. A deficiency of plasma carnitine has not been identified in PSSM1 horses (Valberg unpublished

data; plasma free carnitine in PSSM1 horses ranged from 10.24 – 27.11 μM, with a reference interval of 13.20–25.63 μM; however, plasma carnitine does not always reflect muscle carnitine concentrations).

Rest

- Duration of stall confinement should be less than 48 hours after an episode of acute rhabdomyolysis for most cases, and then turnout in paddocks of gradually increasing size provided. Over time, as much free exercise as possible on pasture is beneficial.
- A grazing muzzle may be needed if pasture is lush.[17]
- Excitable horses may require tranquilization initially before turn-out to avoid excessive activity.
- Hand-walking of horses should be limited to less than 5 minutes at a time because when initially recovering from an episode of PSSM more than 5 to 10 minutes may trigger another episode of rhabdomyolysis.

Exercise

Both a low-starch fat supplemented diet and a regular incremental exercise program are needed for optimal prevention of further episodes of ER.[20,30] Important principles to follow when starting exercise programs in horses with PSSM include

1. If the horse has experienced a moderate to marked episode of rhabdomyolysis recently, 2 weeks of turn-out and diet change are often beneficial before recommencing training exercise.
2. Duration of exercise, not the intensity, is of primary importance in reintroducing exercise.
3. Exercise should be gradually introduced and then consistently executed and consecutive days of rest avoided.
4. Advancing exercise volume too quickly can result in an episode of rhabdomyolysis and repeated frustration for the owner.
5. Minimize any days without some form of exercise and subsequent mild ER episodes should only result in a few days off exercise at the most.

Initial warm-up exercise should be very relaxed, and the horse should achieve a long, low-frame without collection. For many horses this is most readily done in a round pen or on a lunge-line but can be done under saddle if needed. A gradual increase in exercise might be achieved as follows.

- Apply a successive daily addition of 2-min intervals of walk and trot beginning with only 4-min of exercise and working up to 30-min after 3 weeks.
- If the horse had minor elevations in 4-h postexercise CK with the 15-min exercise test, the exercise program may commence with 15-min of exercise.
- After 3 weeks, workload can be increased by adding 2-min intervals of collection or canter to the initial relaxed warm-up period of walk and trot.

Reevaluating serum CK activity is not helpful for the first month in PSSM horses unless an episode of ER occurs. This is because it is very common to have subclinical elevations in CK activity when exercise is reintroduced and a return to normal values often requires 4 to 8 weeks of gradual exercise.

Medications

PSSM horses with ER that cannot be controlled by diet and exercise changes alone may benefit from the administration of 2 mg/kg of dantrolene orally 60 minutes before exercise (and given with food) as they are reintroduced to exercise for the first 2 weeks or before exercise that is likely to induce rhabdomyolysis. Withdrawal times should be followed before competitions.

Expectations of Polysaccharide Storage Myopathy Management Changes

With adherence to both the diet and exercise recommendations 70% to 75% of Quarter Horses show notable improvement of their clinical signs and many of them return to acceptable levels of performance.[17,20] Horses homozygous for the PSSM1 mutation and PSSM1 horses that concurrently have the mutation for MH, do not respond as well to diet and exercise recommendations and horses with MH can have a fatal episode of ER.[29]

CLINICS CARE POINTS

- PSSM is a glycogen storage disorder in horses, with two types currently described: PSSM1 and PSSM2: PSSM1 is caused by a mutation in the GYS1 gene, affecting breeds such as draft horses and Quarter Horses.

- PSSM2 includes subsets such as PSSM2-ER, related to glycogen storage, and other forms like myofibrillar myopathy (MFM).

- Clinical signs: PSSM1 can vary from asymptomatic to exertional rhabdomyolysis (ER), muscle soreness, and topline atrophy. Affected horses may show stiffness, pain, elevated serum CK, reluctance to move, and in some cases, myoglobinuria and weakness. Horses may present with chronic performance issues or reluctance to exercise with elevated CK.

- PSSM2-ER horses present similarly, with high serum CK, muscle stiffness and pain after light exercise.

- Diagnosis: PSSM1 is diagnosed through genetic testing for the GYS1 mutation.

- PSSM2-ER is diagnosed through muscle biopsies which show abnormal glycogen storage, but its genetic basis is unclear. Commercial genetic tests for PSSM2 do not accurately correspond with a muscle biopsy diagnosis and are not recommended at this time.

- Management: Both PSSM1 and PSSM2-ER respond well to a low nonstructural carbohydrate (NSC), high-fat diet and regular exercise.

- Acute ER episodes are managed by reducing muscle pain, correcting fluid/electrolyte imbalances, and preventing renal damage.

- Proper management can reduce clinical signs and improve quality of life for affected horses.

DISCLOSURES

A.M. Firshman has no conflicts to declare. S.J. Valberg directs the Valberg Neuromuscular Disease Laboratory (ValbergNMDL.com) and receives remuneration for analyzing muscle biopsies. Her website is sponsored by Kentucky Equine Research, and she receives royalties from the PSSM1 genetic test and the feed products "Releve" and "MFM pellet" developed in association with Kentucky Equine Research.

REFERENCES

1. Valberg SJ, Cardinet GH 3rd, Carlson GP, et al. Polysaccharide storage myopathy associated with recurrent exertional rhabdomyolysis in horses. Neuromuscul Disord 1992;2:351–9.

2. Firshman AM, Valberg SJ, Bender JB, et al. Comparison of histopathologic criteria and skeletal muscle fixation techniques for the diagnosis of polysaccharide storage myopathy in horses. Vet Pathol 2006;43:257–69.
3. Valberg SJ, Macleay JM, Billstrom JA, et al. Skeletal muscle metabolic response to exercise in horses with 'tying-up' due to polysaccharide storage myopathy. Equine Vet J 1999;31:43–7.
4. Valentine BA, Habecker PL, Patterson JS, et al. Incidence of polysaccharide storage myopathy in draft horse-related breeds: a necropsy study of 37 horses and a mule. J Vet Diagn Invest 2001;13:63–8.
5. Valentine BA, McDonough SP, Chang YF, et al. Polysaccharide storage myopathy in Morgan, Arabian, and Standardbred related horses and Welsh-cross ponies. Vet Pathol 2000;37:193–6.
6. McCue ME, Valberg SJ, Miller MB, et al. Glycogen synthase (GYS1) mutation causes a novel skeletal muscle glycogenosis. Genomics 2008;91:458–66.
7. McCue ME, Armien AG, Lucio M, et al. Comparative skeletal muscle histopathologic and ultrastructural features in two forms of polysaccharide storage myopathy in horses. Vet Pathol 2009;46:1281–91.
8. Stanley RL, McCue ME, Valberg SJ, et al. A glycogen synthase 1 mutation associated with equine polysaccharide storage myopathy and exertional rhabdomyolysis occurs in a variety of UK breeds. Equine Vet J 2009;41:597–601.
9. Valberg SJ, Williams ZJ, Finno CJ, et al. Type 2 polysaccharide storage myopathy in Quarter Horses is a novel glycogen storage disease causing exertional rhabdomyolysis. Equine Vet J 2023;55:618–31.
10. Valberg S, McKenzie E, Eyrich L, et al. Suspected myofibrillar myopathy in Arabian horses with a history of exertional rhabdomyolysis. Equine Vet J 2016; 48:548–56.
11. Valberg SJ. Diagnosis and management of myofibrillar myopathy in warmblood performance horses. Proceedings of American Association of Equine Practitioners 2021;67:214–8.
12. Williams ZJ, Valberg SJ. Myofibrillar myopathy. In: McKenzie EC, Valberg SJ, editors. Muscle Disorders of horses: an issue of Veterinary Clinics of North America: Equine Practice. 2025. p. 139–50.
13. Maile C, Hingst JR, Mahalingan K, et al. A highly prevalent equine glycogen storage disease is explained by constitutive activation of a mutant glycogen synthase. Biochim Biophys Acta Gen Subj 2017;1861:3388–98.
14. De La Corte FD, Valberg SJ, MacLeay JM, et al. Developmental onset of polysaccharide storage myopathy in 4 Quarter Horse foals. J Vet Intern Med 2002;16: 581–7.
15. Baird JD, Valberg SJ, Anderson SM, et al. Presence of the glycogen synthase 1 (GYS1) mutation causing type 1 polysaccharide storage myopathy in continental European draught horse breeds. Vet Rec 2010;167:781–4.
16. McCue ME, Anderson SM, Valberg SJ, et al. Estimated prevalence of the type 1 polysaccharide storage myopathy mutation in selected North American and European breeds. Anim Genet 2010;41(Suppl 2):145–9.
17. Patterson-Kane J, Slater J, McGowan C. Equine polysaccharide storage myopathy. Vet Rec 2005;156:456.
18. McCue ME, Ribeiro WP, Valberg SJ. Prevalence of polysaccharide storage myopathy in horses with neuromuscular disorders. Equine Vet J Suppl 2006;36:340–4.
19. Tryon RC, Penedo MC, McCue ME, et al. Evaluation of allele frequencies of inherited disease genes in subgroups of American Quarter Horses. J Am Vet Med Assoc 2009;234:120–5.

20. Firshman AM, Valberg SJ, Bender JB, et al. Epidemiologic characteristics and management of polysaccharide storage myopathy in Quarter Horses. Am J Vet Res 2003;64:1319–27.

21. Naylor R, Luis-Fuentes V, Livesey L, et al. Evaluation of cardiac phenotype in horses with type 1 polysaccharide storage myopathy. J Vet Intern Med 2012; 26:1464–9.

22. McGowan CM, McGowan T, Patterson-Kane J. Prevalence of equine polysaccharide storage myopathy and other myopathies in two equine populations in the United Kingdom. Vet J 2009;180:330–6.

23. Quiroz-Rothe E, Novales M, Aguilera-Tejero E, et al. Polysaccharide storage myopathy in the M. longissimus lumborum of showjumpers and dressage horses with back pain. Equine Vet J 2002;34:171–6.

24. Firshman AM, Baird JD, Valberg SJ. Prevalences and clinical signs of polysaccharide storage myopathy and shivers in Belgian draft horses. J Am Vet Med Assoc 2005;227:1958–64.

25. Naylor RJ, Livesey L, Schumacher J, et al. Allele copy number and underlying pathology are associated with subclinical severity in equine type 1 polysaccharide storage myopathy (PSSM1). PLoS One 2012;7(7):e42317.

26. Bloom B, Valentine B, Gleed R, et al. Postanaesthetic recumbency in a Belgian filly with polysaccharide storage myopathy. Vet Rec 1999;144:73.

27. Herszberg B, McCue ME, Larcher T, et al. A GYS1 gene mutation is highly associated with polysaccharide storage myopathy in Cob Normand draught horses. Anim Genet 2009;40:94–6.

28. Valentine B, Credille K, Lavoie JP, et al. Severe polysaccharide storage myopathy in Belgian and Percheron draught horses. Equine Vet J 1997;29:220–5.

29. McCue ME, Valberg SJ, Jackson M, et al. Polysaccharide storage myopathy phenotype in quarter horse-related breeds is modified by the presence of an RYR1 mutation. Neuromuscul Disord 2009;19:37–43.

30. Ribeiro W, Valberg SJ, Pagan J, et al. The effect of varying dietary starch and fat content on serum creatine kinase activity and substrate availability in equine polysaccharide storage myopathy. J Vet Intern Med 2004;18:887–94.

31. Johlig L, Valberg S, Mickelson JR, et al. Epidemiological and genetic study of exertional rhabdomyolysis in a Warmblood horse family in Switzerland. Equine Vet J 2011;43:240–5.

32. Lewis SS, Nicholson AM, Williams ZJ, et al. Clinical characteristics and muscle glycogen concentrations in warmblood horses with polysaccharide storage myopathy. Am J Vet Res 2017;78:1305–12.

33. Valberg SJ, Williams ZJ, Finno CJ, et al. Type 2 polysaccharide storage myopathy in Quarter Horses is a novel glycogen storage disease causing exertional rhabdomyolysis. Equine Vet J 2022;55(4):618–31.

34. Valberg S, Nicholson A, Lewis S, et al. Clinical and histopathological features of myofibrillar myopathy in Warmblood horses. Equine Vet J 2017;49:739–45.

35. Valentine BA, Cooper BJ. Development of polyglucosan inclusions in skeletal muscle. Neuromuscul Disord 2006;16:603–7.

36. Valberg SJ, Finno CJ, Henry ML, et al. Commercial genetic testing for type 2 polysaccharide storage myopathy and myofibrillar myopathy does not correspond to a histopathological diagnosis. Equine Vet J 2021;53:690–700.

37. Valberg SJ, Henry ML, Herrick KL, et al. Absence of myofibrillar myopathy in Quarter Horses with a histopathological diagnosis of type 2 polysaccharide storage myopathy and lack of association with commercial genetic tests. Equine Vet J 2023;55:230–8.

38. Williams ZJ, Velez-Irizarry D, Petersen JL, et al. Candidate gene expression and coding sequence variants in Warmblood horses with myofibrillar myopathy. Equine Vet J 2021;53:306–15.

39. Valberg SJ, Henry ML, Herrick KL, et al. Absence of myofibrillar myopathy in Quarter Horses with a histopathological diagnosis of type 2 polysaccharide storage myopathy and lack of association with commercial genetic tests. Equine Vet J 2023;55:230–8.

40. Valentine BA, Van Saun RJ, Thompson KN, et al. Role of dietary carbohydrate and fat in horses with equine polysaccharide storage myopathy. J Am Vet Med Assoc 2001;219:1537–44.

41. Borgia L, Valberg S, McCue M, et al. Glycaemic and insulinaemic responses to feeding hay with different non-structural carbohydrate content in control and polysaccharide storage myopathy-affected horses. J Anim Physiol Anim Nutr 2011;95:798–807.

42. Pagan JD, Valberg SJ. The role of nutrition in muscular disorders. In: McKenzie EC, Valberg SJ, editors. Muscle Disorders of horses an issue of Veterinary Clinics of North America: Equine Practice. 2025. p. 151–63.

43. Hua Y, Clark S, Ren J, et al. Molecular mechanisms of chromium in alleviating insulin resistance. J Nutr Biochem 2012;23:313–9.

Myofibrillar Myopathy

Stephanie J. Valberg, DVM, PhD[a], Zoë J. Williams, DVM, PhD[b],*

KEYWORDS

- Skeletal muscle • Myopathy • Myofibrillar • Polysaccharide storage • Equine
- Desmin

KEY POINTS

- Myofibrillar myopathy (MFM), previously grouped under type 2 polysaccharide myopathy, is now recognized as a stand-alone myopathy that is not a glycogen storage disease.
- MFM is diagnosed by the presence of desmin aggregates in muscle biopsy.
- Both Arabian endurance horses and Warmbloods have been diagnosed with MFM but have different clinical presentations.
- MFM is managed with antioxidant and amino acid supplementation and altered exercise regimes.

INTRODUCTION
Skeletal Muscle in Brief

The strategic orientation of muscle fibers allows muscles to generate immense power and motion while maintaining structural integrity. Each myofiber contains parallel alignments of myofibrils composed of myofilaments. These myofilaments (primarily actin and myosin) are organized into contractile units called sarcomeres. The M-line, located at the center of the sarcomere, serves to anchor myosin filaments. Actin is anchored by Z-discs at the end of each sarcomere (**Fig. 1**). The intermediate filament desmin threads through the Z-disc and aligns parallel myofibrils giving skeletal muscle its striated appearance. Desmin also anchors myofibrils to the cell membrane and the positioning of organelles, such as mitochondria. The Z-disc acts as a mechanosensor and mechanotransducer, upregulating gene transcription in response to training and creating exercise adaptations.

Skeletal muscle has 3 contractile fiber types based on the myosin heavy chain. Type 1 fibers, in high proportion in postural muscles, have slower contractile speeds and are highly reliant on oxidative metabolism in mitochondria. Type 2 fibers are fast-twitch fibers that make up a large proportion of locomotor muscles and are composed of 2

[a] Michigan State University, Large Animal Clinical Sciences, College of Veterinary Medicine, East Lansing, MI, USA; [b] Department of Clinical Sciences, College of Veterinary Medicine and Biomedical Sciences, Colorado State University, Fort Collins, CO, USA
* Corresponding author. Colorado State University, 200 West Lake Street, 1621 Campus Delivery, Fort Collins, CO 80523-1621.
E-mail address: Zoe.Williams@colostate.edu

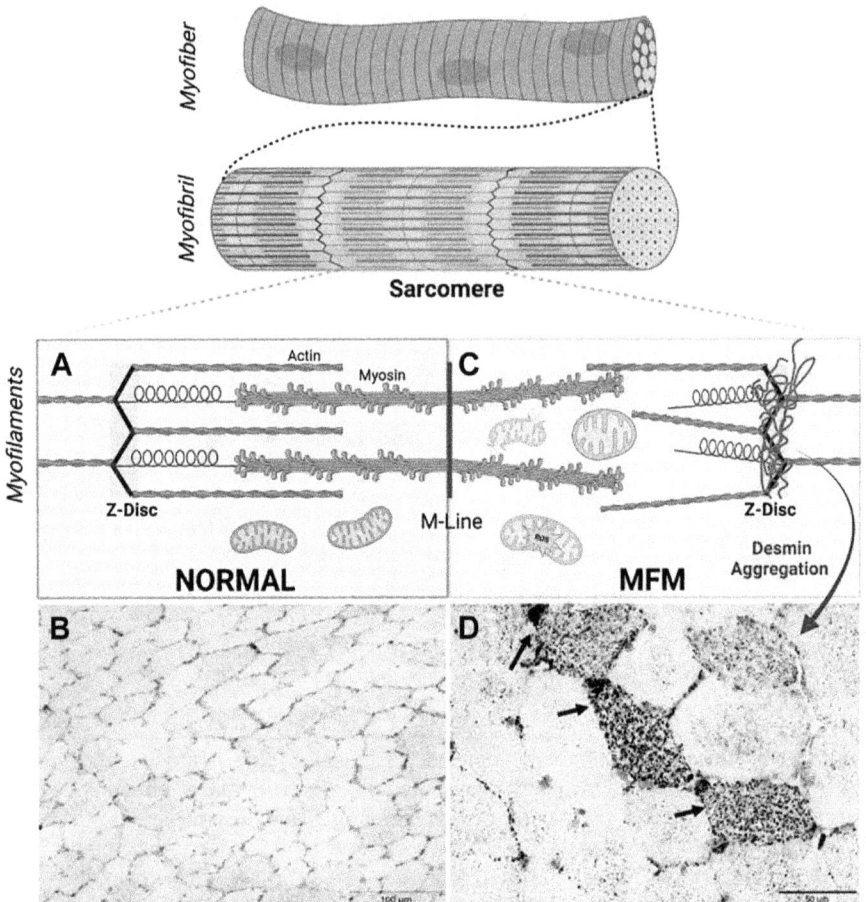

Fig. 1. Myofibers are composed of myofibrils, which contain contractile units called sarcomeres. Each sarcomere is composed of myofilaments that are bordered by Z-discs and centered around the M-line. (*A*) Normal organized myofilaments in a portion of the sarcomere. (*B*) An immunohistochemical stain for desmin in a cross section of gluteal muscle from a healthy horse (20X). (*C*) Depiction of a segment of a sarcomere showing myofibrillar disarray and desmin aggregation. (*D*) An immunohistochemical stain for desmin in a cross section of gluteal muscle from an MFM horse showing 4 muscle fibers (*arrows*) with desmin aggregates (40X). (*Created in* BioRender. Williams, Z. (2025) https://BioRender.com/f39q105.)

subtypes. Type 2A fibers have high oxidative and anaerobic capacity and type 2X fibers have low oxidative and high anaerobic capacity especially in untrained horses.

Disease History

The R309H *GYS1* genetic mutation causes type 1 polysaccharide storage myopathy (PSSM1); however, there are horses that have abnormal polysaccharide evident histologically that do *not* have the R309H *GYS1* genetic mutation.[1] Horses with this phenotype lacking the *GYS1* mutation were initially diagnosed with *type 2* polysaccharide storage myopathy (PSSM2) based on the presence of either abnormal *amylase-resistant glycogen* or *small aggregates of amylase-sensitive glycogen*.[1] A subset of Quarter Horses with exertional rhabdomyolysis and PSSM2 (PSSM2-ER) have been found to have a glycogen storage disease.[2] Further research found that, unlike Quarter Horses, Arabian horses, and Warmblood horses diagnosed with PSSM2 by histology did not have high concentrations of glycogen in their muscle—indicating that Arabians and Warmbloods have another disorder that is not a glycogen storage disease (**Fig. 2**).

Myofibrillar Myopathy

Ultrastructural studies and immunohistochemical stains of skeletal muscle from these Arabian and Warmblood horses identified regions of muscle fibers with myofibrillar disarray and ectopic accumulation of the cytoskeletal protein desmin.[3,4] This discovery led to the renaming of PSSM2 in Arabians and Warmbloods to myofibrillar myopathy (MFM) and the use of immunohistochemical staining for desmin to diagnose MFM (**Figs. 3A–F and 4**). The previous diagnosis of PSSM2 in Arabians with MFM likely arose because small pools of glycogen form between disrupted myofibrils seen on electron microscopy (see **Fig. 4**) which likely gave the false appearance of cytoplasmic aggregates of glycogen in light microscopy.[3]

Arabians and Warmbloods with MFM have distinctive clinical presentations and molecular signatures that share overlapping features of altered mitochondrial complex I and a propensity for low cysteine-based antioxidants.[5] Arabians present with high

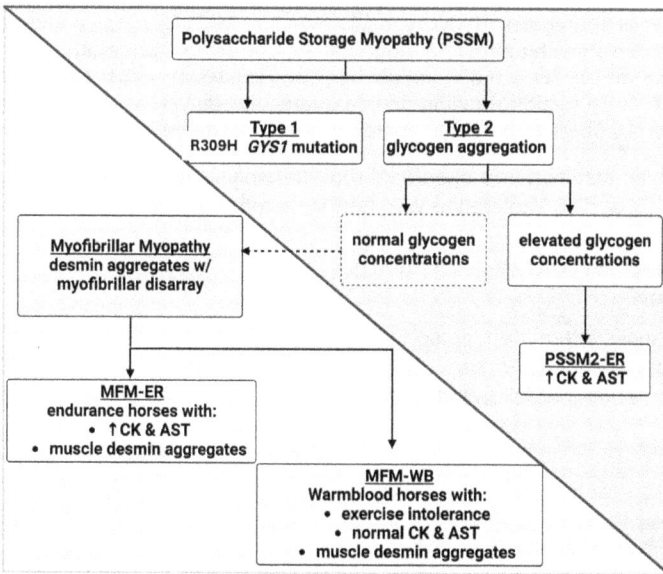

Fig. 2. Polysaccharide storage myopathy can be divided into type 1 (PSSM1) and type 2 (PSSM2) based on the presence of *increased* amylase-sensitive or resistant polysaccharide in skeletal muscle biopsies and result of genetic testing for the glycogen synthase 1 mutation (*GYS1*). Further research has shown that there are 3 forms of what was previously called PSSM2, -based on measurement of serum creatine kinase (CK) activity in conjunction with an episode of muscle stiffness, assessment of glycogen concentrations and immunostaining for desmin in muscle biopsies. PSSM2-ER horses have episodes of exertional rhabdomyolysis (ER), excessive glycogen concentrations and normal staining for desmin in skeletal muscle. MFM-ER horses are often Arabian endurance horses that develop ER and have aggregates of the cytoskeletal protein desmin in skeletal muscle. MFM-WB is often Warmblood horses with exercise intolerance, normal serum CK activity, and aggregates of desmin in muscle biopsies. (*Created in* BioRender. Williams, Z. (2025) https://BioRender.com/o43t769.)

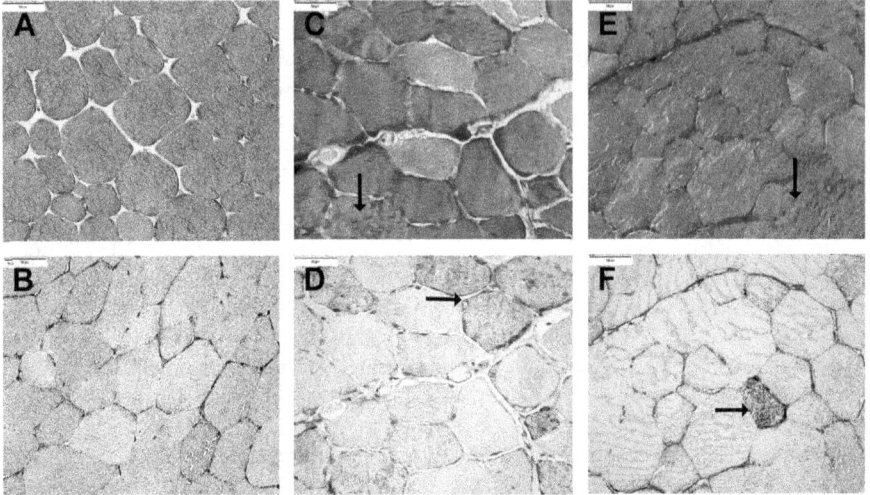

Fig. 3. Periodic acid Schiff's (*top row*) and desmin immunohistochemical (*bottom row*) stains of formalin-fixed cross sections of semimembranosus muscle 40X. (*A*) Normal, even glycogen staining in a healthy horse. (*B*) Normal, even desmin staining in a healthy horse. (*C*) Fibers containing small aggregates of glycogen (*arrow*) in an MFM-ER Arabian endurance horse. (*D*) Serial section showing abnormal aggregates of desmin in numerous fibers (*arrow*) in the MFM-ER Arabian. (*E*) A few small glycogen aggregates in a fiber (*arrow*) in an MFM-WB horse. (*F*) Serial section showing desmin aggregates (*arrow*) in a fiber in an MFM-WB horse. Numerous fibers with desmin aggregates were scattered throughout the sample.

serum muscle enzymes and exertional rhabdomyolysis (MFM-ER) and Warmbloods present with exercise intolerance with normal serum muscle enzymes (MFM-WB).

MYOFIBRILLAR MYOPATHY IN ARABIANS
Clinical Signs

MFM-ER causes intermittent episodes of ER often in older Arabian endurance horses at the end of prolonged endurance rides.[3] Clinical signs are also apparent about 10 km (5 miles) into a ride that follows fit horses being given 2 weeks off work. Horses exhibit

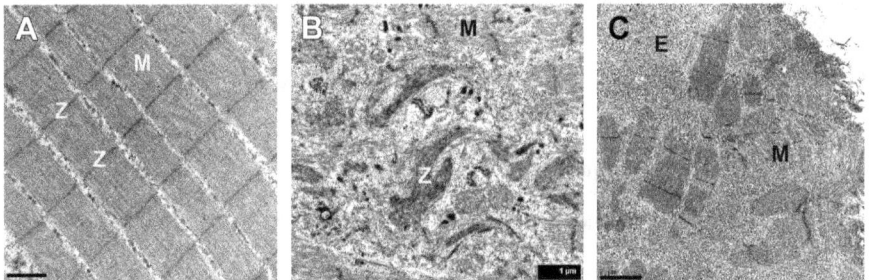

Fig. 4. Electron microscopy of a portion of a muscle fiber. (*A*) Normal organization of myofibrils containing sarcomeres with electron dense Z-discs (Z) and M-lines (M) in a segment of one muscle fiber. (*B*) Severe myofibrillar disruption (M) and ectopic accumulation of electron dense Z-disc material (Z) likely correlating with the desmin aggregation seen on light microscopy. (*C*) Myofibrillar disruption (M) and pooling of granulofilamentous material (E) between the disrupted myofibrils that likely contains desmin, Z-disc material and beta glycogen particles.

muscle stiffness and pain that is not as pronounced as that seen with other causes of ER. Serum CK activity can be markedly elevated from 10,000 to greater than 300,000 U/L, and myoglobinuria may be evident.[3,6] If horses have gone for many years without treatment, clinical signs may become more frequent and evident with lesser amounts of exertion.

Diagnosis

A diagnosis of MFM-ER is established by correlating clinical signs, serum CK activity (after an endurance ride), and histopathology in a muscle biopsy. Immunohistochemical staining of gluteal or semimembranosus muscle for the ectopic accumulation of the cytoskeletal protein desmin is essential (see **Fig. 3**C, D).[3,4] Gluteal or semimembranosus muscle biopsies in some MFM-ER horses can also show internalized myonuclei in mature myofibers and occasionally amylase-resistant polysaccharide in a few fibers.[3]

Pathophysiology

The heart rate and metabolic response to exercise in MFM-ER horses is normal and muscle glycogen concentrations are similar to controls.[6] Transcriptomic and proteomic analyses of skeletal muscle from MFM Arabians highlighted alterations in cysteine synthesis from methionine in postexercise samples, altered expression of complex I subunits in the first step of the mitochondrial respiratory chain, and identified markedly lower content of the cysteine-based antioxidant peroxiredoxin 6.[5] Arabian endurance horses have an innately heightened ability to oxidize fatty acids which produce reactive oxygen species (ROS) during aerobic exercise via complex I.[7] A lack of cysteine-based antioxidants in MFM-ER, combined with a highly aerobic metabolic phenotype is hypothesized to promote oxidative stress, oxidation, and aggregation of structural proteins like desmin and potentially oxidation of the ryanodine receptor (calcium release channel) resulting in ER (**Fig. 5**).[5,8]

Genetic Testing

A familial basis for Arabian MFM is not apparent from pedigree evaluation (Dr S.J. Valberg, personal observation). Rather there seems to be a strong environmental influence for developing MFM in endurance horses. Genetic testing for MFM and PSSM2 is offered by a commercial company; however, research evaluating their P2, P3, and P4 variants found that by chance alone 25% of Arabians will have at least one P variant regardless of whether they have MFM diagnosed by muscle biopsy or are healthy horses with no desmin aggregation.[9] Further, these genetic tests would give a false negative diagnosis in 50% of MFM-ER horses. For these reasons, the commercial genetic tests are not recommended, and muscle biopsy remains the gold standard diagnostic.

Treatment

Treatment of acute rhabdomyolysis is discussed in the article by Valberg on Sporadic and Recurrent Exertional Rhabdomyolysis in this issue.[10]

Management

Diet. Because MFM-ER is not a glycogen storage disease, there is no scientific support for a low nonstructural carbohydrate (NSC) diet. Dietary management is thoroughly described in the article The Role of Nutrition in Managing Muscle Disorders in this issue authored by Pagan and follows the principles of moderate levels of NSC (20%–30% of the concentrate) and fat (6%–8% of the concentrate) and higher levels of protein (12% crude protein) than often fed to endurance horses.[11,12]

Synopsis of altered gene and protein expression in MFM-Arabians

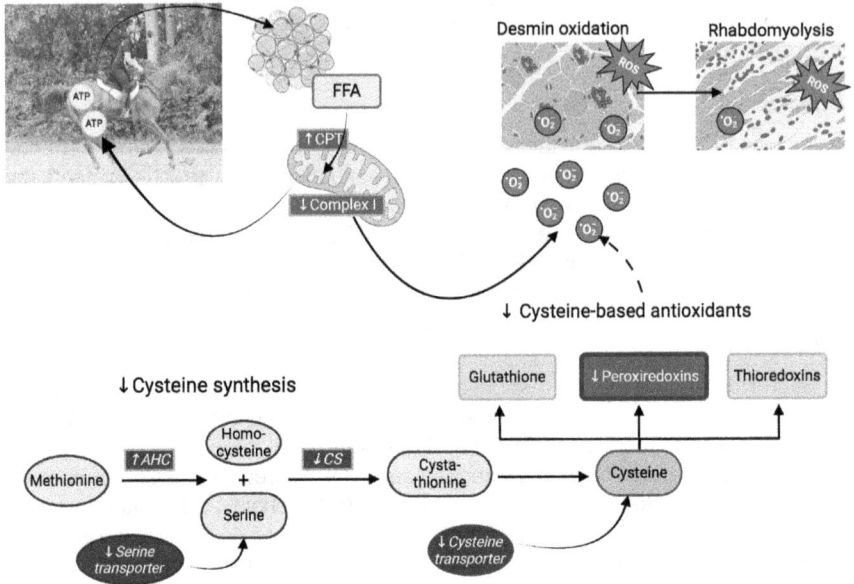

Fig. 5. Proposed pathophysiology of MFM-ER based on transcriptomic and proteomic analysis of gluteal muscle before and after exercise. MFM-ER horses have significantly higher carnitine palmitoyl transferase content which transports fat into mitochondria and lower expression of subunits of mitochondrial complex I, which is a site of ROS production. Oxidation of fat during prolonged endurance rides generates increased ROS. A 4 $\log_2$ fold lower content of cysteine-dependent peroxiredoxin 6 in MFM-ER versus control muscle at rest and altered expression of genes encoding enzymes required to import cysteine or synthesize cysteine from methionine following exercise indicated that the oxidoreductase pathway plays a central role in the pathogenesis of MFM-ER. Protein misfolding, myofibrillar disarray, and aggregation of desmin in MFM-ER endurance horses could arise from protein oxidation due to excessive generation of ROS (O2-) decreased postexercise cysteine synthesis, and depletion of cysteine-dependent antioxidants. Rhabdomyolysis could be a consequence of oxidation of the calcium release channel (RYR1).

Supplements. The most absorbable form of cysteine is N-acetylcysteine, and N-acetylcysteine has been shown in a vertebrate MFM disease model to diminish desmin aggregation.[13] Supplementation of healthy fit thoroughbreds with oral N-acetylcysteine was shown to increase gluteal muscle glutathione (a ubiquitous cysteine-based antioxidant), and therefore, it is being used as an antioxidant to manage MFM horses.[14] A commercial supplement containing N-acetylcysteine and other amino acids (MFM pellet)[a] has been developed for MFM horses, and when fed in amounts that provide 10 g of N-acetylcysteine per day has decreased clinical signs of rhabdomyolysis in endurance horses (Valberg, personal observation).

Coenzyme Q_{10} (CoQ$_{10}$) is another potent antioxidant that may also benefit endurance horses as proteomic analysis shows supplementation with CoQ$_{10}$ enhances flux through complex II rather than complex I, the complex generating the most

---

[a] Kentucky Equine Research, 3910 Delaney Ferry Road, Versailles, KY 40383.

ROS.[15] Whole blood selenium and serum vitamin E should also be tested, and supplementation provided if deficiencies exist.

Rest/Exercise. Regular daily exercise is important in MFM-ER horses as time off tends to increase the risk for ER. At endurance races, housing horses in as large an enclosure as possible is recommended as well as periodic hand walking. After endurance rides, rather than complete time off, some exercise, which can be as little as 5 to 10 minutes of trotting daily, is recommended. Further recommendations on getting horses back to work after an episode of rhabdomyolysis are provided in the article, "Sporadic and Recurrent Exertional Rhabdomyolysis" by Valberg in this issue.[10]

MYOFIBRILLAR MYOPATHY IN WARMBLOODS

Desmin aggregates have also been identified in skeletal muscle of Warmblood horse (see **Fig. 3**E, F). However, the underlying etiology for MFM-WB appears to be more complex than for MFM-ER. Clinical aspects of MFM-WB differ significantly from those of Arabian endurance horses. Warmbloods with MFM:

1. Rarely develop elevations in serum CK or ER.
2. Develop persistent exercise intolerance after very little exercise.
3. Can have a mild shifting hindlimb lameness.
4. Develop mild to moderate muscle atrophy.

Clinical Signs

Horses with MFM-WB often are successful and promising as young horses. At 6 to 8 years of age, clinical signs of an insidious onset of exercise intolerance develop characterized by a lack of stamina, unwillingness to go forward, inability to collect, abnormal canter transitions, and often an inability to sustain a normal canter.[4] Atrophy can be present and is usually mild to moderate affecting the topline and hind quarters. Horses may show signs of stiffness, and moderate muscle pain upon palpation. Although owners often complain that their horses are tying up, serum CK activity is almost always within the normal range. A mild shifting hindlimb lameness that remains unresolved after a thorough orthopedic assessment is also common. Interestingly, the prevalence of gastric ulceration is also higher in this population of Warmblood horses.[16]

Diagnosis

Because the clinical signs exhibited with MFM-WB are typical of exertional pain, other overlapping disorders that cause pain or exercise intolerance should first be eliminated before pursuing muscle biopsy. This includes saddle fit, training issues, equine asthma, gastric ulcers, and orthopedic causes of pain upon exertion (**Fig. 6**). Equine neuroaxonal dystrophy (eNAD) can cause mild ataxia and behavioral changes under saddle which should be ruled out as a potential differential diagnosis through a neurologic evaluation.[17,18] Muscle biopsies of horses greater than or equal to 8 years of age are required to establish a diagnosis of MFM-WB. Gluteal or semimembranosus biopsies from MFM-WB horses contain scattered myofibers with aggregates of desmin (see **Fig. 3**E, F). Because desmin aggregates appear to be a later-stage indicator of MFM they may not be apparent in younger horses with MFM-WB. In horses less than 8 years of age, a diagnosis of MFM-WB may require a treatment trial with the regimen described later to establish a diagnosis. A clinical response is expected within 4 weeks of starting the regimen. If a response is not seen at this time another diagnosis for exercise intolerance should be pursued.

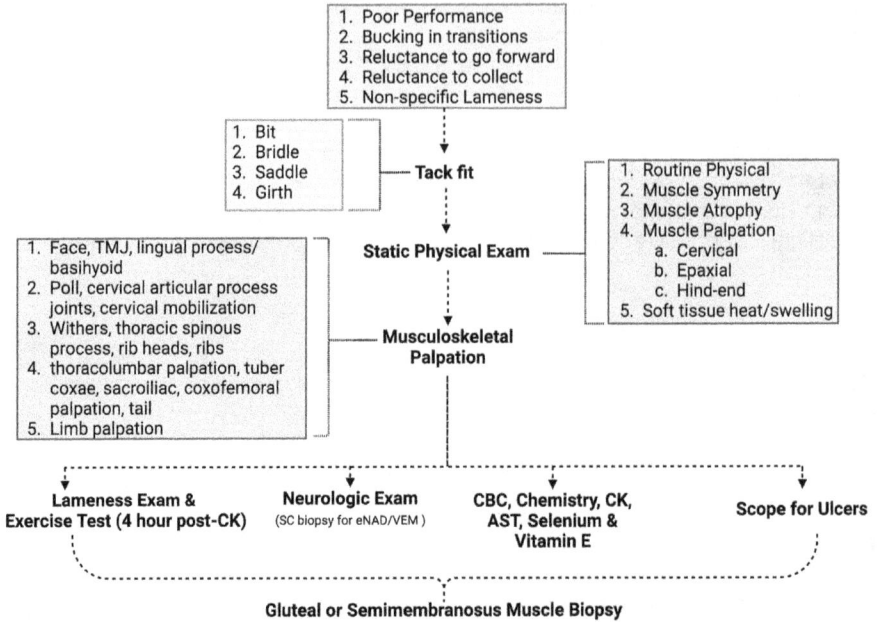

1. Poor Performance
2. Bucking in transitions
3. Reluctance to go forward
4. Reluctance to collect
5. Non-specific Lameness

1. Bit
2. Bridle
3. Saddle
4. Girth

Tack fit

1. Routine Physical
2. Muscle Symmetry
3. Muscle Atrophy
4. Muscle Palpation
   a. Cervical
   b. Epaxial
   c. Hind-end
5. Soft tissue heat/swelling

Static Physical Exam

1. Face, TMJ, lingual process/ basihyoid
2. Poll, cervical articular process joints, cervical mobilization
3. Withers, thoracic spinous process, rib heads, ribs
4. thoracolumbar palpation, tuber coxae, sacroiliac, coxofemoral palpation, tail
5. Limb palpation

Musculoskeletal Palpation

Lameness Exam & Exercise Test (4 hour post-CK)

Neurologic Exam (SC biopsy for eNAD/VEM)

CBC, Chemistry, CK, AST, Selenium & Vitamin E

Scope for Ulcers

Gluteal or Semimembranosus Muscle Biopsy

Fig. 6. A diagnostic workflow for MFM in Warmbloods. Due to their nonspecific signs, a thorough examination is warranted. This is composed of checking tack, a full physical examination with muscle and soft tissue palpation, neurologic examination, and an ortho-pedic examination. If no significant findings are noted, then a dynamic ridden evaluation may be warranted. To rule out rhabdomyolysis, a 4-hour postexercise serum CK sample should be assessed. If eNAD or Vitamin E-responsive myopathy is suspected, a *sacrocaudalis dorsalis* muscle biopsy is recommended. Additionally, routine laboratory work including CK, AST, Vitamin E, and selenium is recommended. Lastly, due to the over-representation of gastric ulcers in Warmbloods with MFM, gastroscopy is also recommended. If no significant findings are identified in these examinations, then a *gluteus medius* or *semimembranosus* muscle biopsy is recommended to diagnose MFM. (*Created in* BioRender. Williams, Z. (2025) https://BioRender.com/x66v595.)

Genetic Testing

Genetic variants in genes that cause MFM in humans have been investigated in MFM Warmbloods and were not found to be associated with MFM-WB.[19] A commercial company offers genetic tests for MFM. Evaluation of the P2, P3, and P4 variants offered as diagnostic tests for MFM found that by chance alone 29% of Warmbloods will have at least one P variant regardless of whether they have MFM diagnosed by muscle biopsy or lack MFM based on the absence of desmin aggregates.[9] P2, P3, and P4 genetic tests would give a false negative diagnosis in 49% of MFM-WB. Based on this research, these tests appear to be for variants common in the genome of hors-es that are unassociated with muscle disease. For these reasons, the authors do not recommend these genetic tests.

Pathophysiology

With MFM-WB, fast twitch oxidative type 2A muscle fibers contain scattered areas of myofibrillar disarray, Z-disc streaming, disruption of the Z-discs, and ectopic accumulation of Z-disc proteins such as desmin.[4] Z-discs contain hundreds of proteins, and some of these are specifically involved in mechanosignaling and mechanotransduction.[20] During mechanosignaling tension created during muscle contractions stimulates specific Z-disc-associated proteins such as cysteine and glycine rich protein 3 (CSRP3) to migrate to the nucleus (**Fig. 7**). There, these Z disc-associated proteins activate transcription of genes (transduction) that produce proteins needed for the training adaptations to occur (see **Fig. 7**).[20] A combined proteomic and transcriptomic analysis of skeletal muscle from MFM-WB and control Warmbloods identified aberrant expression of proteins such as CSRP3 involved in mechanotransduction, decreased mitochondrial complex I expression, and potential for a pro-oxidative cellular environment in the muscle of affected horses (see **Fig. 7**).[21] The gene with the highest expression in MFM-WB was *CHAC1* which encodes an enzyme that degrades the cysteine-based antioxidant glutathione.[21] Thus, MFM in Warmbloods appears to arise from aberrant gene and protein

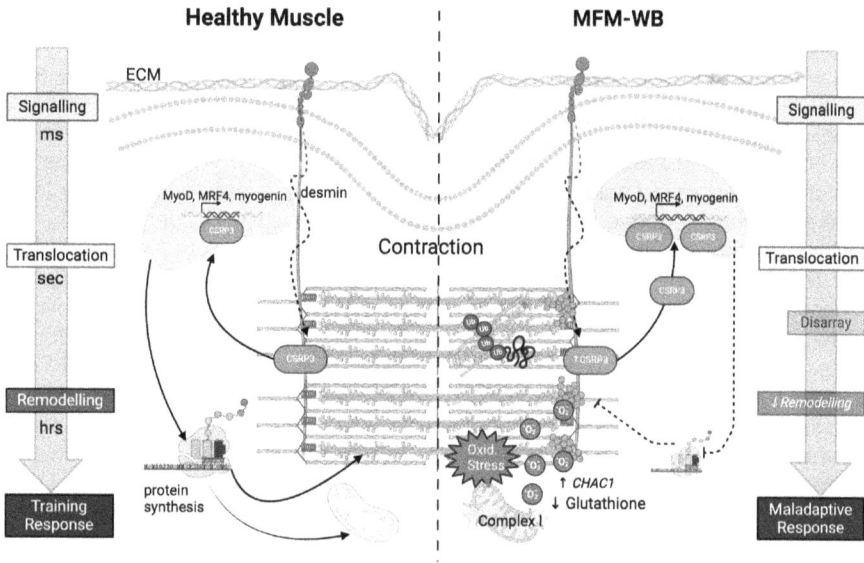

Fig. 7. Left panel: The propagation of events that occur during muscle contraction and the mechanotransduction process induced by CSRP3 in a healthy horse. The molecular partners in this process include crosstalk between the extracellular matrix (ECM—endomysium, perimysium, epimysium, and cell membrane) that connects via integrins to the cytoskeleton at costameres. The cytoskeletal protein desmin connects to the ECM at costameres and anchors parallel arrays of myofibrils at the Z-disc. Of hundreds of proteins in the Z-disc, several including CSRP3 are transduced by mechanical stimuli to migrate to the nucleus. The activated monomeric form of CSRP3 serves as a cofactor for MyoD, MRF4, and myogenin transcription factors and induces protein synthesis and remodeling designed to strengthen the sarcomere for subsequent exercise. Right panel: Proposed mechanism causing MFM-WB based on proteomic and transcriptomic analysis of skeletal muscle from MFM-WB and control Warmbloods. Upregulation of the gene *CHAC1* which encodes a protein that degrades glutathione and decreased expression of complex I mitochondrial subunits could perturb redox homeostasis with downstream effects of oxidative damage to proteins and aggregation of desmin (light brown circles). Exercise could exacerbate an underlying Z-disc instability in MFM-WB. An increase in Z-disc protein CSRP3 and 2 other nuclear cofactors, PDLIM3, SYNPO3 could indicate that the process of signal transduction is abnormally regulated leading to inadequate protein remodeling (ub=ubiquitination), Z-disc instability, and myofibrillar disarray. The overall effect would be an inability to appropriately adapt to training and reluctance to exercise.

expression that impacts the alignment of contractile proteins, mitochondrial proteins that generate ROS, and molecular training adaptations (see **Fig. 7**). MFM is likely caused by complex interactions between the diet, environment, and multiple genes.

Management

Diet. Management of MFM requires altering diet and exercise regimes. Dietary management is thoroughly described in the article, "The Role of Nutrition in Managing Muscle Disorders" by Pagan in this issue.[11] Dietary principles include hay with 12% to 17% NSC and a concentrate with moderate levels of NSC (20%–30%), lower fat (4%–6%), and higher levels of protein (12%–14% CP).[12] If horses have underlying issues with obesity, metabolic syndrome, or laminitis, the concentrate should be adjusted accordingly.

Supplements. For horses with MFM, whey-based protein supplements are recommended because they are rich in cysteine, a key component of many antioxidants that are potentially deficient in MFM horses.[21] Branched chain amino acids such as leucine stimulate protein synthesis in the muscle postexercise, which could be beneficial to MFM horses. A commercial supplement has been developed for MFM horses (MFM Pellet, KER, Versailles, KY)[a] that contains N-acetylcysteine and branched chain amino acids. When fed to MFM horses, it improves exercise tolerance particularly in those horses in earlier stages of disease.[22] Coenzyme Q_{10} is a key component of the first step in the mitochondrial electron transport chain that is impacted by MFM and can be provided as an additional antioxidant to enhance the production of NADH which reduces oxidized glutathione.[15] Provision of N-acetylcysteine and CoQ_{10} has been shown to increase the important cysteine-rich antioxidant glutathione in muscle following exercise in healthy Thoroughbred horses.[14]

Rest/Exercise. Unlike ER, Warmbloods with MFM require days off training during the week to recover. The number of days per week varies with each horse, however, 3 days of 20 to 45 minutes of work then 2 days rest works well for many horses (Valberg, personal observation). A warm-up on the lunge-line in both directions in a long, low frame for 10 to 15 minutes can improve ridden work. Hill work, cavaletti, small jumps, and core strengthening exercises can be used to build strength. As much daily turnout as possible in an area where the horse is encouraged to move about is recommended.

Behavior. Many Warmblood horses have strong, reactive temperaments and can develop behavioral issues such as refusing to go forward under saddle and bucking even after painful conditions like MFM have been resolved. In these cases, groundwork that re-establishes relaxation, trust, and leadership and the help of a professional trainer experienced with difficult horses may be required to safely ensure forward movement without protestation.

In summary, breed-specific research into PSSM2 has evolved, and there appears to be several muscle disorders previously grouped under the term PSSM2. These include PSSM2-ER in Quarter Horses, a true glycogen storage disease, MFM-ER in Arabians, and MFM-WB in Warmbloods. MFM Arabians and Warmbloods both have desmin aggregates in muscle and evidence of oxidative stress with a lack of cysteine-based antioxidants in skeletal muscle. MFM-ER appears to be largely due to oxidative stress at the end of long endurance rides associated with a lack of cysteine-based antioxidants. MFM-WB appears to be more complex than MFM-ER and in addition to a lack of cysteine-based antioxidants, also involves aberrant training adaptations.

CLINICS CARE POINTS

- Arabians and endurance horses can have MFM with exertional rhabdomyolysis.
- Warmblood horses don't usually present with exertional rhabdomyolosis, but rather pain-associated behavioral issues.
- MFM appears to result from oxidative stress and training maladaptations.
- Horses with MFM may benefit from antioxidant supplementation of vitamin E, CoQ10, and/or N-acetylcysteine.

DISCLOSURE

S.J. Valberg directs the Valberg Neuromuscular Disease laboratory (ValbergNMDL. com) and receives remuneration for analyzing muscle biopsy as well as royalties from the PSSM1 genetic test, the feed Re-Leve, and MFM pellet sold by Kentucky Equine Research. Z.J. Williams reports no conflict of interest.

FUNDING

Z.J. Williams was funded by the NIH Veterinary Research Student Training Program grant number 5T32OD011167-14 during her PhD for this work. Contents are the author's sole responsibility and do not nessecarily represent NIH official views.

REFERENCES

1. McCue ME, Armién AG, Lucio M, et al. Comparative skeletal muscle histopathologic and ultrastructural features in two forms of polysaccharide storage myopathy in horses. Vet Pathol 2009;46(6):1281–91.
2. Valberg SJ, Williams ZJ, Finno CJ, et al. Type 2 polysaccharide storage myopathy in Quarter Horses is a novel glycogen storage disease causing exertional rhabdomyolysis. Equine Vet J 2023;55(4):618–31.
3. Valberg SJ, McKenzie EC, Eyrich LV, et al. Suspected myofibrillar myopathy in Arabian horses with a history of exertional rhabdomyolysis. Equine Vet J 2016; 48(5):548–56.
4. Valberg SJ, Nicholson AM, Lewis SS, et al. Clinical and histopathological features of myofibrillar myopathy in Warmblood horses. Equine Vet J 2017;49(6):739–45.
5. Valberg SJ, Perumbakkam S, McKenzie EC, et al. Proteome and transcriptome profiling of equine myofibrillar myopathy identifies diminished peroxiredoxin 6 and altered cysteine metabolic pathways. Physiol Genom 2018;50(12):1036–50.
6. McKenzie EC, Eyrich LV, Payton ME, et al. Clinical, histopathological and metabolic responses following exercise in Arabian horses with a history of exertional rhabdomyolysis. Vet J 2016;216:196–201.
7. Prince A, Geor R, Harris P, et al. Comparison of the metabolic responses of trained Arabians and Thoroughbreds during high- and low-intensity exercise. Equine Vet J Suppl 2002;34(34):95–9.
8. Pessah IN. Ryanodine receptor acts as a sensor for redox stress. Pest Manag Sci 2001;57(10):941–5.
9. Valberg SJ, Finno CJ, Henry ML, et al. Commercial genetic testing for type 2 polysaccharide storage myopathy and myofibrillar myopathy does not correspond to a histopathological diagnosis. Equine Vet J 2021;53(4):690–700.

10. Valberg SJ. Sporadic and recurrent exertional rhabdomyolysis. In: McKenzie EC, Valberg SJ, editors. Muscle disorders of horses: Veterinary Clinics of North America: equine practice. 2025. p. 111–24.

11. Pagan JD, Valberg SJ. The role of nutrition in muscular disorders. In: McKenzie EC, Valberg SJ, editors. Muscle Disorders of horses an issue of Veterinary Clinics of North America: Equine Practice. 2025. p. 151–63.

12. Joe D, Pagan SJV. Feeding performance horses with myopathies. In: Pagan JD, Valberg SJ, editors. 66th Annual Connvention of the America Association of Equine Practitioners, vol. 66. San Antonio (TX): American Associan of Equine Practitioners; 2020. p. 66–74.

13. Dowling JJ, Arbogast S, Hur J, et al. Oxidative stress and successful antioxidant treatment in models of RYR1-related myopathy. Brain 2012;135(Pt 4):1115–27.

14. Henry ML, Velez-Irizarry D, Pagan JD, et al. The impact of N-acetyl cysteine and coenzyme Q10 supplementation on skeletal muscle antioxidants and proteome in fit thoroughbred horses. Antioxidants 2021;10(11). https://doi.org/10.3390/antiox10111739.

15. Henry ML, Wesolowski LT, Pagan JD, et al. Impact of coenzyme Q10 supplementation on skeletal muscle respiration, antioxidants, and the muscle proteome in thoroughbred horses. Antioxidants 2023;12(2). https://doi.org/10.3390/antiox12020263.

16. Williams ZJ, Bertels M, Valberg SJ. Muscle glycogen concentrations and response to diet and exercise regimes in Warmblood horses with type 2 Polysaccharide Storage Myopathy. PLoS One 2018;13(9):e0203467.

17. Finno CJ, Johnson AL. Equine neuroaxonal dystrophy and degenerative myeloencephalopathy. Vet Clin N Am Equine Pract 2022;38(2):213–24.

18. Young AE, Finno CJ. Current insights into equine neuroaxonal dystrophy/equine degenerative myeloencephalopathy. Vet J 2024;305:106129.

19. Williams ZJ, Velez-Irizarry D, Petersen JL, et al. Candidate gene expression and coding sequence variants in Warmblood horses with myofibrillar myopathy. Equine Vet J 2021;53(2):306–15.

20. Germain P, Delalande A, Pichon C. Role of muscle LIM protein in mechanotransduction process. Int J Mol Sci 2022;23(17). https://doi.org/10.3390/ijms23179785.

21. Williams ZJ, Velez-Irizarry D, Gardner K, et al. Integrated proteomic and transcriptomic profiling identifies aberrant gene and protein expression in the sarcomere, mitochondrial complex I, and the extracellular matrix in Warmblood horses with myofibrillar myopathy. BMC Genom 2021;22(1):438.

22. Valberg SJ. Diagnosis and management of myofibrillar myopathy in Warmblood performance horses. In: Proceedings of the American Association of Equine Practitioners, Nashville TN, vol 67, 2021, 214-218.

The Role of Nutrition in Managing Muscle Disorders

Joe D. Pagan, MS, PhD[a],*, Stephanie J. Valberg, DVM, PhD[b]

KEYWORDS

- Skeletal • Muscle • Tying up • Rhabdomyolysis • Myopathy • Atrophy
- N-acetylcysteine

KEY POINTS

- Horses with exertional rhabdomyolysis caused by types 1 and 2 polysaccharide storage myopathy (PSSM1 and PSSM2-ER) benefit from low nonstructural carbohydrate (NSC) diets and supplementary fat as a metabolizable form of energy.
- Horses with recurrent exertional rhabdomyolysis can be managed by lowering NSC, but not to the extremes of PSSM, and then replacing needed calories with fat.
- Arabian horses with myofibrillar myopathy (MFM-ER) can be managed with moderate NSC, supplementary fat, amino acids, and antioxidants N-acetylcysteine and coenzyme Q10.
- Warmblood horses with myofibrillar myopathy (MFM-WB) benefit from a similar diet to MFM-ER horses but with less additional fat.

INTRODUCTION

In combination with exercise, nutrition is an essential component of managing horses with myopathies. The optimal feeding program for an individual is tailored to the diagnosis of a specific underlying myopathy.

Classification of Exertional Myopathies

Exertional myopathies cause muscle pain and impaired performance during or after exercise. Exertional rhabdomyolysis (ER) represents a subset of exertional myopathies characterized by muscle fiber degeneration and elevations in serum creatine kinase (CK) and aspartate transaminase (AST) activities. Polysaccharide storage myopathy (PSSM) was one of the first specific causes of ER identified and is

[a] Kentucky Equine Research, Versailles, KY 40383, USA; [b] Department of Large Animal Clinical Sciences, Michigan State University, East Lansing, MI 48824, USA
* Corresponding author. Kentucky Equine Research, 3910 Delaney Ferry Road, Versailles, KY 40383.
E-mail address: pagan@ker.com

Vet Clin Equine 41 (2025) 151–163
https://doi.org/10.1016/j.cveq.2024.11.007
0749-0739/25/© 2024 Elsevier Inc. All rights are reserved, including those for text and data mining, AI training, and similar technologies.

Abbreviations	
AST	aspartate transaminase
CK	creatine kinase
DE	digestible energy
EMND	equine motor neuron disease
ER	exertional rhabdomyolysis
FFA	free fatty acid
MFM	myofibrillar myopathy
MH	malignant hyperthermia
NRC	National Research Council
NSC	nonstructural carbohydrate
PSSM	polysaccharide storage myopathy
RER	recurrent exertional rhabdomyolysis
US	United States
VEM	vitamin E-responsive myopathy
WSC	water-soluble carbohydrate

characterized by the presence of abnormal muscle glycogen staining in muscle biopsies.[1] Genetic discoveries led to the subdivision of PSSM into type 1 PSSM (PSSM1), which indicates horses with a mutation in glycogen synthase 1, and PSSM2, indicating horses with abnormal glycogen stains lacking the PSSM1 mutation.[2,3] With a lack of information on the cause of PSSM2, the low-nonstructural carbohydrate (NSC), high-fat PSSM1 diet was universally recommended for all horses diagnosed with PSSM regardless of whether PSSM1 or PSSM2.[4] Recommendations for feeding PSSM2 horses, however, have now evolved according to breed-based research into muscle glycogen concentrations, histologic markers, and molecular approaches that better subclassify PSSM2.[5–10]

Forms of ER now include PSSM1, PSSM2 with ER (PSSM2-ER), malignant hyperthermia (MH), recurrent exertional rhabdomyolysis (RER), and myofibrillar myopathy (MFM-ER) in Arabians.

Other exertional myopathies do not cause ER and elevations in serum CK and AST activities with exercise.[8] Although previously grouped under the heading PSSM2, research into Warmblood horses with exercise intolerance, reluctance to go forward, collect, and engage the hindquarters led to the identification of another form of myofibrillar myopathy in this breed, MFM-WB.[7,11]

Deficiencies in vitamin E can impact performance by causing muscle atrophy and loss of strength. Short-term deficiencies affect skeletal muscle, causing vitamin E-responsive myopathy (VEM), and long-term deficiencies are neuropathic, causing equine motor neuron disease (EMND).[12,13] These disorders and nutritional requirements are covered in Carrie Finno and Erica C. McKenzie's article, "Vitamin E and Selenium Related Manifestations of Muscle Disease," in this issue.[14]

MANAGEMENT OF CHRONIC EXERTIONAL MUSCLE DISORDERS

Altering diet and exercise regimes to compensate for underlying defects is often the best available strategy to assist horses with exertional myopathies. Identifying and eliminating any known factors that trigger ER are also important in preventing further episodes. Controlled treatment trials have been performed to validate management strategies for PSSM1 and RER.[4,15,16] Less evidenced-based information is available with regard to management of PSSM2-ER and MFM. Recommendations for these disorders are based largely on retrospective studies or clinical impressions.[5,17,18]

FEEDING PROGRAMS FOR HORSES WITH MYOPATHIES

A nutritionally balanced diet with appropriate caloric intake and adequate protein, vitamins, and minerals is a core element in treating all forms of exertional myopathies. As with all classes of horses, the development of a ration includes a series of steps.

1. Determine daily nutrient requirements. A horse's nutrient requirements depend on age, breed, body size, growth rate, level of exercise, and other considerations. The National Research Council (NRC) last published its recommendations for horses in 2007.[19] NRC requirements are often considered minimums for many nutrients. Recommendations that are more commonly used in practice are also available in commercially available software such as MicroSteed[a] or Feed XL[b].
2. Select type and intake of forage. Forage should be the foundation of every equine feeding program, so it is important to establish the type and expected intake of forage before choosing concentrates or supplements.
3. Select energy sources in concentrate. One of the keys to managing exertional myopathies is controlling the source of energy in a ration. Energy requirements in the United States are expressed in terms of megacalories (Mcal) of digestible energy (DE). DE can be supplied from nonstructural carbohydrates (NSCs), fat, structural carbohydrates (fiber), and protein. NSC is the sum of water-soluble carbohydrates (WSCs) (sugars) and starch. Most concentrates fed to ER horses are low in NSC and high in fat. Unfortunately, determining the NSC content of commercial concentrates is not easy, as these nutrients rarely appear as guarantees on feed tags or bags. The American Association of Feed Control Officials (AAFCO) does not have an agreed-upon method for measuring WSC and starch. Therefore, many state regulatory agencies do not allow these nutrients to appear with other nutrient analyses such as protein, fat, or crude fiber. Feed manufacturers often supply this information in supporting literature or on the internet, but these figures are not regulated by any governmental agency. Most feed manufacturers use Equi-Analytical in Ithaca, New York,[c] to determine WSC and starch values in feeds, and horse owners and veterinarians can also send feeds and forages to this laboratory for analysis.
4. Calculate intake of concentrate to meet energy requirement. The quantity of concentrate required by a horse equals the DE requirement of the horse minus the DE supplied by forage. The DE requirement depends on the activity level and the current energy status of the horse. DE requirements will vary depending on whether the horse needs to lose, gain, or maintain its body weight.
5. Calculate intake of other nutrients (protein, minerals, vitamins) provided from forage and concentrate. Most commercial concentrates are formulated to meet nearly all the protein, mineral, and vitamin requirements of the horse if fed at a typical level of intake as recommended on the feed bag. Often a horse will be fed below this expected range of intake, and additional fortification will be required. This is particularly true when horses are fed high-quality forage or if they need to lose weight.
6. Supplement required nutrients not provided by forage and concentrate. Supplements are often necessary to provide nutrients not found in the forage and

---

[a] MicroSteed Ration Evaluation Software, Kentucky Equine Research, Versailles, KY 40383.

[b] Feed XL Nutrition Software, available at feedxl.com.

[c] Equi-Analytical, Ithaca, New York 14850.

concentrate, either because of low concentrate intakes or to supply levels of nutrients that are greater than typically added to commercial feeds. Electrolytes, amino acids, vitamin E, and other antioxidants fall into this category for horses suffering from myopathies.

EXERTIONAL RHABDOMYOLYSIS

A general approach to designing a ration for horses with primary clinical signs of exertional rhabdomyolysis is outlined in **Fig. 1**.

Sporadic Exertional Rhabdomyolysis

Total nutrient requirements will vary depending on the horse's size, breed, discipline, and level of activity. DE requirements will vary from near maintenance to twice maintenance.

Because low forage intake may contribute to sporadic bouts of ER, horses should be provided adequate quantities of high-quality forage. Performance horses will typically consume 1.5% to 2% of body weight per day of hay. Good-quality grass or grass-legume mixed hays (55%–65% NDF, 10%–12% CP, 10%–17% NSC) are preferable.

A concentrate with moderate levels of soluble carbohydrate (20%–30% NSC), fat (4%–8%), and fiber (20%–30% NDF) is appropriate. Horses with sporadic ER do not necessarily benefit from increased dietary fat, so addition of fat should depend on caloric needs.

Concentrate intake will depend on the horse's DE requirement and the quality and quantity of forage. If low concentrate (<3 kg/d) is required, supplemental protein,

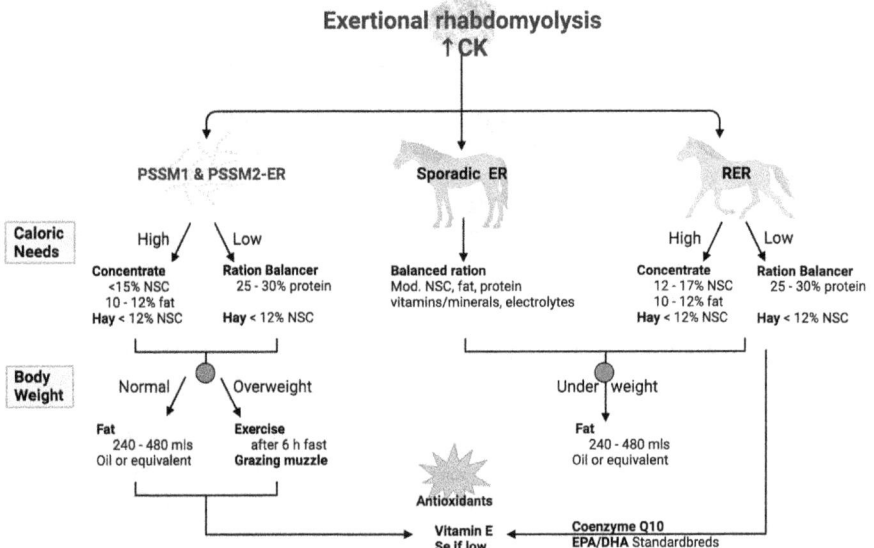

Fig. 1. An approach to managing horses with clinical signs of ER characterized by muscle stiffness, sweating, reluctance to move, and increased serum CK activity. Decisions should be based on the underlying myopathy, the horse's caloric needs, and current body weight. NSC, nonstructural carbohydrate; Omega 3s: EPA, eicosapentaenoic acid; DHA, docosahexaenoic acid. (*Created in* BioRender. Valberg, S. (2025) https://BioRender.com/w15q798.)

minerals, and vitamins may be required. This is best accomplished with appropriately fortified ration balancer pellets. Underweight horses may benefit from additional vegetable oil (120–240 mL) or stabilized rice bran (0.5–1 kg).

Electrolyte imbalances and deficiencies are a common cause of sporadic ER. Horses should have free-choice access to a salt block and be supplemented with salt or a commercial electrolyte at levels to meet requirements. This can vary from 30 to 60 g per day with light sweating and up to 120 to 150 g per day with heavy sweating. Furosemide administration (5 cc) results in around 20 g of sodium and 35 g chloride loss in urine in the first 4 hours after administration.[20]

Selenium and vitamin E status should be evaluated. Low serum concentrations of either nutrient warrant supplementation. Natural-source vitamin E is more bioavailable than synthetic sources, and either micellized[d] or nanodispersed[e] sources rapidly restore serum status.[21,22]

Recurrent Exertional Rhabdomyolysis

As with sporadic ER, RER nutrient requirements will vary depending on the horse's size, breed, discipline, and level of activity. DE requirements will vary from near maintenance to twice maintenance. Signs of RER occur most frequently in Thoroughbred and Standardbred racehorses that have DE requirements of 30 to 35 Mcal DE per day.

Thoroughbred horses do not appear to show the same significant increase in serum insulin concentrations in response to consuming hay with an NSC of 17% as seen in Quarter Horses.[23] This fact, combined with the high caloric requirements of racehorses, suggests that it is not as important to select hay with very low NSC content in RER Thoroughbreds as it is in PSSM horses. Anecdotally, some trainers find horses with RER have more frequent episodes of ER when consuming alfalfa hay, in which case it should be avoided on an individual basis. The nervous disposition of some RER horses may predispose them to gastric ulcers, and thus frequent provision of hay with a moderate NSC and mixed alfalfa content may be indicated.

Substitution of fat for NSC in an energy-dense ration significantly reduces muscle damage in exercising RER horses. A controlled trial using a specialized feed[f] developed for RER showed that NSC should provide no greater than 20%, and fat should provide between 20% and 25%, of daily DE intake for optimal management of RER horses requiring high DE intakes (>30 Mcal DE/d).[15] The benefit of a high-fat diet for RER does not appear to be from a change in muscle metabolism. Pre- and postexercise muscle glycogen and lactate concentrations are the same in RER horses fed a low-starch, high-fat diet compared with a high-starch diet.[15,24] Rather, low-NSC, high-fat diets in RER horses may decrease muscle damage by assuaging anxiety and excitability, which are tightly linked to developing rhabdomyolysis in susceptible horses. High-fat, low-NSC diets fed to fit RER horses produce lower glucose, insulin, and cortisol responses and led to a calmer demeanor and lower pre-exercise heart rates.[15,25] Neurohormonal changes may develop in response to high serum glucose, insulin, and cortisol concentrations, resulting in an anxious demeanor.

Racehorses in full training typically consume 6 to 7 kg per day of concentrate. Racehorse concentrates for RER horses should contain 12% to 18% NSC and 10% to 13%

---

[d] Elevate WS, Kentucky Performance Products, Versailles, KY 40383.

[e] Nano-E, Kentucky Equine Research, Versailles, KY 40383.

[f] Re-Leve, Kentucky Equine Research, Versailles, KY 40383.

fat by weight. To maintain high energy densities (3.2–3.4 Mcal DE/kg), they should also contain sources of highly digestible fiber such as beet pulp or soy hulls. The beneficial effect of low-NSC, high-fat rations appears to be more directly related to the glycemic and insulinemic nature of the feeds rather than their absolute NSC and fat content. Therefore, the ingredients used in a concentrate also affect its suitably as an RER feed. Water-soluble carbohydrates (WSCs) produce higher glycemic responses than starch. Molasses is extremely glycemic in horses,[26] but added fat greatly reduces glycemic response, even in high-NSC feeds.[27,28] Glycemic response is also affected by rate of intake and rate of gastric emptying.[28,29] Although a calm demeanor is desired during training, some racehorse trainers feeding low-NSC, high-fat feeds prefer to supplement with a titrated amount of grain 3 days before a race to potentially boost liver glycogen and increase a horse's energy availability during the race.

As with sporadic ER, concentrate intakes less than 3 kg per day may not provide adequate amounts of protein, minerals, or vitamins, and a balancer pellet may be required.

Studies in RER horses show that significant reductions or normalization of postexercise serum CK activity occurs within a week of commencing a low-starch, high-fat diet.[15] Days of no training and standing in a stall are discouraged, because postexercise CK activity is higher after 2 days of rest compared with values observed when performing consecutive days of the same amount of submaximal exercise.[15]

The gluteal muscle of RER-susceptible Standardbreds is characterized by perturbation of pathways for calcium regulation, cellular/oxidative stress, and inflammation weeks after an episode of rhabdomyolysis.[30] Supplementation with vitamin E, vitamin C, and Coenzyme Q10 may help reduce oxidative stress[15,24,31,32] Additionally, supplementation with Omega−3 long-chain polyunsaturated fatty acids (EPA and DHA) may be useful in mitigating long-term inflammation.[33,34]

Type 1 Polysaccharide Storage Myopathy and Type 2 Polysaccharide Storage Myopathy with Exertional Rhabdomyolysis

PSSM1 and recently PSSM2 in Quarter Horses with ER (PSSM2-ER) have been found to be glycogen storage diseases.[1,5] Dietary recommendations for PSSM1 are based on controlled trials, whereas recommendations for PSSM2-ER are based on owner surveys.[4,5]

Meeting the horse's caloric requirements for an ideal body weight is the most important consideration in designing a ration for PSSM1 and PSSM2-ER, as many horses with PSSM are easy keepers and may be overweight at the time of diagnosis. Adding excessive calories in the form of fat to the diet of an obese horse may produce metabolic syndrome and is contraindicated. If necessary, caloric intake should be reduced by using a grazing muzzle during turnout, feeding hay with a much lower NSC content at 1% to 1.5% of body weight, providing a low-calorie ration balancer, and gradually introducing daily exercise. Rather than provide dietary fat to an overweight horse, fasting for 6 hours before exercise can be used to elevate plasma free fatty acids (FFAs) before exercise and alleviate any restrictions in energy metabolism in muscle.

Quarter Horses develop a significant increase in serum insulin concentrations in response to consuming hay with an NSC of 17%, whereas insulin concentrations are fairly stable when fed hay with 12% or 4% NSC content.[16] Because insulin stimulates the already overactive enzyme glycogen synthase in the muscle of PSSM1 horses, selecting hay with 12% or less NSC is advisable. The degree to which the NSC content of hay should be restricted below 12% NSC depends on the caloric requirements of the horse. Feeding a low-NSC (<5%), high-fiber (>65% NDF) hay provides room to add an adequate amount of fat to the diet of easy keepers without exceeding the daily caloric requirement and inducing excessive weight gain. For example, a 500-kg lightly exercised horse generally requires 18 Mcal DE per day. A mixed-grass hay (12% NSC, 55% NDF, 2.0 Mcal DE/kg) fed at 9 kg per day meets the horse's daily caloric requirement. In contrast, 8 kg of 4% NSC hay (1.7 Mcal DE/kg) would provide 13.6 Mcal DE per day, which would allow a reasonable addition of 4.4 Mcal DE from fat per day (530 mL of vegetable oil).

A high-NSC diet increases the propensity to develop muscle pain with aerobic exercise in PSSM1 and PSSM2-ER horses.[4,35] A high-NSC diet results in enhanced glycogen synthase activity, which may impair oxidative metabolism of substrates such as pyruvate and fatty acids.[36] PSSM1 horses consuming high-NSC diets have low plasma non-esterified FFA concentrations, possibly because of suppression of lipolysis by high insulin.[4] Low dietary starch and fat supplementation facilitate muscle fat metabolism in PSSM1 horses.

Concentrates for PSSM1 and PSSM2-ER horses should be low in NSC (<15% by weight) and low glycemic. High-fat (10–12%) concentrates can be included in the diet but, if daily intake is low (<2 kg/d), then additional fat supplementation may be required from added vegetable oil (120–240 mL) or stabilized rice bran. Hydrated, rinsed beet pulp produces a very low glycemic response and can be used as a carrier for added vegetable oil.[26] One kilogram of beet pulp (prehydrated weight) and 1 cup (240 mL) of vegetable oil and 500 g of a balancer pellet (to meet protein, mineral, and vitamin requirements) would provide around 6.0 Mcal DE, which is equivalent to the DE supplied by 2 kg of a typical commercial concentrate.

Myofibrillar Myopathy in Arabian Endurance Horses

Whereas some excitable endurance horses present with signs of RER early in races, other seasoned endurance horses develop signs of muscle stiffness, cramping, myoglobinuria, and high serum CK at the end of long endurance races. Muscle biopsies from the latter horses recently found glycogen concentration to be normal. Rather, myofibrillar disarray and characteristic aggregates of the cytoskeletal protein desmin were identified, leading to the term myofibrillar myopathy with ER (MFM-ER) being applied to endurance horses with desmin aggregates and high serum CK activity.[6,37] This subset of horses was previously classified as PSSM2 because of glycogen pooling in regions of broken myofilaments.[11,37] Transcriptomic and proteomic studies implicate a pro-oxidant environment and low cysteine-based antioxidants as potential causes of MFM-ER and led to a new approach to managing MFM-ER.[9]

Endurance riders feed low-protein rations because they are concerned that high-protein diets may increase body heat, urine production, and water needs. Although this level of protein intake may meet crude protein requirements in normal horses, it may be deficient in specific amino acids such as lysine, methionine, and threonine needed for muscle repair and generation of cysteine-based antioxidants in MFM-ER. Leucine stimulates protein synthesis in the muscle after exercise,[38] which would be beneficial to MFM-ER horses. Arabian endurance horses are typically fed higher-fat diets, as Arabians depend more on fat oxidation than Thoroughbreds during exercise.[39] However, because MFM in Arabian endurance horses is related to oxidative stress resulting from fat oxidation, it is questionable whether these horses need extremely high levels of fat intake (>15% total DE intake). Because oxidative stress is likely involved in the degenerative process, antioxidants or precursors of antioxidants are additionally important to support the mitochondrial respiratory chain, the major source of reactive oxygen species in exercising muscle.

MFM-ER horses will typically consume 1.5% to 2% of body weight per day of hay. Good-quality grass or grass-legume mixed hays (55%–65% NDF, 10%–12% CP, 10%–17% NSC) are preferable.

In a survey of US endurance riders, concentrate intake averaged 2.27 kg per day, with an average protein content of 10% CP (range 6.2%–15.7% by weight).[32] Concentrates for MFM-ER horses should include higher levels of protein (12%–14% CP) containing high-quality amino acids and moderate levels of NSC (20%–30%) and fat (4%–8%).

Supplements

Whey-based proteins are recommended because they are rich in cysteine. Cysteine is a key component of many antioxidants, and MFM-ER Arabian horses appear to have an increased cysteine requirement following exercise.[9] The most absorbable form of cysteine is N-acetylcysteine, and supplementation with N-acetylcysteine has been shown to increase gluteal muscle glutathione (a ubiquitous cysteine-based antioxidant) in healthy fit Thoroughbreds.[40]

Coenzyme Q10 (CoQ10) is a key component of the first step - Complex I - in the mitochondrial electron transport chain, which generates reactive oxygen species. MFM-ER Arabians have altered expression of subunits of complex I.[9] When fed to healthy horses, CoQ10[9] supplementation enhanced electron transfer capacity via complex II, which could decrease reactive oxygen species formation and enhance fat metabolism. CoQ10 is used in human muscle disorders and is now being trialed as a supplement for MFM horses.

EXERTIONAL MYOPATHIES
Myofibrillar Myopathy in Warmblood Horses

Research into a subset of Warmbloods with PSSM2 found normal muscle glycogen concentrations, myofibrillar disarray, and desmin aggregation leading to a reclassification as MFM-WB.[7] Based on this new finding and transcriptomic and proteomic analyses of muscle, a new dietary approach was developed for MFM-WB horses.[10] This new diet outlined in **Fig. 2** is informed by indicators that myofibrillar instability, Z-disc signaling, aberrations in cysteine-based antioxidants, oxidative stress, and the mitochondrial respiratory chain are key drivers of MFM-WB.[10] A diagnosis of MFM-WB is based on muscle biopsy and not commercial genetic tests for PSSM2 or MFM that have not been scientifically validated through peer-reviewed publication.[41–43] Many horses with signs of exercise intolerance are initially managed with a low-NSC, high-fat diet with limited relief of exercise intolerance. It seems sensible to assume that if horses have not responded satisfactorily to this diet, a trial period of 6 to 8 weeks on the MFM-WB diet would be warranted provided other causes of exercise intolerance have been investigated and ruled out (see **Fig. 2**).

Because Warmblood horses diagnosed with MFM have normal glycogen concentrations, the rationale for a low-NSC diet in these breeds appears lacking.[11,37] The presence of muscle sarcomere breakdown and atrophy indicates that rations should focus on providing quality protein and specific amino acids as described for MFM-ER to aid in sarcomere regenesis. Additionally, because oxidative stress is likely involved in the degenerative process, antioxidants or precursors of antioxidants are important to reduce oxidative stress and support the mitochondrial respiratory chain, the major source of reactive oxygen species in exercising muscle.

---

[9] Nano-Q10, Kentucky Equine Research, Versailles, KY 40383.

Warmbloods
Exercise intolerance, normal CK

Rule out saddle fit, gastric ulcers, orthopedic lameness etc

< 8 yrs

Dx Diet trial

muscle biopsy

> 8 yrs

Myofibrillar myopathy

Overweight, Metabolic
Dark glycogen stain

Hay: < 12% NSC

Ration balancer
25 - 30% protein

Supplement:
Amino acids +
N-acetylcysteine

Normal Weight
Normal glycogen stain

Hay: 12 -15% NSC

Concentrate
20 - 30% NSC
4 - 8% fat
10 - 12% protein
Supplement:
Amino acids +
N-acetylcysteine

Antioxidants

Coenzyme Q10
Vitamin E
Se if low

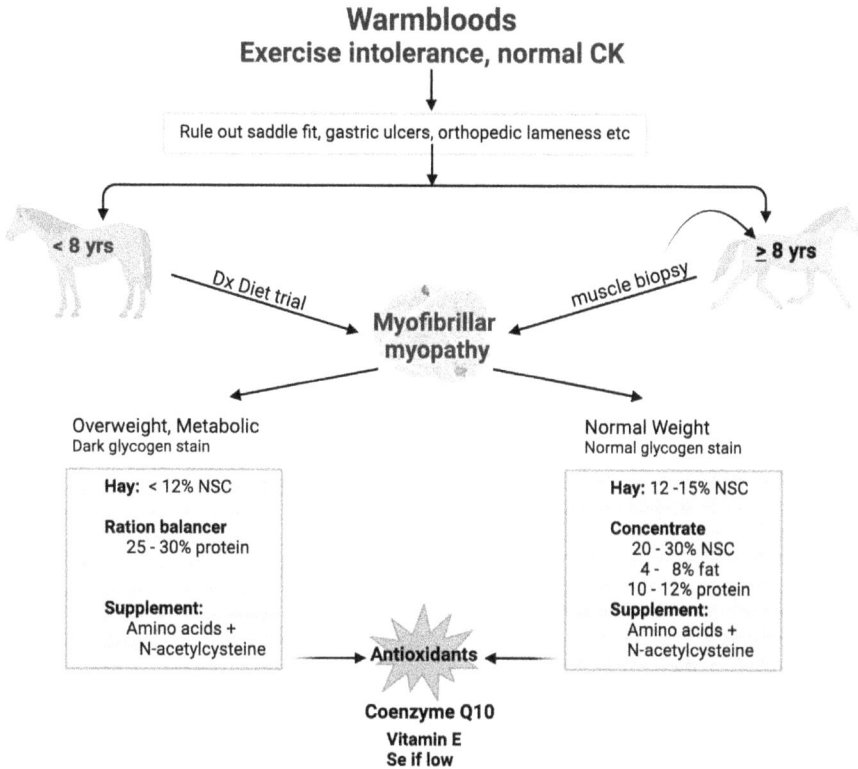

Fig. 2. An approach to managing MFM-WB horses with clinical signs of exertional myopathy characterized by exercise intolerance and normal to mildly increased serum CK activity. To conclude a myopathy is responsible for exercise intolerance, other common causes should first be ruled out. Because the diagnostic feature of desmin aggregation may lag behind clinical signs, muscle biopsies from young horses can give false-negative results; therefore a treatment trial for 4 weeks looking for a clinical response may be the best diagnostic option for young horses. Horses that are overweight or have evidence of equine metabolic syndrome are fed a diet lower in NSCs than normal-weight horses. (*Created in* BioRender. Valberg, S. (2025) https://BioRender.com/l64f863.)

MFM horses will typically consume 1.5% to 2% of body weight per day of hay. Good-quality grass or grass-legume mixed hays (55%–65% NDF, 10%–12% CP, 10%–17% NSC) are preferable.

In the United States, the trend for feeding Warmbloods has been toward low-NSC, high-fat diets. This is not the case in Europe. Elite European sport horses consume feeds that are higher in NSC (25%–35%) and more moderate in fat (4%–6%).[44] There is no evidence that extremely low-NSC, high-fat diets are needed by Warmbloods with MFM-WB unless horses have metabolic disease, excess adipose cells, or dark muscle glycogen stains in muscle biopsies. In addition, there does not appear to be a scientific reason why additional fat, a potential source of oxidative stress, would be of benefit to Warmbloods with MFM.

Concentrates for MFM-WB horses should include higher levels of protein (12%–14% CP by weight) containing high-quality amino acids and moderate levels of NSC (20%–30%) and fat (4%–8%). This level of protein intake will provide specific amino acids such as lysine, methionine, and threonine needed for muscle repair and generation of cysteine-based antioxidants. Leucine stimulates protein synthesis in the muscle after exercise,[38] which would be beneficial to MFM-WB horses.

Supplements

For horses with symmetric topline muscle atrophy and horses with MFM, amino acid supplements are currently recommended.[8,45] Whey-based proteins are recommended, because they are rich in cysteine. The top upregulated gene in MFM-WB horses is *CHAC1,* and the CHAC1 enzyme degrades the cysteine-based antioxidant glutathione. Because of this, supplementation with N-acetylcysteine is recommended. N-acetylcysteine can increase postexercise gluteal muscle glutathione.[40]

Horses with MFM have altered expression of genes and proteins involved in mitochondrial complex 1 and glutathione degradation in their muscle.[10] Coenzyme Q10 is a key component of the first step in the mitochondrial electron transport chain and a potent antioxidant, and has been recommended for MFM-WB.

A survey of 50 owners of MFM-WB horses feeding the recommended diet (17 responses) found that 92% of horses improved after 4 weeks, with hindlimb engagement and reluctance to work being the clinical signs to show the most improvement (Valberg unpublished observation, 2023).

SUMMARY

In combination with exercise, nutrition is an essential component of managing horses with myopathies. The type of diet needed depends on the specific myopathy in question. ER represents a subset of exertional myopathies characterized by elevations in serum CK and AST activities. Several forms of ER including PSSM1, PSSM2-ER, and RER require low-NSC diets. If extra exergy is also required, then supplemental fat may also be beneficial. MFM horses do not require low-NSC, high-fat diets. Instead, they respond to protein and amino acid supplementation to rebuild muscle and antioxidants such as N-acetylcysteine, CoQ10, and vitamin E.

CLINICS CARE POINTS

- In order to best manage horses with myopathies it is important to distinguish between those with exertional rhabdomyolysis by measuring serum CK and those with normal serum CK and exercise intolerance due to myofibrillar myopathy.
- An exercise challenge test with CK measured 4 h after exercise can be of benefit to make this distinction.
- While horses with exertional rhabdomyolysis are fed diets with lower nonstructural carbohydrates and fat supplementation, horses with myofibrillar myopathy are fed moderate amounts of nonstructural carbohydrates, less fat, and increased amino acids with N-acetylcysteine and antioxidants.

DISCLOSURES

J.D. Pagan is the founder and owner of Kentucky Equine Research, which owns Microsteed Ration Evaluation Software, Nano-E, Re-Leve, MFM Pellet, and Nano-Q10. S.J. Valberg directs the Valberg Neuromuscular Disease Laboratory (ValbergNMDL.com) and receives remuneration for analyzing muscle biopsies. Her website is sponsored by Kentucky Equine Research, and she receives royalties from the PSSM1 genetic test and the feeds Re-Leve and MFM Pellet developed in association with Kentucky Equine Research.

REFERENCES

1. Valberg SJ, Cardinet GH 3rd, Carlson GP, et al. Polysaccharide storage myopathy associated with recurrent exertional rhabdomyolysis in horses. Neuromuscul Disord 1992;2:351–9.

2. McCue ME, Valberg SJ, Miller MB, et al. Glycogen synthase (GYS1) mutation causes a novel skeletal muscle glycogenosis. Genomics 2008;91:458–66.

3. McCue ME, Armién AG, Lucio M, et al. Comparative skeletal muscle histopathologic and ultrastructural features in two forms of polysaccharide storage myopathy in horses. Vet Pathol 2009;46:1281–91.

4. Ribeiro WP, Valberg SJ, Pagan JD, et al. The effect of varying dietary starch and fat content on serum creatine kinase activity and substrate availability in equine polysaccharide storage myopathy. J Vet Intern Med 2004;18:887–94.

5. Valberg SJ, Williams ZJ, Finno CJ, et al. Type 2 polysaccharide storage myopathy in Quarter Horses is a novel glycogen storage disease causing exertional rhabdomyolysis. Equine Vet J 2023;55:618–31.

6. Valberg S, McKenzie E, Eyrich L, et al. Suspected myofibrillar myopathy in Arabian horses with a history of exertional rhabdomyolysis. Equine Vet J 2016; 48:548–56.

7. Valberg SJ, Nicholson AM, Lewis SS, et al. Clinical and histopathological features of myofibrillar myopathy in Warmblood horses. Equine Vet J 2017;49:739–45.

8. Valberg SJ. Muscle conditions affecting sport horses. Vet Clin N Am Equine Pract 2018;34:253–76.

9. Valberg SJ, Perumbakkam S, McKenzie EC, et al. Proteome and transcriptome profiling of equine myofibrillar myopathy identifies diminished peroxiredoxin 6 and altered cysteine metabolic pathways. Physiol Genom 2018;50:1036–50.

10. Williams ZJ, Velez-Irizarry D, Gardner K, et al. Integrated proteomic and transcriptomic profiling identifies aberrant gene and protein expression in the sarcomere, mitochondrial complex I, and the extracellular matrix in Warmblood horses with myofibrillar myopathy. BMC Genom 2021;22:438.

11. Lewis SS, Nicholson AM, Williams ZJ, et al. Clinical characteristics and muscle glycogen concentrations in warmblood horses with polysaccharide storage myopathy. Am J Vet Res 2017;78:1305–12.

12. Finno CJ, Valberg SJ. A comparative review of vitamin E and associated equine disorders. J Vet Intern Med 2012;26:1251–66.

13. Bedford HE, Valberg SJ, Firshman AM, et al. Histopathologic findings in the sacrocaudalis dorsalis medialis muscle of horses with vitamin E–responsive muscle atrophy and weakness. J Am Vet Med Assoc 2013;242:1127–37.

14. McKenzie EC, Finno CJ. Vitamin E and selenium related manifestations of muscle disease. Muscle disorders of the horses. Veterinary Clinics of North America: Equine Practice; 2025. p. 77–93.

15. McKenzie EC, Valberg SJ, Godden SM, et al. Effect of dietary starch, fat, and bicarbonate content on exercise responses and serum creatine kinase activity in equine recurrent exertional rhabdomyolysis. J Vet Intern Med 2003;17:693–701.

16. Borgia L, Valberg S, McCue M, et al. Glycaemic and insulinaemic responses to feeding hay with different non-structural carbohydrate content in control and polysaccharide storage myopathy-affected horses. J Anim Physiol Anim Nutr (Berl) 2011;95:798–807.

17. Hunt LM, Valberg SJ, Steffenhagen K, et al. An epidemiological study of myopathies in Warmblood horses. Equine Vet J 2008;40:171–7.

18. Williams ZJ, Bertels M, Valberg SJ. Muscle glycogen concentrations and response to diet and exercise regimes in Warmblood horses with type 2 Polysaccharide Storage Myopathy. PLoS One 2018;13:e0203467.

19. National Research Council of the Academies. Nutrient requirements of horses. Washington, DC: The National Academies Press; 2007.

20. Pagan JD, Waldridge BM, Whitehouse C, et al. Furosemide administration affects mineral excretion and balance in non-exercised and exercised Thoroughbreds. J Equine Vet Sci 2013;329:329.

21. Pagan JD, Lennox M, Perry L, et al, Form of α-tocopherol affects vitamin E bioavailability in Thoroughbred horses 1st Nordic Feed Science Conference, 2010, 112–113.

22. Brown JC, Valberg SJ, Hogg M, et al. Effects of feeding two RRR-alpha-tocopherol formulations on serum, cerebrospinal fluid and muscle alpha-tocopherol concentrations in horses with subclinical vitamin E deficiency. Equine Vet J 2017;49:753–8.

23. Borgia LA. Resistance training and the effects of feeding carbohydrates and oils on healthy horses and horses with polysaccharide stroage myopathy. College of Veterinary Medicine. Pro Quest. Ann Arbor (MI): University of Minnesota; 2010.

24. MacLeay JM, Valberg SJ, Pagan JD, et al. Effect of diet on thoroughbred horses with recurrent exertional rhabdomyolysis performing a standardised exercise test. Equine Vet J Suppl 1999;(30):458–62.

25. Finno CJ, McKenzie E, Valberg SJ, et al. Effect of fitness on glucose, insulin and cortisol responses to diets varying in starch and fat content in Thoroughbred horses with recurrent exertional rhabdomyolysis. Equine Vet J Suppl 2010;(38):323–8.

26. Groff L, Pagan J, Hoekstra K, et al. Effect of preparation method on the glycemic response to ingestion of beet pulp in Thoroughbred horses. Proc. 17th Equine Nutr Physiol Soc Symp, Lexington, Kentucky, May 31-June 2, 2001.

27. Pagan JD, Rotmensen T, Jackson SG. Responses of blood glucose, lactate and insulin in horses fed equal amounts of grain with or without added soybean oil. In: Pagan JD, editor. Advances in Equine Nutrition. Nottingham, England: Nottingham University Press; 1995. p. 49–56.

28. Geor R., Harris P., Hoekstra K., et al., Effect of corn oil on solid-phase gastric emptying in horses. In: Proc Forum Amer Coll Vet Inter Med. 2001. 853.

29. Vervuert I, Coenen M, Factors affecting glycaemic index of feeds for horses. In: Proc Eur Equine Nutr Health Congress, 2006.

30. Valberg SJ, Velez-Irizarry D, Williams ZJ, et al. Enriched pathways of calcium regulation, cellular/oxidative stress, inflammation, and cell proliferation characterize gluteal muscle of standardbred horses between episodes of recurrent exertional rhabdomyolysis. Genes 2022;13:1853.

31. Clarkson PM, Thompson HS. Antioxidants: what role do they play in physical activity and health? Am J Clin Nutr 2000;72:637S–46S.

32. Henry ML, Wesolowski LT, Pagan JD, et al. Impact of coenzyme Q10 supplementation on skeletal muscle respiration, antioxidants, and the muscle proteome in thoroughbred horses. Antioxidants 2023;12:263.

33. Calder PC. Polyunsaturated fatty acids, inflammation, and inflammatory diseases. Am J Clin Nutr 2006;83:1505S–19S.

34. Wesolowski LTS, JL, Pagan JD, et al. Impacts of exercise and DHA/EPA/GLA supplementation on plasma cytokines in Thoroughbreds. Comparative Exercise Physiology 2022;18:S30.

35. Firshman AM, Valberg SJ, Bender JB, et al. Epidemiologic characteristics and management of polysaccharide storage myopathy in Quarter Horses. Am J Vet Res 2003;64:1319–27.
36. Valberg SJ, McCue ME, Mickelson JR. The interplay of genetics, exercise, and nutrition in polysaccharide storage myopathy. J Equine Vet Sci 2011;31:205–10.
37. McKenzie EC, Eyrich LV, Payton ME, et al. Clinical, histopathological and metabolic responses following exercise in Arabian horses with a history of exertional rhabdomyolysis. Vet J 2016;216:196–201.
38. Zhang S, Zeng X, Ren M, et al. Novel metabolic and physiological functions of branched chain amino acids: a review. J Anim Sci Biotechnol 2017;8:1–12.
39. Prince A, Geor R, Harris P, et al. Comparison of the metabolic responses of trained Arabians and Thoroughbreds during high-and low-intensity exercise. Equine Vet J 2002;34:95–9.
40. Henry ML, Velez-Irizarry D, Pagan JD, et al. The impact of N-acetyl cysteine and Coenzyme Q10 supplementation on skeletal muscle antioxidants and proteome in fit thoroughbred horses. Antioxidants 2021;10:1739.
41. Valberg SJ, Finno CJ, Henry ML, et al. Commercial genetic testing for type 2 polysaccharide storage myopathy and myofibrillar myopathy does not correspond to a histopathological diagnosis. Equine Vet J 2021;53:690–700.
42. Valberg SJ, Henry ML, Herrick KL, et al. Absence of myofibrillar myopathy in Quarter Horses with a histopathological diagnosis of type 2 polysaccharide storage myopathy and lack of association with commercial genetic tests. Equine Vet J 2023;55:230–8.
43. Williams ZJ, Velez-Irizarry D, Petersen JL, et al. Candidate gene expression and coding sequence variants in Warmblood horses with myofibrillar myopathy. Equine Vet J 2021;53:306–15.
44. Pagan J, Phethean E, Whitehouse C, et al. A comparison of the nutrient composition of European feeds used at the 2010 and 2018 FEI World Equestrian Games. J Equine Vet Sci 2019;76:86.
45. Graham-Thiers P, Kronfeld D. Amino acid supplementation improves muscle mass in aged and young horses. J Anim Sci 2005;83:2783–8.

Anesthesia and Myopathies of Horses

Douglas Castro, DVM, MSc, DSc[a],*,
Stuart Clark-Price, DVM, MS, EMBA[a,b]

KEYWORDS

- Muscle disorder • Equine anesthetic-associated myopathy
- Hyperkalemic periodic paralysis • Malignant hyperthermia

KEY POINTS

- Anesthetic drugs can influence skeletal muscle functions and with surgical stress, can potentially trigger clinical signs of muscle disorders.
- Equine anesthetic associated myopathy (EAAM) is linked to inadequate padding, improper positioning, prolonged procedures, and hypotension.
- Hyperkalemic periodic paralysis (HYPP) and malignant hyperthermia (MH) may present similar clinical signs such as fasciculation, rigidity, sweating, hyperthermia, tachycardia, hypertension, hypercapnia, and arrhythmias.
- Horses with a suspected inherited myopathy should have a diagnosis confirmed prior to any elective anesthetic event.

INTRODUCTION

Anesthesia of horses with pre-existing or developing muscle disorders poses distinctive challenges and considerations for veterinarians providing anesthesia to equine patients. Clinical signs of these disorders can be subtle, and in some instances, an intrinsic muscle disease might not have been previously diagnosed. Therefore, general anesthesia or the stress associated with a surgical procedure can potentially trigger development of clinical signs of muscle disease, which may only be observed during or after anesthesia. This unpredictability underscores the importance of thorough pre-anesthesia assessment and vigilant monitoring throughout the perioperative period to promptly address any emerging complications.

[a] Department of Clinical Sciences, Auburn University College of Veterinary Medicine, 1130 Wire Road, Auburn, AL 36849, USA; [b] College of Veterinary Medicine, 1220 Wire Road, Auburn, AL 36849, USA
* Corresponding author. Department of Clinical Sciences, Auburn University College of Veterinary Medicine, 1130 Wire Road, Auburn, AL 36849.
E-mail address: dzc0087@auburn.edu

Vet Clin Equine 41 (2025) 165–180
https://doi.org/10.1016/j.cveq.2024.11.008
0749-0739/25/© 2024 Elsevier Inc. All rights reserved, including those for text and data mining, AI training, and similar technologies.

Abbreviations	
AST	aspartate aminotransferase
CK	creatine kinase
EAAM	equine anesthetic-associated myopathy
HYPP	hyperkalemic periodic paralysis
IV	intravenous
MAP	mean arterial pressure
MH	malignant hyperthermia
NSAIDs	nonsteroidal anti-inflammatory drugs
RMP	resting membrane potential
TP	threshold potential

Anesthetic drugs exert both direct and indirect effects on skeletal muscle function, primarily through their modulation of voltage-gated ion channels. For instance, propofol, local anesthetics, and inhalant anesthetics are known to enhance sodium current decay within muscle cells, potentially leading to effects akin to those of neuromuscular blocking agents.[1,2] Additionally, anesthetic agents may impact contractile function by inhibiting cholinergic neurotransmission.[3]

While anesthetic drugs can impact metabolic and contractile functions of skeletal musculature, the foremost concern during general anesthesia in horses lies in the potential for reduced cardiac output, vasodilation, and consequent hypotension. These physiologic changes induced by anesthesia may result in decreased blood flow, particularly affecting dependent muscles under pressure. Muscles, sensitive to pressure and influenced by force-to-surface area ratios, become particularly susceptible in such circumstances. This compromised blood flow can precipitate tissue ischemia and subsequent complications.[4–9] The detailed effects of individual drugs used in premedication, induction, and maintenance of general anesthesia are outside the scope of this article and are discussed elsewhere.[10]

EQUINE ANESTHETIC-ASSOCIATED MYOPATHY

Equine anesthetic-associated myopathy (EAAM) represents a prevalent and significant skeletal muscle complication associated with general anesthesia. This condition can affect even apparently healthy horses, despite the care of experienced clinicians and within well-equipped hospital facilities.

Approximately 2 decades ago, postanesthetic myopathy accounted for roughly 7% of equine deaths.[11] However, over time, advancements in inhalant anesthetics and clinical management during anesthesia have led to a decline in the prevalence to roughly 2% of equine anesthetic deaths.[12,13] Despite the overall reduction in prevalence, EAAM continues to have elevated risk in certain procedures, such as MRI, with approximately 2.3% of cases reported,[14] and transvenous electrical cardioversion, where it has been reported in 9.2% of cases.[15] Subclinical or unrecognized EAAM occurs after anesthesia at an unknown rate; however, in one study, 50% of horses undergoing anesthesia had a postanesthetic creatine kinase (CK) activity of greater than 1000 U/L, meeting the researchers' definition of EAAM even without overt clinical signs.[16]

Pathophysiology

Factors such as inadequate padding, inappropriate limb positioning, prolonged anesthesia and/or recovery periods, inadequate blood pressure management, and hypoxemia are considered known predisposing factors for muscle injury during anesthetic events.[13,17] Additionally, large body mass may be a relevant risk factor, as evidenced by a study in which approximately 6% of draft horses under general anesthesia developed neuromuscular complications.[18]

EAAM shares striking similarities with the pressure stretch myopathy described in human literature, commonly known as "crush syndrome," induced by prolonged and continuous pressure on the limb during recumbency.[19] Resulting from sustained pressure ischemia and hypoxia, the muscle cell membrane experiences substrate depletion and a reduction in pH. This, in turn, affects the functionality of calcium, sodium, potassium, and chloride ion channels, thereby disrupting electrochemical gradients. The accumulation of sarcoplasmic and mitochondrial calcium due to dysfunctional ion pumps leads to an autolytic process and cellular damage.[19]

Intracompartmental pressure, or the pressure within fascial planes of muscle, may increase in dependent musculature in horses during prolonged recumbency such as during anesthesia. In a study investigating the infusion of autologous plasma into canine muscle, findings indicated that when intracompartmental pressure exceeds 30 mm Hg, there is an increased risk of muscle damage due to reduced blood flow.[20] Pressures surpassing this threshold have been consistently observed in dependent limbs during general anesthesia in horses across multiple studies.[21–24]

The reduction of muscle perfusion is one of the consequences of general anesthesia in horses,[25] with the dependent limb typically more affected than the upper limb. Dependent muscles demonstrate a depressed but relatively stable microflow of blood whereas upper limb muscles have a greater average microflow but a high degree variability.[26] Thus, abnormal positioning or angles of the upper limbs in relation to the trunk that impede blood flow may result in EAAM. Reduction in perfusion leads to a reduction in cellular pH in the muscle, affecting the activity of adenosine triphosphate and disrupting cellular homeostasis.[23] Reperfusion exacerbates this damage, resulting in the production of oxygen free radicals, inflammation, and edema.[19]

Numerous studies have identified the association of EAAM with hypotension, prompting suggestions to maintain mean arterial pressure (MAP) at or above 70 mm Hg.[5,16] While this measure may not entirely prevent myopathy, it is believed to reduce the clinical severity of the condition.

Clinical Presentation

Clinical presentation of EAAM typically corresponds to the location and amount of musculature that is affected. Horses in lateral recumbency commonly exhibit issues in the dependent quadriceps, triceps, and masseter muscles. Conversely, horses positioned in dorsal recumbency often develop damage to the gluteal and longissimus dorsi muscles.[27] Additionally, adductor muscles, situated proximal to the biceps femoris, can be bilaterally affected in horses placed in dorsal recumbency during prolonged anesthesia procedures. Reduced blood flow from the medial circumflex femoral artery is believed to contribute to the involvement of adductor muscles.[28]

Clinical signs related to EAAM are typically observed during recovery, although they may manifest hours after anesthetic events. Common signs include prolonged recumbency, difficulty standing, weakness or reduced weight-bearing on limbs, fasciculation, signs of distress, sweating with pain, as well as swelling and firmness of the affected musculature on palpation. In severe cases, pigmenturia (myoglobinuria) may occur.[17,27,29]

Most commonly, for horses in lateral recumbency, the triceps of the dependent limb develops the most damage. In this scenario, observations may include the inability to bear weight on the thoracic limb presenting with a "dropped elbow" appearance accompanied by signs of distress and pain (**Fig. 1**). Additionally, neuropathy or

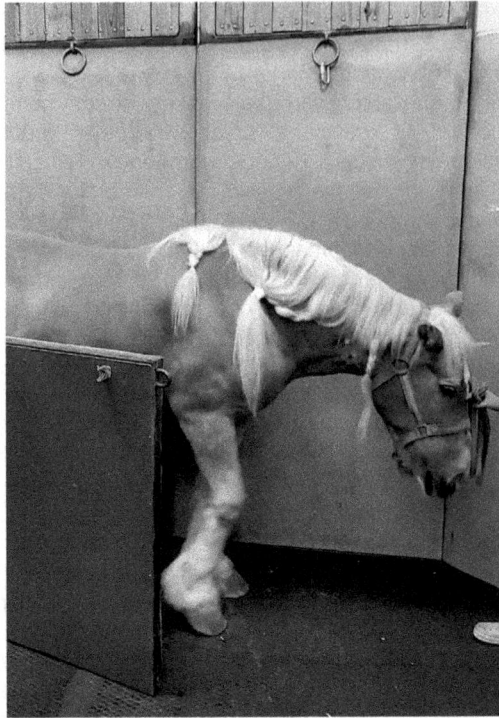

Fig. 1. A horse demonstrating inability to utilize the triceps muscle group of the right thoracic limb resulting in a "dropped elbow" appearance. This may occur from EAAM or neuropraxia of the radial nerve.

neuropraxia of the brachial or radial nerve may occur. Differentiation between muscle and nerve damage can be observed through lack of pain and swelling of the triceps muscle observed with neuropathy/neuropraxia, especially when associated with plasma CK activity within expected reference intervals.[30] However, it is important to note that a combination of both disorders can occur. Inability to stand due to weakness or pain in the pelvic limbs can be indicative of adductor or gluteal myopathy. Horses may exhibit a base-wide, crouched posture, with the pelvic limbs lower than the thoracic limbs. The horse may bear its weight on the toes of the pelvic limbs, resulting in flexion of the stifle, hocks, and fetlocks.[28] Additionally, nerves such as the sciatic and/or femoral may also be affected, and limited signs of pain are typically observed in such cases.[31] Furthermore, back pain and inability to walk can be associated with damage to the longissimus dorsi and/or gluteal muscles.

Destruction of the cellular structure of skeletal muscle, such as associated with EAAM, leads to an elevation in serum CK activity, typically showing a mild increase after anesthesia (approximately 1000–5000 U/L), followed by a significant rise over the next 24 to 48 hours.[16,17] In severe cases of myopathy, myoglobinuria may be observed, typically characterized by a dark brown or red wine coloration of urine. Aspartate aminotransferase (AST) is less volatile than CK and can provide an indication of severity of prior recent muscle damage, particularly when CK activity is declining or has normalized.[32]

Assessment of serum electrolyte concentrations is valuable in severe cases of myopathy since disturbances are common and may require correction.[10] Ultrasonographic imaging can be utilized to evaluate and monitor localized swelling, edema, and changes in muscle architecture.[33] Given the potential for progression of muscle damage, particularly in the first 24 to 48 hours, it is advisable to conduct serial measurements of biochemical variables including blood urea nitrogen, creatinine, CK, AST, serum electrolytes, and acid–base status.[10] Serial urinalysis including pH determination may be of benefit to monitor frank and occult myoglobinuria, acid–base status, and for indications of renal injury.

Treatment

In cases of suspected EAAM, it is crucial to initiate treatment promptly to alleviate pain, distress, muscle swelling, and electrolyte imbalances. Moreover, steps should be taken to mitigate potential renal damage caused by circulating myoglobin. For horses that have difficulty standing or that remain recumbent, providing support to help them obtain a standing position is a critical priority. The longer a horse remains recumbent after anesthesia, their prognosis for full recovery likely decreases; recumbency can continue to detrimentally affect muscle blood flow and the ability for clinicians to deliver effective treatment. Therefore, horses demonstrating prolonged recumbency should be encouraged to stand. Head and tail ropes may aid in recovery, but some horses may require hoisting in a sling to achieve a standing position. It may be necessary for horses to remain in a sling even after standing for support. Applying wraps to the distal limbs and removing shoes may help to minimize the risk of leg wounds in recumbent or struggling horses.

Large volume fluid therapy, preferably intravenous (IV), is recommended to minimize myoglobin pigment nephropathy via dilution and increased renal clearance. Additionally, fluid therapy will assist normalization of any electrolyte abnormalities and acid–base disturbance. In cases of blood pH less than 7.2 or urine pH less than 7.0, addition of bicarbonate to IV fluid therapy may provide benefit and may help reduce the nephrotoxicity of myoglobin.[34]

Mannitol may offer some therapeutic benefit as an osmotic diuretic to help decrease swelling and edema within muscle cells and help restore normal function.[19] However, mannitol should not be administered while pigment nephropathy is still a concern as it may increase the chances of acute renal injury.[35]

Cryotherapy with ice packs or cold water (hydrotherapy) applied to affected musculature may reduce pain and edema. Additionally, oral dantrolene 2 to 4 mg/kg every 8 to 12 hours may provide benefits for horses experiencing diffuse or severe focal rhabdomyolysis by reducing muscle spasm and stiffness and muscle necrosis related to high intracellular calcium concentration.[36]

In exceptionally severe cases, surgical fasciotomy to alleviate pressure within affected muscle compartments may be necessary. Elevated pressure in these compartments due to swelling can hinder blood flow, resulting in tissue ischemia and potential damage to peripheral nerves. Fasciotomy entails making incisions in the fascia surrounding the affected muscle compartments to release the accumulated pressure.[10]

Multimodal analgesia is recommended in cases of EAAM. While nonsteroidal anti-inflammatory drugs (NSAIDs) can be used, such as flunixin meglumine (1 mg/kg IV) or phenylbutazone (2.2 mg/kg IV), caution is advised in cases with azotemia or suspected renal compromise.[37] However, once normalization of renal status is achieved, NSAIDs should be provided. Acepromazine (0.04 mg/kg IV) is commonly utilized in cases of EAAM for anxiolytic, muscle relaxant, and vasodilator effects that may improve perfusion of affected muscle groups.[38] Acepromazine may also potentiate the effects of analgesic medications. Opioids such as morphine, hydromorphone, or butorphanol can also be employed either intermittently or as continuous rate infusions. Fentanyl patches are well tolerated in horses and result in good absorption of fentanyl systemically. Anecdotal reports indicate an antinociceptive effect in horses with inflammatory pain. However, in healthy research horses, there appears to be minimal antinociception with thermal or mechanical models of pain.[39] Adverse effects from the use of opioids include excitement, compulsive walking, reduced gastrointestinal motility, and urinary retention. Other medications that may provide analgesia include lidocaine and ketamine administered as constant rate infusions.[40]

For cases of EAAM localized to the hind limbs, placement of an epidural catheter provides a convenient method for drug delivery, requiring lower doses due to the proximity of receptors in the spinal cord (**Fig. 2**). Opioids (morphine or methadone at

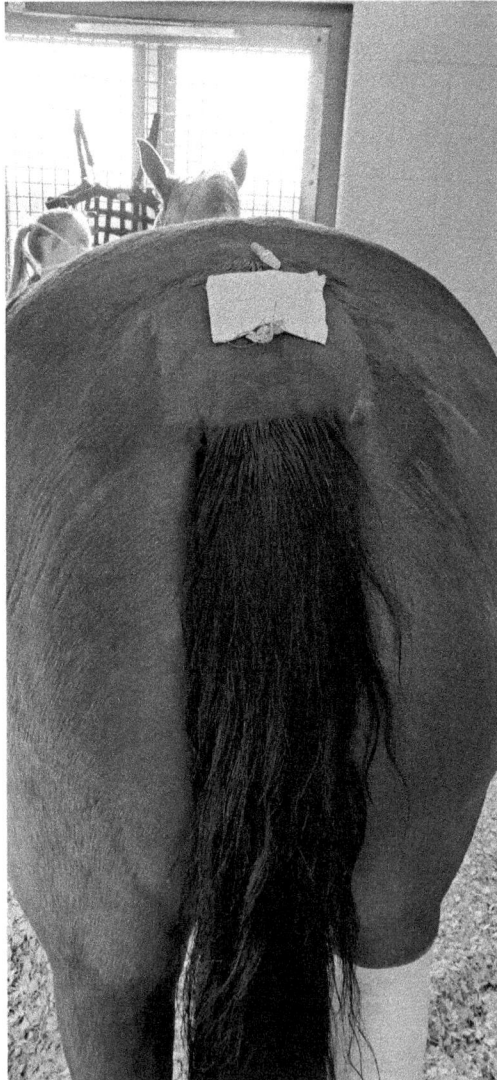

Fig. 2. An epidural catheter placed to manage pain in the pelvis and pelvic limbs.

0.1 mg/kg), often combined with alpha 2 agonists such as xylazine (0.17 mg/kg) or detomidine (20 µg/kg), can provide segmental analgesia to the pelvic limbs while minimally affecting motor function. Increasing the total volume of injection can extend analgesia to the thoracic limbs as well.[41]

Prevention

The consequences from EAAM can be devastating to a horse and its owner. Therefore, clinicians anesthetizing horses should have a primary focus on prevention of this condition. A combination of approaches should be employed to minimize the occurrence of EAAM. Ensuring adequate limb and body positioning, providing adequate padding, minimizing anesthesia duration, and effectively managing blood pressure appear to be effective strategies.[16]

Thick and soft padding should be utilized to ensure distribution of the horse's body weight across the surface, effectively reducing localized pressure on smaller areas of the body. In cases of lateral recumbency, gently pulling the dependent thoracic limb forward helps alleviate pressure on the triceps muscle and nerve bundle. Additionally, arranging the upper limbs on pads or supports in a neutral horizontal position reduces the chances for obstructed blood flow and enhances postanesthesia comfort. Similarly, during dorsal recumbency, padding can be strategically placed in the lateral region of the pelvic limbs, in contact with the biceps femoris, to minimize abduction. This precautionary measure helps prevent reduced blood flow to the adductor muscles, consequently reducing the risk of myopathy or neuropathy, as previously described. It is important to reassess the position of the horse over time, especially if anesthesia is prolonged. Typically, during recovery, horses are placed in the same lateral recumbency as on the surgery table, utilizing a thick mat or adequate padding for support. Alternatively, air mattresses, pools, and rope systems can serve as additional options to the recovery process. The dependent front limb should be pulled forward to reduce pressure on the triceps muscles as well as the radial nerve. Duration of time a horse can be expected to remain in lateral recumbency after anesthesia is dependent on many factors including length of anesthesia, procedure performed, physiologic status, administered drugs, presence of hypotension during anesthesia, and recovery environment.[42] In general, horses receiving inhalant anesthesia show signs of awakening by 30 to 45 minutes after discontinuation and make a first attempt to stand by 90 minutes.[42] Horses that are taking longer than 2 hours to make a first attempt to stand or those that have made several attempts but appear weak or unable to use one or more limbs should be further examined to identify any underlying causes.[42]

Balanced anesthesia techniques with meticulous blood pressure monitoring appear to mitigate the risk of myopathy. Typically, maintaining a MAP of at least 70 mm Hg is recommended.[9] In instances of hypotension, assessing anesthetic depth should take precedence. Clinicians should decide to increase the volume of crystalloid delivery (fluid bolus), along with considering the use of sympathomimetic agents such as dobutamine to improve MAP. Dobutamine primarily acts on $\beta 1$ receptors, enhancing cardiac contractility and thus increasing cardiac output at a dose of approximately 1.7 µg/kg/min.[43] Depending on the dose, dobutamine can affect systemic vascular resistance, potentially producing vasodilation and improving muscle perfusion.[9]

The utilization of dantrolene prior to anesthesia can serve as a preventive measure for EAAM in horses deemed at high risk of developing the condition. However, it is important to note that this drug may have adverse effects, including a decrease in cardiac output and the potential development of hyperkalemia in horses under isoflurane anesthesia and therefore monitoring of serum potassium during anesthesia is recommended in treated horses.[44]

HYPERKALEMIC PERIODIC PARALYSIS

Hyperkalemic periodic paralysis (HYPP) is a hereditary muscle disease initially described in Quarter horses, the predominant breed affected by this condition due to a prestigious ancestor carrying the trait. However, other breeds such as American Paint horses, Palominos, Appaloosas, and Quarter horse crossbreeds are also susceptible.[45]

Initial reports of HYPP in horses emerged in the 1980s detailing clinical manifestations of periodic episodes of muscle fasciculation, spasms, weakness, and occasionally recumbency, frequently accompanied by hyperkalemia.[46,47] The causative genetic mutation for HYPP is observed in approximately 4.4% of the Quarter horse population. However, its prevalence is much higher in specific groups and was reported at 55% in a genetic survey of elite Halter horses.[48] This mutation has been positively selected for because of the characteristically enhanced muscle mass observed in horses that carry it.[45]

Pathophysiology

The pathogenesis of HYPP in horses is linked to a genetic mutation within the *SCN4A* gene, responsible for encoding the alpha subunit of the voltage-gated sodium channel (NaV1.4), predominantly expressed in skeletal muscle cells.[49] In healthy horses, resting membrane potential (RMP) of skeletal muscle is typically maintained around -70 mV. However, in horses with this mutation in the sodium channel, this RMP is perturbed, decreasing to approximately -55 mV. This alteration renders the muscle cell more susceptible to depolarization as the RMP approaches the threshold potential (TP). Under normal physiologic conditions, sodium channels close upon membrane depolarization, while potassium channels open, facilitating potassium efflux for membrane repolarization. However, in HYPP affected horses, the mutated sodium channel fails to close properly after depolarization, leading to a sustained influx of sodium ions and a reduction in membrane potential. Consequently, this disruption in ion flow triggers involuntary muscle fasciculation and weakness during clinical events.[50] The intense muscle activity resulting from the disruption of sodium channels also elevates the extracellular concentration of potassium resulting in hyperkalemia. Hyperkalemia can directly affect cardiac electrophysiology by increasing the excitability of myocardial cells. This occurs through the reduction of the gradient between the RMP and TP, which can lead to serious cardiac arrhythmias.[51,52]

Clinical Presentation

Clinical episodes of HYPP typically occur during the first few years of a horse's life and are often triggered by their first episode of general anesthesia. The recovery phase of anesthesia seems to be a common time for clinical signs to be recognized in anesthetized horses.[52,53] Nonspecific signs, including prolonged anesthesia recovery and unsuccessful attempts to stand can be observed. However, severe clinical indicators such as fasciculation, rigidity, sweating, tachycardia, hypertension, hypercapnia, and cardiac arrhythmias may also occur, and may be confused with signs of malignant hyperthermia (MH).[53,54] Arrhythmias resulting from hyperkalemia can occur and require immediate intervention. Observations of the electrocardiogram during anesthesia may reveal widening and decreased amplitude of the P wave, elongation of the P–R interval and increased amplitude of the T wave.[55]

Treatment

Anesthetic events induce a stress response and may trigger HYPP in susceptible individuals. The primary concern lies in the elevation of plasma potassium concentrations

(>5.5 mEq/L), which can lead to life-threatening arrhythmias. Homozygous individuals can also develop acute upper respiratory obstruction related to laryngeal weakness. In horses that carry the HYPP gene, it is crucial to conduct frequent blood sampling to monitor serum potassium concentrations before anesthesia, during the procedure, and if necessary, during the recovery phase.[45,56] Prompt intervention is essential in cases of hyperkalemia. This may include cardiac protection with calcium gluconate, appropriate ventilation to minimize respiratory acidosis, administration of crystalloid solutions with negligible potassium concentrations, and the use of glucose, insulin, sodium bicarbonate, and diuretics to decrease plasma potassium concentrations (**Fig. 3**).

Prevention

For breeds that are predisposed to HYPP or for suspected HYPP horses, genetic testing for the causative mutation can be performed with whole blood or plucked hair samples. Additionally, testing for other genetic conditions common to Quarter horse breeds can be performed using the same sample.[48] Elective anesthesia in horses suspected or confirmed to be HYPP positive requires careful planning to minimize the potential for a clinical episode. Prior to anesthesia, horses should be placed on a low-potassium diet and given a potassium-wasting diuretic such as acetazolamide (a carbonic anhydrase inhibitor) at a dose of 2 to 4 mg/kg orally every 8 to 12 hours for at least 1 week prior to the anesthetic event.[57] Monitoring blood gases during anesthesia provides valuable information regarding ventilation status and plasma potassium concentration as well as acid–base balance. Metabolic acidosis can be a potential side effect of acetazolamide due to its inhibition of carbonic anhydrase, leading to decreased proximal tubular reabsorption of bicarbonate in the kidneys, and low pH can shift potassium out of the cell.[56] Additionally, acclimatizing the horse to the

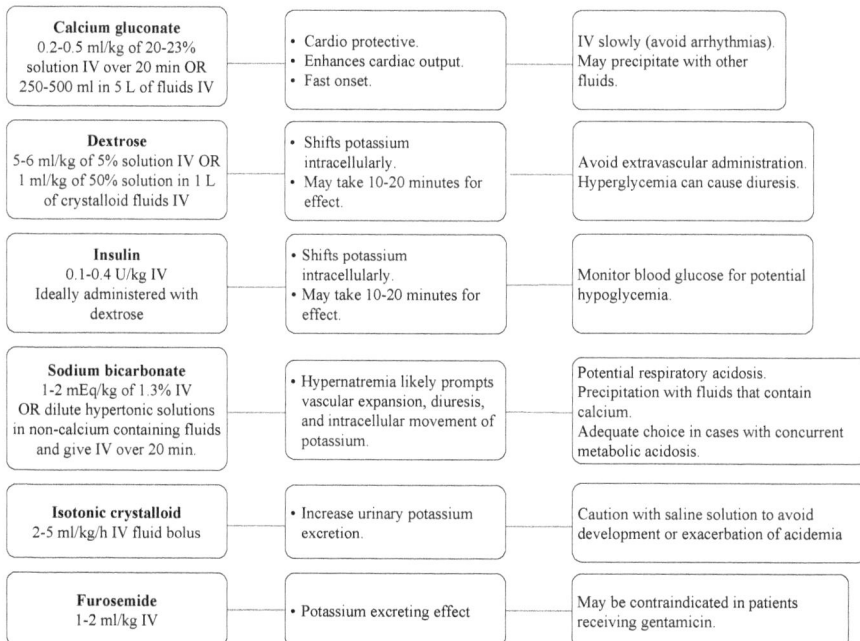

Calcium gluconate 0.2-0.5 ml/kg of 20-23% solution IV over 20 min OR 250-500 ml in 5 L of fluids IV	• Cardio protective. • Enhances cardiac output. • Fast onset.	IV slowly (avoid arrhythmias). May precipitate with other fluids.
Dextrose 5-6 ml/kg of 5% solution IV OR 1 ml/kg of 50% solution in 1 L of crystalloid fluids IV	• Shifts potassium intracellularly. • May take 10-20 minutes for effect.	Avoid extravascular administration. Hyperglycemia can cause diuresis.
Insulin 0.1-0.4 U/kg IV Ideally administered with dextrose	• Shifts potassium intracellularly. • May take 10-20 minutes for effect.	Monitor blood glucose for potential hypoglycemia.
Sodium bicarbonate 1-2 mEq/kg of 1.3% IV OR dilute hypertonic solutions in non-calcium containing fluids and give IV over 20 min.	• Hypernatremia likely prompts vascular expansion, diuresis, and intracellular movement of potassium.	Potential respiratory acidosis. Precipitation with fluids that contain calcium. Adequate choice in cases with concurrent metabolic acidosis.
Isotonic crystalloid 2-5 ml/kg/h IV fluid bolus	• Increase urinary potassium excretion.	Caution with saline solution to avoid development or exacerbation of acidemia
Furosemide 1-2 ml/kg IV	• Potassium excreting effect	May be contraindicated in patients receiving gentamicin.

Fig. 3. Treatment options, dosages, purpose, and precautions for hyperkalemia in horses.

hospital environment a few days before anesthesia can help reduce stress, which may trigger clinical signs of the disease.

MALIGNANT HYPERTHERMIA

MH is a rare and life-threatening pharmacogenetic disorder characterized by a hypermetabolic state of skeletal muscles, resulting in severe rhabdomyolysis due to excessive muscle contraction and heat production. It can be triggered by exposure to certain drugs, such as halogenated inhalation anesthetics (halothane, isoflurane, sevoflurane, desflurane, and so forth), the depolarizing muscle relaxant, succinylcholine, as well as stress and exercise. In Quarter horses specifically, MH has been linked to a mutation in the gene encoding skeletal muscle ryanodine receptor gene (RyR1).[54,58] The initial description of MH in horses dates back to 1975.[59] Since then, numerous descriptions have emerged across various breeds.[60–62] Notably, a single point mutation (C7360G) in exon 46 of the RyR1 gene was identified in 1 Quarter horse that developed the syndrome when exposed to inhalant halothane.[54] The propensity of horses carrying the genetic mutation to develop MH is unknown; however, mortality in horses that carry the gene and that develop signs under general anesthesia is reported to be extremely high.[63]

Pathophysiology

The pathophysiology of MH involves dysregulation of intracellular calcium flux, mediated in Quarter horses by a genetic defect in RyR1 receptors, which play a pivotal role in excitation-contraction coupling homeostasis. In other breeds, a causative mutation has not been demonstrated. Under normal circumstances, RyR1 receptors serve as a regulator of calcium, facilitating the release of calcium ions from the sarcoplasmic reticulum into the cytoplasm in response to electrical impulses during muscle contraction. However, in MH-susceptible individuals, there is dysfunction of the RyR1 receptor, leading to an excessive release of calcium ions into the cytoplasm. This abnormal calcium release triggers the activation of troponin C, accelerating the interaction between actin and myosin to generate sustained muscle contraction, increased metabolism, and heat production.[58,64]

Clinical Presentation

During anesthesia, the initial clinical observation includes a progressive increase in end-tidal and arterial partial pressures of CO_2 ($Paco_2$), despite aggressive controlled mechanical ventilation, which correlates with the elevation in body temperature. Additionally, signs such as tachypnea, hypertension, and tachycardia may accompany these changes. Excessive sweating, extrusion of the third eyelid, muscle rigidity, and fasciculations are also commonly observed. Notably, myoglobinuria and violent recovery have been reported in affected cases.[58,62] Hemoconcentration, hyperkalemia, hypercalcemia or hypocalcemia, hyperphosphatemia or hypophosphatemia, hyperlactatemia, hypoxemia, and mixed metabolic and respiratory acidosis, along with potential elevations in CK and AST can be observed in clinicopathological investigations. Some of these findings may only become evident in the advanced phase of MH.[63] While multiple changes can be detected in blood gas analysis prior to acute death, alterations in serum muscle enzyme activity may be imperceptible due to rapid onset of disease. Additionally, the anesthesia circuit becomes noticeably warm to the touch, and carbon dioxide absorption can be rapidly exhausted.[58] It is important to recognize that hypercarbia, elevated body temperature, and hyperkalemia can also manifest as clinical signs of HYPP, another differential for these clinical signs in horses under anesthesia.[52] The clinical presentation of MH is usually very severe with death ensuing quickly after clinical signs start. Cases where horses show hyperthermia under anesthesia and survive are therefore considered unlikely to result from MH; these horses should be examined for other conditions that can elevate body temperature.

Treatment

Early identification of clinical signs such as hypercarbia, cardiac arrhythmias, acidosis, elevation in body temperature, and muscle fasciculations under anesthesia are common in cases of MH and can occur with HYPP. Recognizing these signs early improves the chances of providing appropriate treatment, though mortality is likely in MH. Since MH is a rare condition, signs such as tachycardia and muscle fasciculations may be mistaken for a light plane of anesthesia.[34] When MH is suspected, the initial step should be to promptly discontinue halogenated anesthetics. If feasible, transition the horse to a different anesthesia machine with a breathing circuit devoid of residual halogenate anesthetic. If another anesthetic machine is not available, change the circuit and rebreathing bag and flush the machine with copious amounts of oxygen to remove as much inhalant anesthetic as possible. Once transitioned to breathing circuit free of inhalant anesthetic agent, provide mechanical ventilation with 100% oxygen while adjusting minute ventilation to help manage hypercapnia. Provide injectable anesthetics to maintain anesthesia and allow for elimination of inhalant anesthetic.[34] Emergent measures should be taken to address acid–base abnormalities and hyperkalemia, and to actively lower body temperature. Dantrolene, a direct-acting skeletal muscle relaxant, is the drug of choice in MH cases[65]; however, the availability of intravenously administered formulations that are most practical for treating anesthetized patients is limited in veterinary medicine (**Table 1**).

If the horse responds positively to the treatment intraoperatively, it should be carefully moved to a safe recovery environment and monitored for violent or prolonged recovery. To prevent trauma, a thick mat or soft pad should be utilized, and recovery assistance can be provided with ropes and head protection. After standing, a treatment plan should be implemented similar to management for EAAM.[10]

Table 1
Emergency management of suspected malignant hyperthermia in anesthetized horses

Action	Comments
Stop triggering agent	Discontinue halogenated inhalant anesthetic exposure Change the machine with another one with no residual agent in the circuit Rapidly transition to injectable anesthesia
Mechanical ventilation with 100% oxygen	Adjust the tidal volume and ventilation rate accordingly to reduce CO_2
Administration of dantrolene	Intravenous 1 mg/kg Nasogastric tube 4 mg/kg
Monitoring core body temperature and active cooling	Ice packs, alcohol bath, cool water bath, gastric lavage, cool water enema, cool intravenous crystalloid fluids, and fans
Serial blood gas analysis	Correct any substantial acid–base or electrolyte abnormalities, particularly hyperkalemia

Prevention

Suspected horses should undergo testing for both the MH and HYPP mutations due to similarities in clinical presentation.[66,67] In the event of a previous MH episode and the necessity for a second anesthesia, trigger agents should be avoided. Total intravenous anesthesia can serve as a suitable alternative in such cases. While dantrolene may be used as a premedication, there is currently no evidence that specifically describes this drug as a preventative measure for MH in horses. However, it has been highly effective for this purpose in other species and appears to reduce muscle damage in horses with exertional rhabdomyolysis and prevented muscle damage in a clinical trial where horses underwent general anesthesia with deliberately induced hypotension.[44,68]

SUMMARY

In conclusion, acquired and genetic muscle disorders can significantly impact horses under anesthesia, potentially leading to life-threatening situations if not promptly recognized and addressed, or prophylactically managed. It is imperative for clinicians working with equine anesthesia to have a thorough understanding of the pathophysiology and clinical presentation of the relevant disorders. Anticipating anesthetic complications is crucial during the anesthetic protocol, as well as knowing how to promptly identify issues, which equipment provides essential information, and how to address problems in a timely manner. By prioritizing these aspects, clinicians can enhance patient safety and improve outcomes during equine anesthesia procedures.

CLINICS CARE POINTS

- Equine anesthetic associated myopathy (EAAM) should be considered a potential problem in any horse undergoing general anesthesia.
- Proper positioning, padding, and maintaining mean blood pressure greater than 70 mm Hg reduces the risk of equine anesthetic associated myopathy (EAAM).
- Postponing elective procedures and performing genetic testing on horses with suspected inherited myopathies is recommended when appropriate.
- Anesthetic plans for horses undergoing general anesthesia should include preventative measures for development of adverse events associated with myopathies.
- Clinicians should be familiar with the clinical signs associated with development of different myopathies during anesthesia so that timely and appropriate interventions can be applied.

DISCLOSURE

None.

REFERENCES

1. Mounsey JP, Patel MK, Mistry D, et al. Protein kinase C co-expression and the effects of halothane on rat skeletal muscle sodium channels. Br J Pharmacol 1999; 128:989-98.
2. Haeseler G, Piepenbrink A, Bufler J, et al. Structural requirements for voltage-dependent block of muscle sodium channels by phenol derivates. Br J Pharmacol 2001;132:1916-24.

3. Wiklund CU, Lim S, Lindsten U, et al. Relaxation by sevoflurane, desflurane and halothane in the isolated Guinea-pig trachea via inhibition of cholinergic neurotransmission. Br J Anaesth 1999;83:422–9.
4. Trim CM, Mason J. Post-anaesthetic forelimb lameness in horses. Equine Vet J 1973;5:71–6.
5. Grandy JL, Steffey EP, Hodgson DS, et al. Arterial hypotension and the development of postanesthetic myopathy in halothane-anesthetized horses. Am J Vet Res 1987;48:192–7.
6. Serteyn D, Lavergne L, Coppens P, et al. Equine post anaesthetic myositis: muscular post ischaemic hyperaemia measured by laser Doppler flowmetry. Vet Rec 1988;123:126–8.
7. Lindsay WA, Robinson GM, Brunson DB, et al. Induction of equine postanesthetic myositis after halothane-induced hypotension. Am J Vet Res 1989;50:404–10.
8. Raisis AL, Young LE, Blissitt KJ, et al. Effect of a 30-minute infusion of dobutamine hydrochloride on hind limb blood flow and hemodynamics in halothane-anesthetized horses. Am J Vet Res 2000;61:1282–8.
9. Raisis AL. Skeletal muscle blood flow in anaesthetized horses. Part II: effects of anaesthetics and vasoactive agents. Vet Anaesth Analg 2005;32:331–7.
10. McKenzie E, Clark-Price S. Anesthetic Management for muscular conditions. In: Price Clark-, Khursheed M, editors. Equine anesthesia and co-existing disease. 1st edition. New Jersey: Wiley Blackwell; 2022. p. 159–94.
11. Johnston GM, Eastment JK, Wood JLN, et al. The confidential enquiry into perioperative equine fatalities (CEPEF): mortality results of Phases 1 and 2. Vet Anaesth Analg 2002;29:159–70.
12. Johnston GM, Eastment JK, Taylor PM, et al. Is isoflurane safer than halothane in equine anaesthesia? Results from a prospective multicentre randomized controlled trial. Equine Vet J 2004;36:64–71.
13. Dugdale AHA, Raylor PM. Equine anaesthesia-associated mortality: where are we now? Vet Anaesth Analg 2016;43:242–55.
14. Franci P, Leece EA, Brearley JC. Post anesthetic myopathy/neuropathy in horses undergoing magnetic resonance imaging compared to horses undergoing surgery. Equine Vet J 2006;38:497–501.
15. Bellei MH, Kerr C, Kimberly M, et al. Management and complications of anesthesia for transvenous electrical cardioversion of atrial fibrillation in horses: 62 cases (2002-2006). J Am Vet Med Assoc 2007;231:1225–30.
16. Duke T, Filzek U, Read MR, et al. Clinical observations surrounding an increased incidence of postanesthetic myopathy in halothane-anesthetized horses. Vet Anaesth Analg 2006;33:122–1227.
17. Ayala I, Rodríguez JM, Aguirre C, et al. Postanesthetic brachial triceps myonecrosis in a Spanish-bred horse. Can Vet J 2009;50:189–93.
18. Kraus BM, Parente EJ, Tulleners EP. Laryngoplasty with ventriculectomy or ventriculocordectomy in 104 draft horses (1992-2000). Vet Surg 2003;32:530–8.
19. Odeh M. The role of reperfusion-induced injury in the pathogenesis of the crush syndrome. N Engl J Med 1991;324:1417–22.
20. Hargens AR, Akeson WH, Mubarak SJ, et al. Fluid balance within the canine anterolateral compartment and its relationship to compartment syndromes. J Bone Jt Surg 1978;60:499–505.
21. Lindsay WA, McDonell W, Bignell W. Equine postanesthetic forelimb lameness: intracompartmental muscle pressure changes and biochemical patterns. Am J Vet Res 1980;41:1919–24.

22. Lindsay WA, Pascoe PJ, McDonell WN, et al. Effect of protective padding on fore-limb intracompartmental muscle pressures in anesthetized horses. Am J Vet Res 1985;46:688–91.
23. Norman WM, Dodman NH, Court MH. Interstitial pH and pressure in the dependent biceps femoris muscle of laterally recumbent anesthetized horses. Vet Surg 1988;17:234–9.
24. White NA, Suarez M. Change in triceps muscle intracompartmental pressure with repositioning and padding of the lowermost thoracic limb of the horse. Am J Vet Res 1986;47:2257–60.
25. Weaver BMQ, Lunn CEM, Staddon GE. Muscle perfusion in the horse. Equine Vet J 1984;16:66–8.
26. Serteyn D, Mottart E, Michaux C. Laser Doppler flowmetry: muscular microcirculation in anaesthetised horses. Equine Vet J 1986;18:391–5.
27. Clark-Price SC, Guiterrez-Nibeyro SD, Santos MP. Anesthesia case of the month. J Am Vet Med Assoc 2012;240:40–4.
28. Dodman NH, Williams R, Court RMH, et al. Postanesthetic hind limb adductor myopathy in five horses. J Am Vet Med Assoc 1988;193:83–6.
29. Friend SC. Postanesthetic myonecrosis in horses. Can Vet J 1981;22:367–71.
30. Auckburally A, Flaherty D. Recovery from anaesthesia in horses. What can go wrong? Practice 2009;31:340–7.
31. Dyson S, Taylor P, Whitwell K. Femoral nerve paralysis after general anaesthesia. Equine Vet J 1988;20:376–80.
32. Appell LH, Blythe LL, Lassen ED, et al. Adverse effects of rapid intravenous DMSO administration in horses. J Equine Vet Sci 1992;12:215–8.
33. Walmsley EA, Steel CM, Richardson JL, et al. Muscle strain injuries of the hindlimb in eight horses: diagnostic imaging, management and outcomes. Aust Vet J 2010;88:313–21.
34. Waldron-Mease E, Correlation of post-operative and exercise-induced equine myopathy with the defect malignant hyperthermia. In Proceedings, Annual Meeting of the American Association of Equine Practitioners, St. Louis, 24:1978, 95-99.
35. Somagutta MR, Pagad S, Sridharan S, et al. Role of bicarbonates and mannitol in rhabdomyolysis: a comprehensive review. Cureus 2020;14. https://doi.org/10.7759/cureus.9742.
36. McKenzie EC, Garrett RL, Payton ME, et al. Effect of feed restriction on plasma dantrolene concentrations in horses. Equine Vet J Suppl 2010;38:613–7.
37. Cook VL, Blikslager AT. The use of nonsteroidal anti-inflammatory drugs in critically ill horses. J Vet Emerg Crit Care 2015;25:76–88.
38. Norman WM, Williams R, Dodman NH, et al. Postanesthetic compartmental syndrome in a horse. J Am Vet Med Assoc 1989;195:502–4.
39. Reed RA, Berghaus LJ, Reynolds RM, et al. The pharmacokinetics and pharmacodynamics of fentanyl administered via transdermal patch in horses. Front Pain Res 2024;5:1373759. https://doi.org/10.3389/fpain.2024.1373759.
40. Sanchez LC, Robertson SA. Pain control in horses: what do we really know? Equine Vet J 2014;46:517–23.
41. Natalini CC. Spinal anesthetics and analgesics in the horse. Vet Clin N Am Equine Pract 2010;26:551–64.
42. Clark-Price SC. Recovery of horses for anesthesia. Vet Clin N Am Equine Pract 2013;29:223–42.
43. Donaldson LL. Retrospective assessment of dobutamine therapy for hypotension in anesthetized horses. Vet Surg 1988;17:53–7.

44. McKenzie EC, Concetto SD, Payton ME, et al. Effect of dantrolene premedication on various cardiovascular and biochemical variables and the recovery in healthy isoflurane-anesthetized horses. Am J Vet Res 2015;76:293–301.

45. Naylor JM. Equine hyperkalemic periodic paralysis-review and implications. Can Vet J 1994;35:279–85.

46. Cox JH. An episodic weakness in four horses associated with intermittent serum hyperkalemia and the similarity of the disease to hyperkalemic periodic paresis in man. Proc Am Assoc Equine Practitioners 1985;21:383–91.

47. Steiss JE, Naylor JM. Episodic muscle tremors in a quarter horse: resemblance to hyperkalemic periodic paralysis. Can Vet J 1986;27:332–5.

48. Tryon RC, Penedo MCT, McCue ME, et al. Evaluation of allele frequencies of inherited disease genes in subgroups of American Quarter Horses. J Am Vet Med Assoc 2009;234:120–5.

49. Naylor JM, Nickel DD, Trimino G, et al. Hyperkalaemic periodic paralysis in homozygous and heterozygous horses: a co-dominant genetic condition. Equine Vet J 1999;31:153–9.

50. Pickar JG, Spier SJ, Snyder JR, et al. Altered ionic permeability in skeletal muscle from horses with hyperkalemic periodic paralysis. Am J Physiol 1991;233–60.

51. Cannon SC, Brown RH, Corey DP. A sodium channel defect in hyperkalemic periodic paralysis: potassium-induced failure of inactivation. Neuron 1991;6:619–26.

52. Bailey JE, Pablo L, Hubbell JA. Hyperkalemic periodic paralysis episode during halothane anesthesia in a horse. J Am Vet Med Assoc 1996;208:1859–65.

53. Baetge CL. Anesthesia case of the month. Hyperkalemic periodic paralysis. J Am Vet Med Assoc 2007;230:33–6.

54. Aleman M, Riehl J, Aldridge BM, et al. Association of a mutation in the ryanodine receptor 1 gene with equine malignant hyperthermia. Muscle Nerve 2004;30:356–65.

55. Carpenter RE, Evans AT. Anesthesia case of the moth. Hyperkalemia. J Am Vet Med Assoc 2005;226:874–6.

56. Fielding L. Potassium homeostasis and derangements. In: Fielding L, Magdesian G, editors. Equine fluid therapy. 1st editoin. Ames: Wiley Blackwell; 2015. p. 27–44.

57. Haskins SC, Munger RJ, Helphrey MG, et al. Effect of acetazolamide on blood acid-base and electrolyte values in dogs. J Am Vet Med Assoc 1981;179:792–6.

58. Aleman M, Brosnan RJ, Williams DC, et al. Malignant hyperthermia in a horse anesthetized with halothane. J Vet Intern Med 2005;19:363–7.

59. Klein LV. A hot horse. Vet Anesth 1975;2:41–4.

60. Hildebrand SV, Howitt GA. Succinylcholine infusion associated with hyperthermia in ponies anesthetized with halothane. Am J Vet Res 1983;44:2280–4.

61. Klein L, Ailes N, Fackelman GE, et al. Postanesthetic equine myopathy suggestive of malignant hyperthermia. A case report. Vet Surg 1989;18:479–82.

62. Manley SV, Kelly AB, Hodgson D. Malignant hyperthermia-like reactions in three anesthetized horses. J Am Vet Med Assoc 1983;183:85–9.

63. Aleman M, Nieto JE, Magdesian KG. Malignant hyperthermia associated with ryanodine receptor 1 (C7360G) mutation in quarter horses. J Vet Intern Med 2009;23:329–34.

64. Mickelson JR, Louis CF. Malignant hyperthermia: excitation-contraction coupling, Ca^{2+} release channel, and cell Ca^{2+} regulation defects. Physiol Rev 1996;76:537–92.

65. Court MH, Engelking LR, Dodman NH, et al. Pharmacokinetics of dantrolene sodium in horses. J Vet Pharmacol Ther 1987;10:218–26.

66. Cornick JL, Seahorn TL, Hartsfield SM. Hyperthermia during isoflurane anaesthesia in a horse with suspected hyperkalaemic periodic paralysis. Equine Vet J 1994;26:511–4.
67. Pang DS, Panizzi L, Paterson JM. Successful treatment of hyperkalaemic periodic paralysis in a horse during isoflurane anaesthesia. Vet Anaesth Analg 2011;38:113–20.
68. McKenzie EC, Valberg SJ, Godden SM, et al. Effect of oral administration of dantrolene sodium on serum creatine kinase activity after exercise in horses with recurrent exertional rhabdomyolysis. Am J Vet Res 2004;65:74–9.

Traumatic Muscle Injuries

Catherine McGowan, BVSc, MANZCVSC, DEIM, Dip ECEIM, PhD, PgCertVBM, FHEA, FRCVS

KEYWORDS

- Delayed-onset muscle soreness • Exercise-induced muscle damage
- Fibrotic myopathy • Muscle strain

KEY POINTS

- Athletic horses can have exercise-induced intrinsic muscle trauma such as delayed-onset muscle soreness and muscle injury such as muscle tears.
- Presentation can range from elevation in serum muscle enzyme activities to overt lameness, and evaluation of muscles should form part of a thorough musculoskeletal examination.
- Treatment and prevention of muscle injuries are optimally performed with a veterinarian-physical therapist multidisciplinary team approach.
- Treatment strategies are usually aimed at reducing pain and restoring maximal function with protection, optimal loading, ice, and compression used rather than rest; even for higher-grade injuries, conservative reintroduction to exercise is recommended to hasten return to function.
- Prevention strategies involve stretching, warming up, and appropriate strength and skill training for the horse's athletic discipline.

INTRODUCTION

Traumatic muscle injuries can present with signs ranging from acute pain and lameness in a localized region to unexplained elevations of muscle enzymes on routine blood tests with or without poor performance. Although any horse can be exposed to external (extrinsic) muscle trauma and muscle damage during procedures such as anesthesia, most other causes of traumatic muscle disease will occur in athletic horses. These traumatic muscle injuries usually involve internal (intrinsic) trauma, and particularly occur in athletic horses exercising at higher intensities, at unaccustomed workloads or performing work requiring sudden acceleration, deceleration, and/or direction changes.

Extrinsic muscle trauma would include open or closed injury caused by impact or falls resulting in contusion or laceration. It also includes damage associated with intramuscular injections, which should not be discounted when evaluating a horse for

Department of Equine Clinical Science, The University of Liverpool, Leahurst Campus, Neston CH64 7TE, UK
E-mail address: cmcgowan@liverpool.ac.uk

Vet Clin Equine 41 (2025) 181–192
https://doi.org/10.1016/j.cveq.2024.11.009
0749-0739/25/© 2024 Elsevier Inc. All rights reserved, including those for text and data mining, AI training, and similar technologies.

muscle pain or muscle enzyme elevations. Anesthetic myopathies are covered in the Douglas Castro and Stuart Clark-Price's article, "Anesthesia and Myopathies of Horses," in this issue.[1] Therefore, this article focuses on intrinsic traumatic muscle injuries in the athletic horse.

Intrinsic traumatic muscle injuries in human athletes are well known and can be broadly divided into exercise-induced muscle damage, including delayed-onset muscle soreness (DOMS) and muscle injury, including muscle and musculotendinous tears.[2,3] Although far less studied, there is evidence that similar intrinsic traumatic muscle injuries occur in equine athletes.[4,5]

Presentation of exercise-induced muscle damage in horses is often vague. Although some horses may show overt stiffness and diffuse muscle pain on palpation, others may show poor performance, and others show no apparent clinical signs. Some horses are diagnosed following routine blood testing, where mild, unexplained elevations of creatine kinase (CK) and aspartate aminotransferase (AST) activities are recognized. Other possible causes of elevated muscle enzyme activity combined with mild generalized muscle pain including recurrent exercise-associated myopathies (see Stephanie J. Valberg's article, "Sporadic and Recurrent Exertional Rhabdomyolysis," in this issue) and nonexertional myopathies such as viral myalgia should be ruled out.[6]

Presentation of muscle injury depends on the severity and location, but often presents as lameness associated with focal intense pain in the associated muscle. Severe, high-grade injuries may present with swelling and palpable deficits in the muscle.[5]

This article discusses intrinsic traumatic muscle injuries in the horse, with review of relevant equine literature and reference to relevant literature in other species.

GENERAL RESPONSE OF MUSCLE TO INTRINSIC TRAUMA: DAMAGE AND HEALING

Unlike extrinsic or external muscle trauma, intrinsic muscle injuries result from excessive stresses or strains on skeletal muscle without direct impact.[3] Stresses can be defined as force per unit of tissue, and strains as the relative length change or deformation of muscle tissue under stress.[3,7] There are well-known risks for intrinsic muscle injuries such as the anatomy and orientation of muscles, the fiber type, and the type of exercise, in particular stress during lengthening or eccentric exercise,[3] which will be discussed. Most of what is known about muscle injury and repair has been derived from two animal models of muscle injury: eccentric contraction injury models and contusion models.[3]

The pathophysiology of muscle injury involves initial degeneration and necrosis, retraction of the ends of the myofibers, followed by infiltration of inflammatory cells, regeneration and repair, and finally remodeling, revascularization, reinnervation, and fibrosis.[8,9] In higher-grade injuries, there will be rupture of surrounding blood vessels leading to hematoma and hypoxia resulting in full fiber necrosis.[3] Muscle fibers have remarkable regenerative capacity, especially when satellite cells (a type of stem cell) can migrate from their usual site between the muscle sarcolemma and basement membrane to the site of necrosis.[9] Muscle can usually repair focal damage intrinsically via myonuclei, but requires satellite cell migration for new myofibers following full myofiber necrosis[3] (**Fig. 1**). If satellite cells are absent, repair can be characterized by the accumulation of fat and fibrous tissue instead of myofibers.[3] Basement membrane damage also results in more extensive fibrosis that can impede revascularization and reinnervation.[9] Unimpeded muscle regeneration is usually mostly complete 3 to 4 weeks after injury, but can take up to several months.[3,9,10]

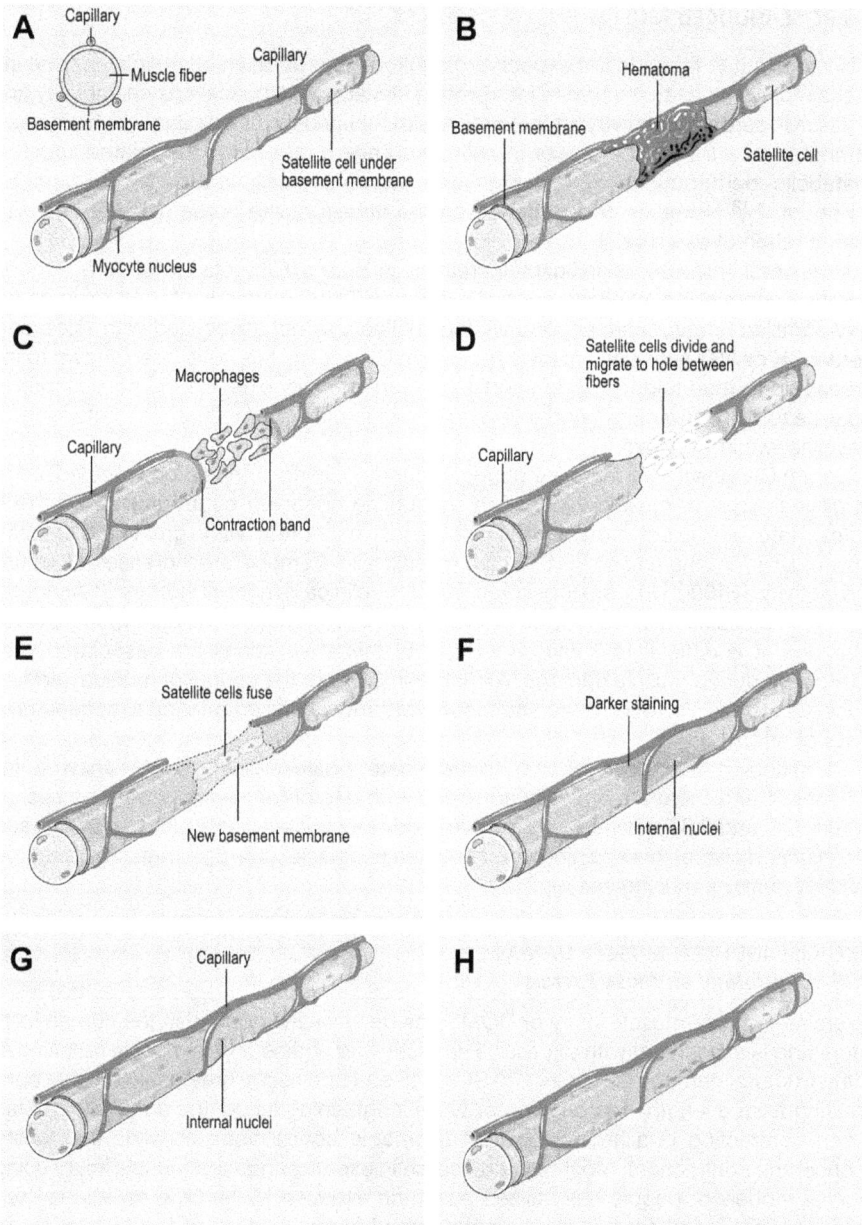

Fig. 1. Repair and regeneration in muscle following damage and disease. (*A*) Normal muscle fiber surrounded by a basement membrane that covers the occasional satellite cell together with a rich network of capillaries. (*B*) Damage causes myofiber disruption that may or may not involve the basement membrane and hematoma formation, depending on severity. (*C*) Myofiber stumps retract and the ends become plugged with the contraction band, made of sarcomeric proteins. Macrophages migrate into the (remnants of the) basement membrane cylinder within the first 24 hours and engulf and remove damaged tissue. (*D*) Satellite cells become activated (12 to 24 hours following injury), proliferate, differentiate into myoblasts and migrate to the damaged region. By days 2 to 3, satellite cells align and bridge the gap,

EXERCISE-INDUCED MUSCLE ENZYME RELEASE

It is important to factor in the expected magnitude and duration of muscle enzyme increase following exercise before interpreting elevations in muscle enzyme activity. Increases in serum CK activity after exercise without intrinsic muscle damage have been attributed to a transient increase in cell membrane permeability associated with the metabolic perturbations of exercise, and values typically return to baseline by 24 hours.[11,12] However, this depends on the fitness of the horse and the intensity and duration of exercise.

In general, clinically significant increases in serum CK activity following short-duration submaximal exercise are not expected. Trotting exercise for 40 minutes on a treadmill at 5 meters per second without incline was not associated with increased serum CK or AST activities.[13] However, serum CK activity has have been shown to increase up to threefold following short-term high-intensity exercise in Thoroughbreds on a treadmill[11] or racing[14] and following showjumping competition,[13,15] returning to baseline within 24 hours.

Serum CK activity will increase during endurance riding competition in the absence of clinical signs of muscle injury, with a doubling observed by around 20 km (12.5 miles) into an event and further increases expected with greater distances covered.[16,17] At the end of 80.5 km (50 miles), mild-to-moderate increases of serum CK activity (<4000 U/L) are observed in many clinically normal horses.[18] Although horses in these studies were apparently healthy, and without significant metabolic alterations, it is difficult to know how many of these elevations are associated with exercise-induced muscle damage. A decline in CK over the course of multiday endurance events has also been observed, potentially suggesting adaptation to consecutive days of effort.[17]

Conditioning has been shown to attenuate postexercise muscle enzyme increases,[11] and there are typically no residual effects of training in normal horses on serum CK and AST activities.[12] However, individuals can display increases caused by injury, disease, overtraining, or cumulative muscle damage that can become evident during a training season.[4,12]

EXERCISE-INDUCED MUSCLE DAMAGE
Pathophysiology and Risk Factors

Exercise-induced muscle injury or DOMS has been well-described in the human literature and is associated with excessive stresses and strains on the muscle resulting in ultrastructural damage and pain.[19,20] Stresses and strains are greatest in muscle contracting from a lengthened position or while lengthening (eccentric contraction) than when contracting in a neutral position (isometric contraction), or while shortening (concentric contraction). Most of the research in exercise-induced muscle injury using animal models or people has utilized eccentric exercise.[3] When the muscle is contracting while lengthened, it is at greater risk of injury because of the biophysics of the myosin cross-bridge interaction with actin filaments.[3] Injury is first observed as

---

fusing between the fiber stumps (*E*). The process continues over the next week as narrower, more differentiated myotubes with internally located nuclei form (*F*) followed by more mature myotubes (*G*). Nuclei return to the normal subsarcolemmal location over several months (*H*). (*Reproduced (with permission) from Piercy RJ, Rivero JL. Muscle disorders of equine athletes. In: Hinchcliff KW, Kaneps AJ, Geor RJ. Equine sports medicine and surgery: basic and clinical sciences of the equine athlete. 2nd edition. 2014:109-143.*)

a disruption in the normal striations of muscle on electron microscopy, in particular at the Z disc, often called Z-band streaming, and is greatest in type II muscle fibers, which have the narrowest and weakest Z-bands, as well as greater force production.[20,21] The disruption is concurrently associated with disruption of the intermediate filament protein, desmin, which unlinks the sarcomere from the rest of the myofiber (**Fig. 2**).[3] Inflammation follows the disruption of the sarcomeres, causing pain and elevated serum CK activity, which peaks 24 to 72 hours following the exercise bout and lasts up to 5 days.[21]

It is important to note that, despite the name, DOMS does not just cause soreness but is well established to result in a sustained loss of muscle force production capacity, which happens immediately after exercise, before the onset of muscle pain.[19] Reported decrements in force production in human athletes with DOMS are between 50% to 65% of baseline.[2,19,22] In people, force generation has also been observed to recover when muscle pain is still at its most severe.[19] Translated to the athletic horse, while mild pain may not be readily apparent, loss of force production could result in poor performance and elevated CK.

Delayed-Onset Muscle Soreness in Horses

DOMS is virtually unreported in the veterinary literature but is likely to occur in athletic horses as it does in people and animal models. In people, as bipeds, eccentric exercise is often performed as downhill running or stepping down (affecting the quadriceps muscle group). However, in quadrupeds such as the horse, each gallop stride involves a mixture of concentric and eccentric muscle contractions. Consider the lengthened position of the triceps muscles and biceps femoris on ground contact during galloping or when landing or taking off from a jump; these muscles contract to stabilize the limb while the muscles are still extended (lengthened) and then further contract to provide the force for the next stride. Unaccustomed exercise that could potentially cause

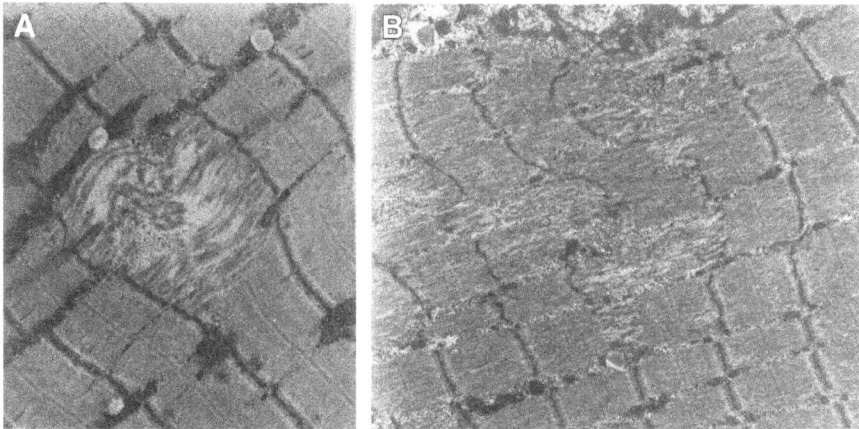

Fig. 2. Electron microscopy images of human muscle following eccentric exercise (magnification x19,000). (*A*) Focal area of disruption immediately after eccentric contractions affecting 1 sarcomere and 2 adjacent myofilaments. The myofilaments are disorganized, and there is displacement of the z-lines. (*B*) Extensive area of sarcomere disruption. (*Reproduced (with permission) from* Newham DJ, McPhail G, Mills KR, Edwards RH. Ultrastructural changes after concentric and eccentric contractions of human muscle. Journal of the neurological sciences. 1983;61(1):109-22.)

soreness can include backing (such as during training of young horses) and introduction of a new exercise such as jumping.

There have been unexplained elevations of muscle enzymes reported in 2-year-old Thoroughbreds commencing training for the first time that were hypothesized to be caused by DOMS.[4] These increases were greatest when the intensity of exercise increased (canter and galloping introduced) and were detected as increased serum activities of AST on monthly samples. Based on these data, DOMS might be occurring in horses starting a new exercise or activity, increasing in level of work effort, or exercising when compensating for lameness.

Overtraining and Cumulative Muscle Damage

Intrinsic exercise-induced muscle damage may also be associated with long-term training or overtraining. Increases in serum activities of AST have been reported in horses that were overtrained[23] and correlated with cumulative training days.[4] These increases are mild, with serum AST activity 2 to 4 times baseline values, and may be reflective of chronic low-grade cumulative muscle damage. This could also be reflective of intermittent episodes of muscle damage, either caused by changes in workload (unaccustomed exercise), or other factors such as compensation for lameness increasing recruitment of alternative muscle groups. Overtraining may also cause incoordination and susceptibility to injury, which could lead to increase stresses or strain on muscles.[23]

MUSCLE INJURY

Muscle ruptures (tears) result from excessive stresses (force per unit of tissue) and/or strains (a measure of deformation of the tissue or relative length change) that exceed the load-bearing capacity of the muscle tissue, leading to damage.[3] Muscle tears are remarkably common in human athletes, constituting approximately one-third of all injuries in soccer and football.[2] It has been shown in human athletes that risk factors for muscle tears are muscles that cross multiple joints (because of the relatively short fibers in these muscles), such as the hamstring, gastrocnemius and rectus femoris, and the presence of type II fibers.[2,3] Intrinsic muscle injury in human athletes often occurs near the musculotendinous junction but also at the origin and insertion of the muscle.[3]

The classic classification system of acute muscle injuries is[24]

1. Grade I injury (often called muscle strains) involving only a few fibers
2. Grade II injury or partial tears
3. Grade III injury or complete tears or rupture of the muscle

Other classification systems have been proposed in human athletes, taking into consideration the location of the injury, the grade, and the mechanism of the injury. In particular, it is determined if the lesion involves the muscle belly, insertion or origin, or musculotendinous junction, since injuries involving the tendinous portions often have longer recoveries and greater reccurence.[24,25] One proposed system is called the MLG-R mechanism, location, grading and reinjury for human athletes.[25] However, based on the relatively limited literature and characterization of muscle injury in horses, the traditional classification system combined with the location or structure involved is likely to be most useful.

Muscle Injury in Horses

Despite how common intrinsic muscle injury is in people, reports of muscle tears and ruptures are relatively scarce in horses.[5,26,27] This is most likely because of a lack of recognition and the difficulty in diagnosis, especially in lower grades of injury. In a retrospective study of 1,512 horses that had undergone scintigraphy of the pelvis in 1 institution over a 7-year period, 128 horses had increased radiopharmaceutical uptake, and 34 (26.6%) had uptake that involved the skeletal muscle.[28] Of these, 9 involved a focal area of uptake in the middle gluteal and in 3 the semimembranosus and semitendinosus suggestive of a discrete muscle tear.[28]

The most common muscles affected with intrinsic muscle injury in athletic horses depend on the type of exercise performed. In 1 study, 5 of the 8 cases occurred in racehorses in race training involving the gluteus medius (3 horses), gracilis (1 horse) and semitendinosus (1 horse) muscles.[5] In 1 of these cases (with a partial tear of the semitendinosus muscle), a diagnosis was only made on scintigraphy of the pelvis.[5] In another case series, 2 barrel racing horses presented with gracilis muscle tears, both occurring during turning around a barrel during competition.[27] Another study reported muscle tears causing lameness in 14 horses of a variety of breeds and disciplines, but 11 of these had a history of extrinsic trauma, and 3 of them had suspected extrinsic muscle trauma.[26] As a result, no pattern of muscle involvement was found for fore or hindlimb muscles, likely reflecting the inciting cause (extrinsic trauma).

Diagnosis of Muscle Tears in Horses

Muscle injury should be a differential diagnosis for lameness in horses, especially intrinsic injury when there is hind limb lameness in athletic horses. Careful history taking might reveal a point of onset during exercise.[27] Palpation of the hamstring muscles and medial thigh as well as the middle gluteal muscles should form part of a routine lameness assessment. DOMS is an important differential diagnosis for grade I injuries (muscle strain injury), but muscle injuries resulting in grade I tears are more localized on palpation and likely to be asymmetric. Grade II and III partial and complete muscle tears may present with localized swelling, pain, or even a palpable defect.[5,26,27] Depending on when the tear occurred, serum muscle enzyme activities may be increased; this is inconsistent, however, and in many cases increases are mild.[5,26,27]

Ultrasonography is an effective imaging technique for muscle injuries, to help confirm the presence and establish a grade, although if the injury occurs at the origin or insertion of a muscle, radiography should also be considered to help determine if there has been an avulsion fracture at the site of the injury.[26] Identification of the location of the injury, especially determining involvement of the musculotendinous junction, will aid in determining recovery times, as injuries involving this region will have longer recovery times.[25] Nuclear scintigraphy, if available, can also identify muscle tears,[5,28] and conversely, increased radiopharmaceutical uptake in the skeletal muscles of horses being investigated for lameness should prompt further investigation for intrinsic muscle injury. This might include thorough palpation, serum muscle enzyme assessment, muscle ultrasound, and potentially muscle biopsy.[5]

Fibrotic Myopathy

Despite the scarcity of reports regarding acute intrinsic muscle injury in horses, one chronic consequence, fibrotic myopathy, has been commonly reported.[29] Typically affecting the semitendinosus, semimembranosus, and gracilis muscles of Quarter Horses performing exercise involving turning and sliding stops using the hindlimbs, fibrotic myopathy produces a characteristic gait, observed during the swing phase, involving a shortened cranial phase and a rapid caudal movement of the limb during the caudal phase where the affected hindlimb appears to slap to the ground.[29] One report has documented the progression from acute muscle tear in a barrel racing

Quarter Horse to fibrotic myopathy over a 3-month period.[27] Although often reported to occur after repeated muscle injury, this report[27] followed a single severe (grade III) muscle tear, which, based on the severity of damage, likely resulted in fibrotic repair.[3]

TREATMENT OF INTRINSIC TRAUMATIC MUSCLE INJURY

Treatment of intrinsic muscle injury in horses has largely been translated from treatment of human athletes because of the limited data available for horses. Treatment is optimally performed with a veterinarian-physical therapist multidisciplinary team approach.

Exercise-Induced Muscle Damage

Following exercise-induced muscle damage, treatment strategies are usually aimed at reducing pain and restoring maximal function, but many of the treatments can also be used to prevent DOMS.[21] These include cryotherapy, stretching, nonsteroidal anti-inflammatory drugs (NSAIDS), compression, and massage.[21] Use of NSAIDS has been studied extensively in people with DOMS, both as a treatment and preventive strategy. However, there have been conflicting results, with very high doses shown to delay recovery.[21] In horses, NSAIDS should be used for analgesia as required at analgesic doses. Exercise can also be used as a treatment to reduce pain,[21] and although intense and unaccustomed exercise is not recommended, continuation of light controlled exercise and muscle loading during recovery is recommended (see Melissa R. King and Sandro Colla's article, "Muscle Rehabilitation Techniques and Prevention of Injury," in this issue).

Muscle Injury

Treatment of intrinsic muscle injury depends on the grade and location. In general, recovery is rapid with low-grade injuries, and similar principles to the treatment of DOMS can be applied. Treatment strategies in human athletes can be defined by the acronym POLICE (protection, optimal loading, ice, compression and elevation).[8] An earlier acronym RICE, with the R indicating rest, has been superseded by evidence showing early exercise therapy and progressive loading through an active approach improve recovery times.[3]

Elevation of the injury is impractical in horses, but the other components of these approaches apply. Application of ice can limit bleeding by promoting vasoconstriction, and reduces edema, swelling, and pain.[2] Ice can be applied 2 to 3 times daily during the first 3 to 5 days.[2] Where compression is practical, it can be applied to limit intramuscular blood flow into the affected area, and hence edema and swelling.[2]

There remains a lack of evidence for the optimal balance in mechanical stimuli to promote recovery, although in people, pain (or pain-free exercise) is commonly used to guide rehabilitation programs.[3] This may not be as easily translatable to the horse, especially for milder pain in the later stages of recovery that does not reliably manifest as lameness, or in horses receiving analgesic drugs, so conservative reintroduction to exercise under close observation is recommended.

Treatment programs for traumatic muscle injuries should not only include the affected muscle, but also muscles that work synergistically with that muscle to reduce the work placed on the affected muscle and protect it.[3] Timeframes for recovery of muscle injury depend on injury grade and location but a proposed timeline is

- In the acute phase (0–14 days), the primary goal is to protect the muscle, and treatment will involve stopping aggravating exercise, cryotherapy, and early gentle activation (optimal loading).

- In the repair phase (0–45 days) the goal is to promote muscle repair and avoid injury aggravation. Treatment will involve controlled and progressive return to exercise and optimal loading including strengthening and gentle stretching. Attention should be paid to sensorimotor control, including the affected muscle and activation of synergistic muscles. Physical therapists are specifically qualified to advise on muscle recruitment and activation strategies as well as motor relearning strategies as part of a multidisciplinary team.[30] Return to activities often ranges from 1 week to 3 months, although mean recovery time for higher-grade tears in 1 study was reported to be 20 weeks.[3,26]

Treatment of fibrotic myopathy is well described and involves surgical correction by means of myotomy or tenotomy of the affected muscle.[29]

PREVENTION OF TRAUMATIC MUSCLE INJURY

As for treatment of intrinsic traumatic muscle injuries, prevention of these injuries in horses has also been largely translated from human athletes. However, even translating from one muscle and location to another in the same species is questionable due to variations in morphology, function, and properties,[3] so general principles are discussed. The importance of working in a veterinarian-physical therapist multidisciplinary team approach is emphasized, with physical therapists being specifically qualified to advise on stretching and warm-up for injury prevention strategies as part of a multidisciplinary team.[31,32]

Stretching and Injury Prevention

Stretching is generally recommended before exercise[2] to prevent muscle injury, but the evidence for stretching before exercise for injury prevention remains inconclusive.[3] Part of the reason for this may be the application of stretching for different muscles and activities may require different approaches, likely even more so in the horse. Using first principles, athletic activities can be broadly separated into high-intensity stretch shortening cycles (such as jumping, rapid acceleration) and low-intensity stretch shortening cycles (such as endurance riding or marching).[31] Activities reflecting high-intensity stretch shortening cycles are more likely to result in intrinsic muscle injury, and more likely to benefit from stretching. Controlled stretching creates a more compliant musculotendinous unit which is able to store and release a high amount of elastic energy and absorb the stresses and strains associated with the activity.[31,32] The use of discipline-specific stretching in horses as a training technique and pre-event warm-up technique is highly recommended.[32]

Warming up and Injury Prevention

Warming up is also generally recommended before exercise[2] to prevent muscle injury and improve aerobic performance, but the evidence for warming up to prevent injury in people is still inconclusive.[3] Similar principles apply for warming up as for stretching, with the aim being to increase the range of motion and compliance of the musculotendinous unit before exercise.[2] Although there has been research into warming up in horses, it has had a primary focus on improvements in cardiorespiratory function and not injury prevention.

Training for Fitness (Strength, Skill and Endurance) and Injury Prevention

The mainstay of management of athletic-induced muscle injury is ensuring the horse is fit enough for the exercise it is performing, and that appropriate rest days for the discipline and level of training are incorporated into the training program. This was shown in polo horses, where exercise-induced muscle damage was associated with playing early in the season, a period of rest preceding the exercise, and where the horse was considered not being fit enough for the level of play.[33]

The evidence for muscle strengthening to improve ability to resist injury is greatest for intrinsic muscle injury prevention in people.[3] However, there is little evidence in horses. Strength training involving combinations of sets and repetitions of isolated muscle groups are not applicable to horses, as it is not possible to instruct them to perform these.[32] However, working from first principles, understanding the anatomy and biomechanics of the muscle at risk could be valuable for targeting strengthening specific muscle groups during more global strength training such as the hamstrings (semimembranosus, semitendinosus, and gracilis muscles).[30] For example, use of graded inclines and uphill exercise using poles could be used for strengthening the hamstring hind limb muscles before more skills-based training is introduced. The latter might include turning on the hindquarters and would include development of proprioception, balance, and coordination for specific tasks and should be considered for the specific exercise the horse will be undertaking.

CLINICS CARE POINTS

- Intrinsic traumatic muscle injuries can be broadly divided into exercise-induced muscle damage including DOMS and muscle injury (muscle tears).

- Muscle has a remarkable ability to regenerate without fibrosis provided the basement membrane remains intact and satellite cells can migrate to fill in a defect.

- Generalized intrinsic traumatic muscle injury, such as DOMS, can be suspected in horses presenting after unaccustomed exercise with elevated serum muscle enzyme activities (2 to 3 times baseline), mild generalized muscle soreness, and reduced performance.

- Overtraining and cumulative muscle damage can result in intrinsic exercise-induced muscle damage and remains an important differential diagnosis for unexplained elevations in muscle enzymes in horses.

- Focal intrinsic muscle injury can occur in horses ranging from grade I (rupture of a few fibers) to III (complete tear or rupture).

- Recovery is rapid with low-grade injuries, but high-grade injuries (grade III) resulting in loss of the basement membrane may lead to fibrous tissue instead of muscle regeneration, which may predispose to re-injury, noticeable defects, or contracture.

- Intrinsic muscle injury in Thoroughbred racehorses and barrel racers is most likely to involve the gluteus medius, gracilis, semimembranosus, and semitendinosus muscles.

- Muscle tears should be considered as possible causes of lameness in horses, and lameness evaluation should include palpation of all large muscle groups. Diagnosis of muscle injury is currently best supported using ultrasonography, although gamma scintigraphy can also be used.

- Treatment and prevention are optimally performed with a veterinarian-physical therapist multidisciplinary team approach, as physical therapists are specifically qualified in rehabilitation program development including proprioception techniques for muscle recruitment and activation, motor relearning strategies, appropriate application of ice and compression, and stretching and warm-up protocols.

- Treatment strategies are usually aimed at reducing pain and restoring maximal function with protection, optimal loading, ice, and compression used rather than rest even for higher-grade injuries.

- Prevention strategies involve stretching, warming up, and appropriate strength and skill training for the discipline.

DISCLOSURES

The authors have nothing to disclose.

REFERENCES

1.. Clark S, Castro D. Anesthesia and myopathies of horses. Muscle disorders of horses. St Louis, MO: Veterinary Clinics of North America: Equine Practice; 2024.
2.. Roger B, Guermazi A, Skaf A, editors. Muscle injuries in sport athletes: clinical essentials and imaging findings. Cham, Switzerland: Springer International Publishing; 2017.
3. Edouard P, Reurink G, Mackey AL, et al. Traumatic muscle injury. Nat Rev Dis Prim 2023;9:56.
4. Mack SJ, Kirkby K, Malalana F, et al. Elevations in serum muscle enzyme activities in racehorses due to unaccustomed exercise and training. Vet Rec 2014; 174:145.
5. Walmsley EA, Steel CM, Richardson JL, et al. Muscle strain injuries of the hindlimb in eight horses: diagnostic imaging, management and outcomes. Aust Vet J 2010;88:313–21.
6.. McKenzie E. Clinical examination of the muscle system. Muscle disorders of horses. St Louis, MO: Veterinary Clinics of North America: Equine Practice; 2024.
7. Tidball JG. Mechanisms of muscle injury, repair, and regeneration. Compr Physiol 2011;4:2029–62.
8.. Cianforlini M, Coppa V, Grassi M, et al. New strategies for muscular repair and regeneration. In: Canata GL, d'Hooghe P, Hunt KJ, editors. Muscle and tendon injuries. Evaluation and management. Berlin, Germany: Springer-Verlag GmbH; 2017. p. 145–53.
9.. Piercy RJ, Rivero JL. Muscle disorders of equine athletes. In: Hinchcliff KW, Kaneps AJ, Geor RJ, editors. Equine sports medicine and surgery: basic and clinical sciences of the equine athlete. 2nd edition. Amsterdam, The Netherlands: Elsevier; 2014. p. 109–43.
10. Laumonier T, Menetrey J. Muscle injuries and strategies for improving their repair. J Exp Orthop 2016;3(1):15.
11. Siciliano PD, Lawrence LM, Danielsen K, et al. Effect of conditioning and exercise type on serum creatine kinase and aspartate aminotransferase activity. Equine Vet J 1995;27(S18):243–7.
12. Harris PA, Marlin DJ, Gray J. Plasma aspartate aminotransferase and creatine kinase activities in thoroughbred racehorses in relation to age, sex, exercise and training. Vet J 1998;155(3):295–304.
13. Dos Santos VP, Gonzalez FD, da Costa Castro Jr JF, et al. Hemato-biochemical response to exercise with ergometric treadmill, mount training and competition in jumping horses. Arch Vet Sci 2015;20(Supl 1):1–8.
14. Snow DH, Mason DK, Ricketts SW, et al. Post-race blood biochemistry in Thoroughbreds. In: Snow DH, Persson SGB, Rose RJ, editors. Equine exercise physiology. Cambridge: Granata Editions; 1983. p. 389–99.
15. Assenza A, Marafioti S, Congiu F, et al. Serum muscle-derived enzymes response during show jumping competition in horse. Vet World 2016;9:251–5.
16. Williams CA, Kronfeld DS, Hess TM, et al. Antioxidant supplementation and subsequent oxidative stress of horses during an 80-km endurance race. J Anim Sci 2004;82(2):588–94.

17. McKenzie EC, Esser MM, Payton ME. Serum biochemistry changes in horses racing a multiday endurance event. Comparative Exercise Physiology 2014;10(4): 215–22.

18. Wilberger MS, Mckenzie EC, Payton ME, et al. Prevalence of exertional rhabdomyolysis in endurance horses in the Pacific Northwestern United States. Equine Vet J 2015;47(2):165–70.

19. Newham DJ, Jones DA, Clarkson PM. Repeated high-force eccentric exercise: effects on muscle pain and damage. J Appl Physiol 1987;63(4):1381–6.

20. Newham DJ, McPhail G, Mills KR, et al. Ultrastructural changes after concentric and eccentric contractions of human muscle. J Neurol Sci 1983;61(1):109–22.

21. Cheung K, Hume PA, Maxwell L. Delayed onset muscle soreness: treatment strategies and performance factors. Sports Med 2003;33:145–64.

22. Coratella G, Varesco G, Rozand V, et al. Downhill running increases markers of muscle damage and impairs the maximal voluntary force production as well as the late phase of the rate of voluntary force development. Eur J Appl Physiol 2024;124:1875–83.

23. Tyler-McGowan CM, Golland LC, Evans DL. Haematological and biochemical responses to training and over training. Equine Vet J 1999;30:621–5.

24.. Maffulli N, Aicale R, Tarantino D. Classification of muscle lesions. In: Canata GL, d'Hooghe P, Hunt KJ, editors. Muscle and tendon injuries, Evaluation and management. Berlin, Germany: Springer-Verlag GmbH; 2017. p. 95–103.

25. Valle X, Alentorn-Geli E, Tol JL, et al. Muscle injuries in sports: a new evidence-informed and expert consensus-based classification with clinical application. Sports Med 2017;47:1241–53.

26. Cullen TE, Semevolos SA, Stieger-Vanegas SM, et al. Muscle tears as a primary cause of lameness in horses: 14 cases (2009–2016). Can Vet J 2020;61(4):389.

27. Dabareiner RM, Schmitz DG, Honnas CM, et al. Gracilis muscle injury as a cause of lameness in two horses. J Am Vet Med Assoc 2004;224(10):1630–3.

28. Davenport-Goodall CL, Ross MW. Scintigraphic abnormalities of the pelvic region in horses examined because of lameness or poor performance: 128 cases (1993–2000). J Am Vet Med Assoc 2004;224(1):88–95.

29. Noll CV, Kilcoyne I, Vaughan B, et al. Standing myotomy to treat fibrotic myopathy: 22 cases (2004-2016). Vet Surg 2019;48(6):997–1004.

30. McGowan CM, Hyytiäinen HK. Muscular and neuromotor control and learning in the athletic horse. Comparative Exercise Physiology 2017;13(3):185–94.

31. Hampson B, Stubbs NC, McGowan CM. Stretching for performance enhancement and injury prevention in animal athletes. Veterinarian 2005;12:35–9.

32. Goff L. Equine sports medicine and performance management. In: McGowan CM, Goff L, editors. Animal physiotherapy: assessment, treatment and rehabilitation of animals. 2nd edition. West Sussex, UK: John Wiley & Sons; 2016. p. 329–46.

33. McGowan CM, Posner RE, Christley RM. Incidence of exertional rhabdomyolysis in polo horses in the USA and the United Kingdom in the 1999/2000 season. Vet Rec 2002;150(17):535–7.

Muscle Rehabilitation Techniques and Prevention of Injury

Melissa R. King, DVM, PhD*, Sandro Colla, DVM, MSc

KEYWORDS

- Muscle • Injury • Horse • Rehabilitation • Prevention

KEY POINTS

- Muscle repair is divided into 3 phases: inflammatory, regenerative, and remodeling.
- Focal acute muscle injuries can be treated with anti-inflammatories, specific targeted therapeutic exercises, and different modalities such as ice, laser, therapeutic ultrasound, and pulsed electromagnetic field therapy.
- Chronic muscle injuries are frequently addressed with therapeutic exercises, physical activities, and neuromuscular electrical stimulation.
- Injury prevention includes adequate warm-up before exercise and appropriate conditioning and fitness.
- Tools such as elastic resistance bands, Pessoa training aids, ground poles, limb weights, tactile devices, and proprioceptive balance pads can be helpful in muscular strengthening.

INTRODUCTION

Muscle disorders in horses are relatively common and can be caused by traumatic events, cyclic fatigue, or genetic and/or endocrine disorders. This article will focus on muscular rehabilitation strategies and injury prevention, as therapeutic exercises, diagnostics, traumatic muscle disorders, and genetic diseases are discussed individually in the other articles of this issue.

Mechanism of Injury

External forces

Muscle injuries can be caused by direct trauma resulting in contusion, strain, or laceration. Direct trauma caused by a sudden, heavy, or strong compressive force is called

Department of Clinical Sciences, College of Veterinary Medicine and Biomedical Sciences, Colorado State University, Colorado State University Veterinary Teaching Hospital, Equine Orthopaedic Research Center, 2250 Gillette Drive, Fort Collins, CO 80523, USA
* Corresponding author.
E-mail address: Melissa.king@colostate.edu

Vet Clin Equine 41 (2025) 193–211
https://doi.org/10.1016/j.cveq.2024.11.010
0749-0739/25/Published by Elsevier Inc.

Abbreviations	
BFR	blood flow restriction
COM	center of mass
DME	dynamic therapeutic exercises
FES	functional electrical stimulation
HILT	high-intensity laser therapy
NMES	neuromuscular electrical stimulation
NO	nitric oxide
PTA	Pessoa training aid
SDF	superficial digital flexor muscle
TENS	transcutaneous electrical nerve stimulation

a contusion. Most commonly contusions in horses are caused by kicks, bites, and falls. Lacerations through the skin can cause direct partial or total disruption of muscle tissue.

Internal forces

Muscle strains are more often related to excessive, forced, and frequently abrupt changes in muscle length that can be acute or chronic. A muscle cramp is characterized by repetitive nerve firing that generates a muscle contraction or fasciculation. Mild cases are usually self-limiting, but moderate to severe cramps can be treated with a number of rehabilitation therapies. Hydration and acid-base imbalances should be considered as possible triggering causes, especially in endurance horses.[1]

Muscle atrophy or hypotrophy can be present focally, in 1 or a group of adjacent muscles, or generalized. Focal atrophies can be related to neurogenic causes (nerve impingement, protozoal myelitis, polyneuropathy, and chronic pain) and myogenic causes (pain and poor saddle fit). Generalized muscle atrophy conditions are frequently related to inadequate nutrition/malabsorption disorders (vitamin E responsive myopathy and equine motor neuron disease), genetic causes (immune-mediated myositis and type 1 polysaccharide storage myopathy homozygotes), and endocrinologic causes (pituitary pars intermedia dysfunction and equine metabolic syndrome).[1]

Focal Muscle Pain

Muscle contusions, strains/tears, and lacerations are associated with local inflammation and vascular damage, frequently resulting in localized hemorrhage. Muscle swelling due to the inflammatory process and hemorrhage contained within the myofascia can result in compartment syndrome, which increases pain and results in inadequate blood flow and lymphatic drainage.

Irrespective of the initial cause, if the muscle injury is not appropriately addressed, it can lead to chronic muscle loss, contracture, fibrosis, and dystrophic mineralization.[1]

Classification of Muscle Injury

Muscle injuries can be classified according to their causes, as traumatic (acute) or overuse (chronic) injuries. They can also be classified as mild (first degree), moderate (second degree), or severe (third degree) according to their severity, determined by physical examination and diagnostic imaging (ultrasound, MRI). First degree muscle injuries are defined as strains or contusions represented by tearing of minimal muscle fibers with minor swelling and discomfort accompanied by negligible loss of strength or ability to mobilize. Second degree injures involve a greater degree of muscle fiber damage with a clear loss of function (inability to contract). A third degree injury is characterized by muscle fiber tearing across the entire cross-section of the muscle, which results in complete loss of muscle function (**Fig. 1**).[2]

Process of Muscle Repair

Regardless of the cause of muscle injury, the skeletal muscle repair process involves 3 major phases that function in a coordinated, overlapping fashion starting with the degenerative/inflammatory phase and progressing to the regenerative/fibrosis and remodeling phases. The muscle cell membranes are responsible, among other functions, for controlling the flow of ions between the intracellular and extracellular space.[3] After an injury, the cellular influx, especially of calcium, causes activation of destructive cellular proteases and inhibition of mitochondrial respiration, which leads to additional cell damage and apoptosis, contributing to an extended degenerative phase.[3] After the injury, platelets, neutrophils, and macrophages migrate to the region over a period of 5 days and initiate the inflammatory phase.[3] The regenerative phase is accompanied by an increase in growth factors and satellite cell activation, division, and differentiation into myotubes and myofibers followed by neovascularization and reinnervation.[3] Often, the fibrotic phase occurs simultaneously with the regenerative phase, thus appropriate management and rehabilitation will dictate the rates between functional regeneration and limiting fibrosis.[3]

MUSCLE REHABILITATION TECHNIQUES
Approach to Rehabilitation

The objective of a well-designed rehabilitation program targets shifting the muscle-repair process toward regeneration versus fibrosis, accelerating the recovery time, avoiding recurrence, and promoting return to full athletic performance. Rehabilitation (wheel exercise) after induced muscle injury in rats was associated with a 17% improvement in maximal isometric torque and a 13% increase in the weight of the injured muscle in comparison with the sedentary control group.[4] Given the similarities in muscle structure and function across species, it is reasonable to expect that rehabilitation, including active exercises, would also benefit equine athletes. An appropriate rehabilitation program for muscle disorders in horses should consider the muscle or groups of muscles involved, the cause, type, and classification of the injury, and the specific individual's future athletic demands.

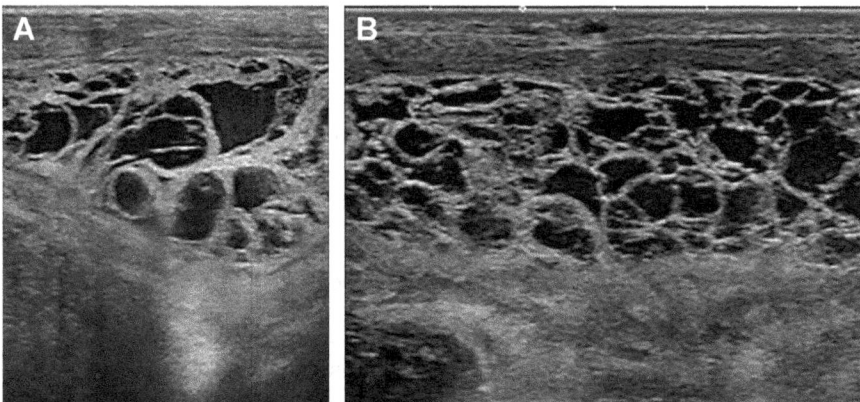

Fig. 1. Ultrasound image of severe muscle tearing within the medial aspect of the right semimembranosus muscle. Note the trabecular pattern due to hemorrhage and inflammatory process. (*A*) Caudal aspect, (*B*) medial aspect (left is lateral or proximal).

Staging of Rehabilitation

Identification of the phase of the reparative process is mandatory for an adequate rehabilitation program design. This information can be obtained from history, physical examination, and diagnostic imaging modalities.[5]

Bayer and colleagues (2017) in a randomized controlled trial involving 50 amateur athletes with acute-muscle strain injury (60% thigh and 40% calf muscles) investigated the effect of early (2 days after injury) versus delayed (9 days after injury) rehabilitation that consisted of static stretching, isometric loading with increasing resistance, and functional exercises combined with heavy strength training. The authors found that the interval between injury and pain-free recovery, as well as injury and return-to-sport, was shorter in the early rehabilitation group without a significant increase in the risk of subsequent injury.[6,7]

For didactic purposes this article divides rehabilitation recommendations into the inflammatory, regenerative, and remodeling phases. However, the overlapping of the phases and individual responses should be considered and frequent reassessments of the patient are strongly recommended.

INFLAMMATORY PHASE REHABILITATION

The acute inflammatory phase of a muscle injury lasts approximately 5 to 10 days depending on the extent of damage and the presence of compartment syndrome. It is characterized by cardinal inflammatory signs, such as focally increased temperature, pain, swelling (edema and hemorrhage), bruising, and reduction in function and mobility. Considering the similarities in muscle composition and physiology, the treatment for horses can follow, with appropriate translation, the most recent human protocol for rehabilitation of an acute muscle injury termed *POLICE* (protection, optimal loading, ice, compression, and elevation).[8] In horses, protection and optimal loading can be achieved with stall rest and progressive, slow, controlled walking sessions, pending the animal's comfort level throughout the inflammatory phase. Elevation and immobilization are techniques rarely possible or recommended for horses with muscle injuries.

Inflammatory Phase Pain Modulation

Cryotherapy
Cryotherapy (ice) should be instituted right after the injury and continued until the acute inflammatory signs resolve. The therapeutic effects of cold therapy are generated through reducing tissue temperatures to 10° to 15°C (50–59 °F).[9] Tissue cooling produces peripheral vasoconstriction and decreases soft-tissue perfusion, which can reduce edema formation and swelling at the site of tissue injury. Cold therapy also mitigates tissue metabolism and apoptosis, inhibits the effect of inflammatory mediators, and abates local enzymatic activity.[10] The application of cold also serves as a form of pain modulation by decreasing nerve conduction velocities in local sensory neurons and by activating descending inhibitory pathways.[11] Cold therapies can penetrate up to 1 to 4 cm in depth, which is dependent on local circulation and adipose tissue thickness.[12] Human studies have documented the analgesic benefits of cryotherapy with a 15 to 20 minute application providing pain relief for 1 to 2 hours.[13,14] Cold therapy for regions within the axial skeleton or for regions inaccessible to ice water immersion may benefit from the application of ice packs or cold packs, use of circulating cryotherapy units without concurrent compression, ice frozen in paper cups, or icing blankets.[11] Optimal duration and frequency of cold therapy are yet to be defined, but a general recommendation is to apply cryotherapy for 20 to 30 minutes every 2 to

3 hours during the first 48 hours after an acute injury and then 2 to 3 times a day for 10 to 14 days post-injury.

Pharmaceuticals
Pain management is critical in this phase and should be cautiously monitored. The use of non-steroidal anti-inflammatory drugs such as systemic phenylbutazone and flunixin meglumine, and topical diclofenac are recommended in the first few days after injury, but they can negatively impact long-term tissue healing.[3,15] Other medications such as muscle relaxants (dantrolene and methocarbamol) and analgesics (gabapentin, pregabalin, acetaminophen, and opioids) can be considered but should be used cautiously to avoid ameliorating the protective effects of pain.

Therapeutic modalities
Transcutaneous electrical nerve stimulation. Transcutaneous electrical nerve stimulation (TENS) can be used as a non-invasive method of pain modulation. TENS uses electrical currents applied via surface electrodes to preferentially stimulate peripheral nerves.[16] The mechanism of pain relief is thought to be through the stimulation of inhibitory interneurons at the spinal cord level or the release of endogenous endorphins within the central nervous system.[16] The *conventional mode* TENS setting is frequently used for more acute pain with a higher frequency (>100 Hz) and lower pulse duration (50 μs), which is thought to modulate pain through the gate control theory (modulation of sensory input from the skin before it evokes pain perception and response).[16] Pain modulation with the conventional TENS mode will be relatively short in duration once the electrodes have been removed. The *acupuncture like mode* TENS setting is used for more chronic pain with a lower frequency (<20 Hz) but a longer pulse duration (200 μs) and relieves pain via release of endogenous opioids, and pain mitigation may persist for 1 to 2 hours.[16] In humans, there is a moderate evidence to support TENS as an effective treatment for managing pain.[17] While there is no evidence of the effectiveness of TENS use in horses, there may be some overlap in the mechanisms of action, clinical indications, and effects reported for electroacupuncture.[18]

TENS units are typically applied for 30 minutes, 2 to 3 times daily. The placement of the electrodes can be on or around the painful region (or associated dermatomes, myotomes, or sclerotomes) over the spinal cord segments that innervate the painful region, or over trigger points. The further apart the electrodes are placed on the equine body, the deeper the penetration. The hair coat may need to be clipped depending on length, but should be cleaned from dirt and debris, wet down, and ample coupling gel applied. For the purpose of pain modulation following muscular injury the authors prefer to place the electrodes over the appropriate spinal cord segments utilizing the chronic pain settings (low frequency/long pulse duration) (**Fig. 2**).

Laser therapy. High-intensity laser therapy (HILT) has become an increasingly popular therapy for the rehabilitation of various equine musculoskeletal injuries. This form of laser therapy is used to treat an impressive assortment of human musculoskeletal conditions ranging from traumatic muscle and overuse injuries to compartment syndrome and neuropathic pain.[19,20] Research in other species demonstrates anti-inflammatory, analgesic, cellular proliferative, and hemodynamic effects. Laser therapy is thought to create photobiomodulation of cellular aerobic respiration and thus can have beneficial effects throughout the stages of injury.[21] The light energy is absorbed at a subcellular level that leads to an increase in ATP production, stabilizing the cell membrane, increasing DNA activity, and the synthesis of RNA and proteins.[21,22] Although not all mechanisms are clearly understood, laser therapy is used as a noninvasive procedure to stimulate cell regeneration, increase angiogenesis,

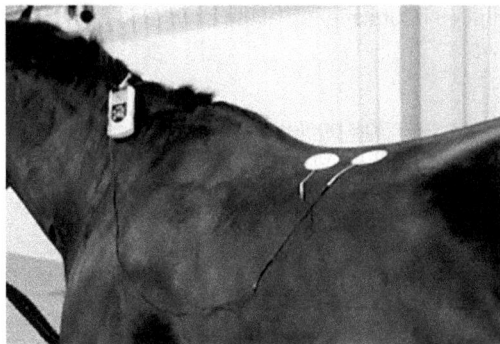

Fig. 2. Transcutaneous electrical stimulation applied on the left thoracic region.

decrease inflammation and myonecrosis, and modulate pain.[23] Laser therapy has also been shown to accelerate tissue healing by improving fibroblast function, enhancing local microcirculation, and oxygen supply, as well as improving collagen fiber alignment within tissues.[24] Human in-vitro and clinical studies demonstrate laser therapy reduces the production of the inflammatory cytokines PGE_2 and TNFα.[23] Laser irradiation of equine bone marrow-derived mesenchymal stem cells exposed to 1064 nm wavelength irradiation with an energy density of 9.77 J/cm^2 and a mean output power of 13.0 W resulted in significant upregulation of IL-10 and VEGF expression.[25] An experimental model of muscle strain in rats demonstrated that laser therapy was effective in improving functional recovery in association with a decrease in inflammatory markers (COX-1, COX-2 and PGE_2,[26]). These investigations provide scientific rationale for the use of HILT to improve the quality of muscle repair tissue, which may in turn reduce the rate of re-injury and improve overall return-to-function.

As with other physical modalities, the exact light wavelength, dosage, and treatment frequency needed for optimal treatment of select muscle injuries or disorders is largely unknown. The effect that occurs in the tissue depends on the wavelength (600–1000 nm) and power that is used, as well as the absorption potential of the tissue itself. Additional treatment parameters to consider include light source delivery as continuous or pulsed, power of the light source (in mWatts or Watts), beam irradiance, duration of treatment per site, tissue or site treated, and the calculated delivered dosage (Joules/treatment site).

Pulsed electromagnetic field therapy. Similar to laser therapy there are many published reviews in humans regarding the efficacy of pulsed electromagnetic field (PEMF) therapy devices to influence tissue repair and modulate pain. PEMF therapy is created when an electrical current is driven through a coiled wire that generates a magnetic field. The magnetic field creates small currents within the target tissue, resulting in various biologic effects. This therapy has been reported to increase microvessel vasomotion, arteriovenous Po_2 difference, number of open capillaries, arteriolar and venular flow volume, as well as to enhance flow rate of red blood cells within the targeted microcirculatory area.[27,28] Improvements in blood flow lead to increases in tissue perfusion, metabolic activity, and muscle relaxation, thereby facilitating cellular repair and diminishing nociception. A number of research studies have demonstrated that exposure to electromagnetic fields upregulates several signaling pathways related to metabolism, circulation, inflammation, and vascular tone.[29] In particular, various PEMF devices have produced a significant increase in the production of nitric oxide (NO) following treatment.[29–31] In addition to its role in stimulating vasodilation,

NO has been associated with reduced inflammatory gene expression, reduction in programmed cell death, and enhanced circulation.[30,31] These outcomes in tissue responses are consistent with reductions in pain, stiffness, and improved function that have been observed clinically in human and canine patients.[32-38] A recent study investigating the use of bio-electromagnetic energy regulation therapy on horses with clinically diagnosed thoracolumbar epaxial muscle pain demonstrated significant improvements in mechanical nociceptive thresholds at all spinal segments tested.[39] This PEMF device also demonstrated significant gains in spinal flexibility and improvements in postural control.[39] Therefore PEMF devices may represent a medication free bio-solution for the management of muscular pain and repair in horses.

Elastic therapeutic tape. Application of elastic therapeutic tape for horses is often used for the management of focal swelling, edema and pain, reduction of myofascial restriction, and for the purposes of improving proprioception and neuromotor control. The mechanism by which the tape potentially affects various physiologic systems is through the ability to interact with the skin and associated cutaneous receptors. Application of the tape to the haired skin is thought to enhance cutaneous proprioceptive stimulation, which increases the activation of alpha motor neurons and timing of associated muscle groups. A functional MRI study conducted in people demonstrated that when elastic therapeutic tape is applied while conducting knee range-of-motion exercises, alterations in muscle activation are appreciated, as well as increases in regional brain perfusion in areas related to motor control and coordination.[40] Additional nociceptive and local tissue fluid dynamic *lifting* mechanisms are considered to be involved in pain modulation and improving edema or lymphatic drainage. When an injury occurs to the skin or underlying muscle, swelling ensues, compressing the lymphatic vessels and local vasculature, as well as compressing nerve endings, causing pain. When elastic therapeutic tape is applied there is a lifting action of the skin and fascia, which *decompresses* the region allowing drainage of fluid away from the injured area, especially in regions in which compression bandaging is not possible (**Fig. 3**). Decreasing swelling and decompressing the region also reduces nerve compression and consequently pain. Pavsek and colleagues demonstrated that in horses with naturally occurring thoracolumbar epaxial muscle pain, the application of elastic therapeutic tape at 30% tension results in significantly improved nociceptive thresholds compared to a control tape application.[41] Unfortunately, there are few controlled clinical trials that clearly assess the efficacy of this form of rehabilitation.[42] Anecdotally, horses seem to respond well to the application of elastic tape suggested by improvements in nociception, edema, proprioception, neuromotor control, stride length, and symmetry of gait patterns.

REGENERATIVE PHASE REHABILITATION

The regenerative phase overlaps the inflammatory phase, and its duration is directly related to the type and extent of the injury, as well as compliance with and response to the treatments. The POLICE principles should be gradually discontinued and substituted by more dynamic exercises. Anti-inflammatory therapies can be discontinued or carefully tailored for each individual patient. Modalities that involve deep tissue heating or those that increase muscle activation and strength can be initiated during this phase and those utilized in the inflammatory phase may be continued (**Table 1**).

Regenerative Phase Thermal Therapy

The topical application of heat increases local circulation, increases tissue extensibility, and induces muscle relaxation and therefore reduces muscle spasms and

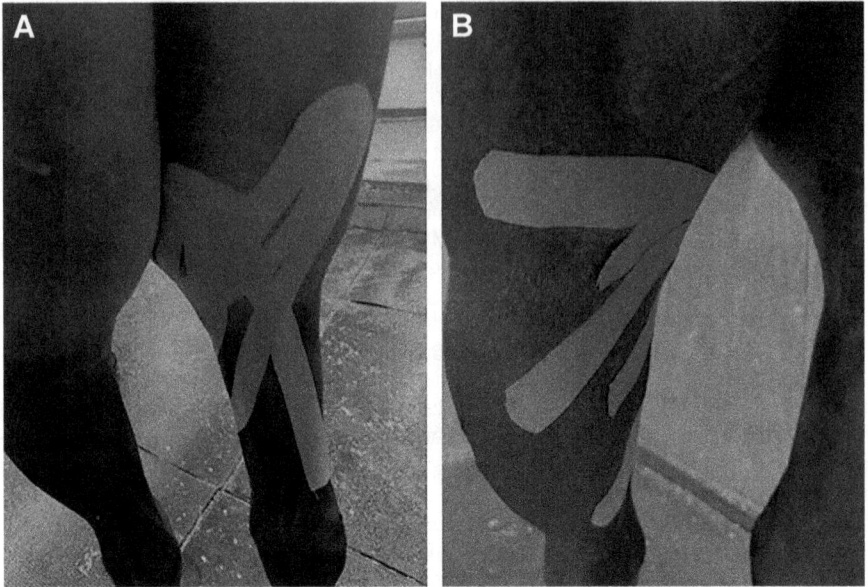

Fig. 3. (*A*, *B*) Elastic therapeutic tape application used to enhance lymphatic drainage, decrease edema, and modulate pain to the right hindlimb after an acute semimembranosus muscle injury.

associated pain. Increased local blood flow mobilizes tissue metabolites and increases tissue oxygenation and the metabolic rate of cells and enzyme systems. Within the clinical setting, the most profound physiological effects of heat occur when tissue temperatures are raised to 40° to 45°C.[43,44] Tissue temperatures above 45°C (113°F) may result in pain and tissue damage. Heat decreases tissue viscosity and increases tissue elasticity, thus facilitating stretching exercises within the rehabilitation setting. Low-load, prolonged stretching of tissues heated between 40° and 45°C results in increased extensibility of tendons, joint capsules, and muscles.[43,44]

Heat is best applied after acute inflammation has subsided. Mechanisms of action for thermal therapies are linked to the depth of penetration and the method used for heating. Superficial heating sources usually penetrate the skin and subcutaneous

Table 1			
Potential therapies to target each phase of skeletal muscle healing			
Modality	Inflammatory Phase	Regenerative Phase	Remodeling Phase
Cryotherapy	√		
Laser Therapy	√	√	√
TENS	√		
Therapeutic Ultrasound Pulsed	√	√	√
Therapeutic Ultrasound Continuous		√	√
PEMF	√	√	√
Elastic therapeutic tape	√	√	√
Radiofrequency diathermy		√	√
Blood flow restriction		√	√

tissue up to a depth of 1 to 2 cm. Deep thermal modalities (eg, therapeutic ultrasound) can rapidly increase tissue temperatures by greater than 4°C at 3 to 5 cm tissue depths. Methods of applying superficial heat in horses include topical hot packs or compresses and circulating warm water heating wraps. For deeper tissues, such as muscle, 15 to 30 minutes is required to elevate tissue temperature to the therapeutic range. When using heat sources warmer than 45°C (ie, chemical hot pack), the sources must be wrapped in several layers of moist towels before application. Heat from these sources is usually applied for 20 to 30 minutes. Although clinical effectiveness for superficial heating in the horse is yet to be demonstrated, it is often recruited in both the training and rehabilitation settings prior to exercise using mounted heating lamps (Solarium).

Radiofrequency diathermy

Human physiotherapists commonly use radiofrequency diathermy units or therapeutic ultrasound in order to heat tissues at deeper depths. Radiofrequency diathermy uses electromagnetic radiation and can be applied for thermal or non-thermal effects. However, a meta-analysis in humans suggested that diathermy's most significant effects on pain and muscle performance were mainly related to its thermal effects,[45] which include increasing cellular metabolism, local vasodilation, increasing the pain threshold, and reducing muscle spasms.[45] Radiofrequency diathermy has been used in humans for conditions such as frozen shoulder,[46] knee osteoarthritis,[47] and cervical and lower back pain with improved pain levels. No studies on the heating ability of diathermy have been performed in horses and a randomized, placebo-controlled study conducted in horses with neck pain, stiffness, and muscle hypertonicity was not able to demonstrate any significant improvement in the functional outcome variables that were assessed.[48] The use of radiofrequency diathermy was ineffective in reducing neck pain and dysfunction using the manufacturer recommended protocols.[48] The ability of this modality to provide a deep heating affect, as well as the specific clinical applications and effective treatment parameters need further investigation in the horse.

Therapeutic ultrasound

Therapeutic ultrasound machines have the capability to produce pulsed or continuous ultrasound emissions to penetrate soft tissues up to 5 cm depth. Pulsed ultrasound waves have non-thermal therapeutic effects, which include increased cellular function, enhanced proliferation of fibroblasts, and increased vascularity.[49] Continuous therapeutic ultrasound waves have deep thermal effects on tissues, which include increased tissue blood flow, enzyme activity, collagen synthesis and extensibility; and decreased pain.[50] In general, pulsed therapeutic ultrasound is used in acute inflammatory conditions where deep heating is contraindicated, and continuous ultrasound is indicated in chronic conditions when deep heating would be beneficial in reducing pain, increasing muscle relaxation, and improving soft tissue extensibility. In humans, therapeutic ultrasound has been widely used for muscle and ligament strains, tendinopathies, osteoarthritis, joint contracture, calcific tendonitis, superficial and chronic wounds, and chronic pain syndromes.[50] In horses, temperature changes in both tendon and muscle have been reported during therapeutic ultrasound application.[51] The superficial digital flexor tendon can be heated to a therapeutic temperature using treatment intensities of 1.0 W/cm^2 and 1.5 W/cm^2 with a 3.3 MHz transducer. A non-therapeutic increase in epaxial musculature temperature of 1.3°C was reported at a depth of 1.0 cm, 0.7°C at 4.0 cm, and 0.7°C at an 8.0-cm tissue depth, respectively, using an ultrasound frequency of 3.3 MHz and an intensity of 1.5 W/cm^2.[51] While tissue temperature changes have been reported in horses, there are currently no studies which demonstrate the clinical efficacy of therapeutic ultrasound. Treatment application is usually performed for 10 to 14 days, once to twice daily. Recommendation is to use immediately prior to range-of-motion or stretching exercises. The potential heating of the tissues will quickly dissipate with 50% of heat loss occurring within the first 10 minutes. For deeper penetration, use a 1 MHz probe (3–5 cm depth of penetration) versus a 3 MHz probe that will only penetrate 1 to 2 cm. Application of heat prior to stretching in people does provide added benefits to stretch related gains appreciated both acutely and sustained.[52]

Regenerative Phase Modality Application

In addition, to the aforementioned inflammatory phase modalities that can be continued into the regenerative phase to promote repair of the tissues, one must also consider how to combat the rapid declines in regional and global muscular strength associated with injury and the prescribed rest period.

Neuromuscular electrical stimulation

Neuromuscular electrical stimulation (NMES) uses a low-level electrical current that, through stimulation of the alpha motor neurons, allows recruitment and muscle contraction after orthopedic or neurologic injury. NMES therapy has been successfully used by human physiotherapists to increase muscle strength, maintain muscle mass during prolonged periods of immobilization, and control edema after injury. This therapy assists neuromuscular function by enhancing the force capacity, or the ability of the muscle to contract, as compared with a true strengthening of the muscle. It is unclear if the role of electrical stimulation in improving muscle function is actually related to increased muscle strength, improved voluntary contractions, restoring motor control, or possibly due to proprioceptive activation within injured or atrophied myofascial tissues.[53,54] The combination of electrical stimulation and exercise has been reported to be effective in alleviating pain and improving voluntary activation in human osteoarthritis patients, but it did not enhance muscle strength or functional performance.[54] The use of NMES can also aid in the reduction of edema and swelling as the direct current drives the charged plasma protein ions within the interstitial spaces to move in the direction of the oppositely charged electrode, facilitating movement into the lymphatic channels.

The difficulty in applying this modality to the horse is the lack of standardized protocols and no validated treatment programs due to large variations in methodology that include treatment parameters, the frequency and duration of treatment, the disease stage and severity, and patient selection. NMES is typically conducted 3 to 5 times a week, inducing 8 to 15 contractions within a treatment session. The electrodes are placed in a bipolar fashion with the muscle at resting length or slightly lengthened at the time of electrode placement. The rest cycle should be 5 to 6 times as long as the contraction, typically in a 1:6 ratio. The hair coat may need to be clipped depending on length, but it should be cleaned from dirt and debris, wet down, and coupling gel applied.

Blood flow restriction training

Low-load exercise training with blood flow restriction (BFR) has transformed how human physical therapists circumvent muscle loss secondary to orthopedic injury, and conditioning experts are utilizing it to maintain peak muscular strength in the absence of damaging loads. This technique uses a specialized tourniquet to temporarily reduce blood flow to an exercising limb. In essence, BFR is being used to increase strength via low-intensity training to a level typically only achieved with mid to high-intensity training. BFR training is being safely used as a progressive clinical rehabilitation tool in the process of return to heavy-load exercise for a variety of human conditions including knee osteoarthritis, soft tissue injuries, and geriatric sarcopenia.[55–58] BFR training is being utilized by equine veterinarians as a rehabilitative aide in selected cases with significant orthopedic injury and subsequent exercise restriction (**Fig. 4**). Even in absence of the ability to safely ambulate, applying intermittent BFR pressure to the limb has been demonstrated to evoke a strong metabolite accumulation that then stimulates beneficial downstream cell signaling pathways that accelerate tendon healing.[59] Accelerated healing in response to BFR training is attributed to the accumulation of key metabolites, specifically pyruvate, lactate, alanine, and succinate.[60] Increases of these metabolites in particular have been implicated as beneficial in muscle regeneration and muscle protein synthesis, giving credence to their pivotal role in improved muscular strength and function with incorporation of BFR.[61,62] Accumulation of succinate and lactate alters beneficial downstream muscle protein synthesis signaling pathways, while alanine and glutamine are markers of muscle catabolism.[60–62] Equine investigations demonstrate that short-term use of BFR (daily for 10 days) significantly increases mitochondrial density and ability to oxidize fuels within the superficial digital flexor muscle (SDF) of the treated limb.[62,63] In addition, prolonged use of BFR (daily for 56 days) had no negative impacts on mechanical strength of the SDF tendon and did not result in forelimb dysfunction.[63,64] Muscle injury and the associated decrease in exercise leads to dramatic declines in muscular strength and function, regardless of primary injury. BFR training may be an additional tool to strengthen supporting musculature and accelerate healing with less intensive exercise.

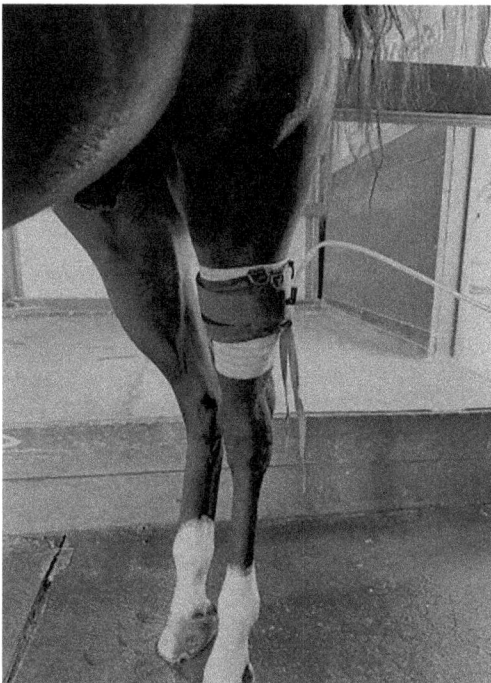

Fig. 4. Blood flow restriction system applied on the left hindlimb.

REMODELING PHASE REHABILITATION

This phase targets a progression of proprioception, muscle use, range-of-motion, muscular strength, and cardiovascular fitness. The addition of various exercises or increased intensity, duration, and frequency of currently prescribed exercises are based on the stability of repair, stage of healing, and ongoing reassessment of patient's ability. Strengthening exercises are incorporated in this phase aiming to restore full muscle function and prevent persistent scar formation. Manual therapies and progression of the earlier discussed therapeutic exercises are essential in this phase of recovery guiding the remodeling of the tissue along the physiological planes of loading and re-establishing mechanical strength and function.

PREVENTION OF MUSCLE INJURY/RE-INJURY

Muscle injury in horses usually occurs either because of a traumatic event (fall and slip) or due to inappropriate exercise activity, such as inadequate warm-up, insufficient training, fatigue, or pre-existing underlying diseases. Specific pathologies in horses are correlated with local muscle atrophy, such as thoracolumbar epaxial muscles in horses with spinous process impingement and gluteus medius atrophy in horses with sacroiliac pain. Efforts to rebuild a strong and functional musculature can be considered one of the key strategies to prevent musculoskeletal injuries and injury recurrence.[65]

Warm-up

Prior to training exercise, a program that involves a *warm-up period* designed to increase blood flow and neuromuscular firing likely decreases the incidence of muscle injuries or re-injury. Muscles can be warmed up with stretching exercises (sternal lifts, lumbosacral tucks, forelimb/hindlimb protraction, and retraction), dynamic mobilization exercises (neck flexion and lateral bending), and focally with heat therapy (hot packs and continuous therapeutic ultrasound). The beginning of the physical activity should be a slow walking session, if under saddle, with a long and low head and neck frame, which can progress to the addition of ground pole exercises, use of tactile stimulators, circles, and different gaits, depending on the individual's fitness and status of the musculature.[66] Exercise is the most potent stimulator of increased core and muscle temperatures.

Conditioning/Resistance/Controlled Exercise

Conditioning the horse or a specific muscle involves progressing increments in workload, in order to increase fitness and ability to perform the intended use, maximizing performance, and maintaining soundness. Any exercise activity should be controlled to avoid excessive overload of unconditioned tissue, and the longer the muscle has been in disuse, the slower and more progressive the conditioning program should be.

Active Assisted Exercises/Tools

Therapeutic exercises discussed earlier can also be used as methods to facilitate changes in limb range-of-motion, neuromotor and proprioceptive development, as well as coordination.

Considering the multifidus muscle is a major stabilizer of the thoracolumbar spine, several physiotherapy approaches, such as dynamic therapeutic exercises (DME) and neuromuscular electrical stimulation (NMES), are indicated for increasing the cross-sectional area of the muscle. A study comparing DME and NMES approaches over a 7-week period showed an increase of 18.7% and 13.4% in the multifidus cross-sectional area after NMES and DME, respectively.[67]

Dynamic mobilization exercises, also known as carrot-baited stretches, consisted of 3 cervical flexions, 1 cervical extension, and 3 lateral bending exercises with 5 repetitions each, 5 days per week for 3 months. This protocol was shown to promote an increase in multifidus cross-sectional area at the levels of T10, T12, T14, T16, T18, and L5 bilaterally.[68] Therapeutic Exercises for Rehabilitation of Muscle Injury by King and Colla in the article of this issue.

Elastic resistance bands are suggested to promote proprioceptive feedback during locomotion, increasing core and hindlimb muscle activity, and consequently improving dynamic stability. A study evaluating the effect of the Equiband® system in a 4-week training (lunge at trot) program showed that the use of the bands reduced mediolateral and rotational movements of the thoracolumbar region at trot.[69] Another study evaluating the effect of the Equiband® system on the multifidus via electromyography showed a reduction in muscle work and peak activity in the thoracolumbar region when using the system compared to without in horses trotting with or without passing over ground poles.[70] A detailed physical examination and an understanding of the stage of rehabilitation are important to better implement the use of this system.

Another system called Pessoa training aid (PTA), which involves ropes and pulleys, and also used in lunge line exercises, was evaluated with high-speed motion capture and inertial measurement units and showed a significant reduction in speed, stride length, head angle, and lumbosacral angle at maximal hindlimb retraction. During use of the PTA system, the highest point of the horse became the neck crest rather than the poll, and dorsoventral displacement of the thoracic spine was greater. It was concluded that the PTA system may improve posture and gait during work and stimulate core musculature.[71]

Therapeutic Modalities

Muscle atrophy due to aging is a consequence of decreased innervation, as well as changes in the distribution of muscle diameter and fiber type. The incorporation of functional electrical stimulation (FES) in horses increases longissimus dorsi muscle mitochondrial density and distribution, as well as increases mean muscle fiber size. Multifidus muscle asymmetry within the thoracolumbar region significantly improved after 8 weeks of FES treatment, compared to no effects in the control group.[72] The use of FES is reported to reduce or reverse muscle decline in aging horses and in those unable to perform physical activities.[73–76]

Postural Stability

Postural stability is necessary to maintain balance and to stabilize and protect the spinal column. Static and dynamic balance control is essential in order to provide a stable platform from which to execute voluntary movements of the axial and appendicular skeleton.[76,77] In addition, postural stability provides the ability to respond appropriately to the numerous destabilizing forces that can occur during functional movement, thereby reducing the chances of injury.[78,79] The evaluation of postural stability during quiet standing has emerged in both the human and equine fields for the evaluation and monitoring of neuromuscular disorders. In both humans and animals, the body establishes static balance by maintaining the center of mass (COM) over the base of support.[80] To accomplish this balance, there is integration of sensory and neuromuscular systems through visual, proprioceptive, and vestibular pathways.[80] The integration of these systems and pathways allows the body to make small adjustments in muscle activity, resulting in slight movements of the COM. These oscillations are known as adjustments in postural sway and are the product of the interplay between the destabilizing forces acting upon the body and the compensatory actions of the postural control system.[81] Disorders that interfere with any component of the postural control system will therefore influence the characteristics of postural sway and affect the body's ability to effectively respond to balance perturbations. The reduced efficiency has consequences in terms of increased postural sway, impaired reaction times, and dysfunctional motor performances.[81] Human athletes that incorporate core balance exercises into their rehabilitation programs are significantly less likely to suffer re-injury during a 12-month period following injury, compared to those individuals with similar injuries that did not emphasize core strength.[82] Horses enrolled in a rehabilitation program for 12 weeks that involved exercises aimed at increasing core strength, improving neuromuscular control and balance (proprioceptive balance pads, dynamic mobilization exercises, aquatic therapy) demonstrated significant increases in the cross-sectional area of the thoracolumbar multifidi muscle at all levels evaluated.[83] In addition, the direct force platform measurement of changes in center of pressure displacement demonstrated profound improvements in postural control and proprioceptive acuity when specifically challenged with conditions requiring increased proprioceptive input for maintaining equilibrium.[83] These findings suggest that an exercise program that includes core strengthening exercises helps improve spinal muscle characteristics and postural stability.

SUMMARY

Muscle injuries are common and can affect horses of all ages, breeds, and physical activity levels. A precise diagnosis based on physical examination and the use of appropriate imaging modalities is fundamental to develop an adequate rehabilitation program. The understanding of the pathophysiology of muscle injury and the phases of the repair process helps to target specific needs for the tissue phase of healing. Prevention of muscle injury or recurrence of a previous injury is another challenge in equine training programs and after a rehabilitation program. Warming up the muscles before exercise is a critical factor in muscle injury prevention. This can be achieved through therapeutic exercises and with the use of therapeutic modalities. Slow and gradual progress in the conditioning of the muscle is strongly recommended and should be guided by individual responses to previous treatments and previous increments of workload. Increasing the multifidus cross-sectional area and, consequently, improvements in postural stability is one of the strategies used to prevent muscle injuries. Effective skeletal muscle repair is unlikely to be achieved from a single intervention; for full functional recovery there is a need to control inflammation, stimulate regeneration, and limit fibrosis.

CLINICS CARE POINTS

- Understanding muscle injury pathophysiology and phases of the repair process is fundamental to develop a proper rehabilitation protocol.
- A critical aspect of a successful rehabilitation program is the appropriate selection of interventions, such as therapeutic modalities and exercises, to target each phase of muscle recovery.
- Proper warm-up and conditioning of the muscles, associated with improvement of postural stability, are key factors in muscle injury prevention.

DISCLOSURES

The authors have nothing to disclose.

REFERENCES

1. Valberg SJ. Muscle conditions affecting sport horses. Vet Clin N Am Equine Pract 2018;34(2):253–76.
2. Järvinen TAH, Järvinen TLN, Kääriäinen M, et al. Muscle Injuries: optimising recovery. Best Pract Res Clin Rheumatol 2007;21(2):317–31.
3. Piercy RJ and Rivero JLL, Muscle disorders of equine athletes, In: Hinchcliff KW, Kaneps AJ, Geor RJ, van Erck-Westergren E, editors. *Equine sports medicine and surgery [Internet]*, 2014, W.B. Saunders; Philadelphia, PA, 109–143. Available at: https://linkinghub.elsevier.com/retrieve/pii/B9780702047718000077 (Accessed 27 July 2024).
4. Aurora A, Garg K, Corona BT, et al. Physical rehabilitation improves muscle function following volumetric muscle loss injury. BMC Sports Sci Med Rehabil 2014; 6(1):41.
5. Haussler KK, King MR, Peck K, et al. The development of safe and effective rehabilitation protocols for horses. Equine Vet Educ 2021;33(3):143–51.
6. Bayer ML, Magnusson SP, Kjaer M, et al. Early versus delayed rehabilitation after acute muscle injury. N Engl J Med 2017;377(13):1300–1.
7. Bayer ML, Hoegberget-Kalisz M, Jensen MH, et al. Role of tissue perfusion, muscle strength recovery, and pain in rehabilitation after acute muscle strain injury: a randomized controlled trial comparing early and delayed rehabilitation. Scandinavian Med Sci Sports 2018;28(12):2579–91.
8. Bleakley CM, Glasgow P, MacAuley DC. PRICE needs updating, should we call the POLICE? Br J Sports Med 2012;46(4):220–1.
9. Petrov R, MacDonald MH, Tesch AM, et al. Influence of topically applied cold treatment on core temperature and cell viability in equine superficial digital flexor tendons. Amer J Vet Research 2003;64:835–44.
10. Algafly AA, George KP. The effect of cryotherapy on nerve conduction velocity, pain threshold and pain tolerance. Br J Sports Med 2007;41:365–9.
11. Sluka KA, Christy MR, Peterson WL, et al. Reduction of pain-related behaviors with either cold or heat treatment in an animal model of acute arthritis. Arch Phys Med Rehabil 1999;80:313–7.
12. Brosseau L, Rahman P, Toupin-April K, et al. A systematic critical appraisal for non-pharmacological management of osteoarthritis using the Appraisal of Guidelines Research and Evaluation II Instrument. PLoS One 2014;9:e82986.
13. Sanchez-Inchausti G, Vaquero-Martin J, Vidal-Fernandez C. Effect of arthroscopy and continuous cryotherapy on the intra-articular temperature of the knee. Arthroscopy 2005;21:552–6.
14. Guillot X, Tordi N, Mourot L, et al. Cryotherapy in inflammatory rheumatic diseases: a systematic review. Expet Rev Clin Immunol 2013;10:281–94.
15. Duchesne E, Dufresne SS, Dumont NA. Impact of inflammation and anti-inflammatory modalities on skeletal muscle healing: from fundamental research to the clinic. Phys Ther 2017;97(8):807–17.
16. Goff LS. Equine therapy and rehabilitation. In: McGowan CM, editor. Animal physiotherapy; assessment, treatment and rehabilitation of animals. Oxford: Blackwell Publishing Ltd; 2007. p. 239–50.

17. Law PP, Cheing GL. Optimal stimulation frequency of transcutaneous electrical nerve stimulation on people with knee osteoarthritis. J Rehabil Med 2004;36(5): 220–5.

18. Shmalberg J, Xie H, Memon MA. Horses referred to a teaching hospital exclusively for acupuncture and herbs: a three-year retrospective analysis. J Acupunct Meridian Stud 2018;12(5):145–50.

19. Dundar U, Turkmen U, Toktas H, et al. Effect of high-intensity laser therapy in the management of myofascial pain syndrome of the trapezius: a double-blind, placebo-controlled study. Laser Med Sci 2015;30:325–32.

20. Alayat MS, Mohamed AA, Helal OF, et al. Efficacy of high-intensity laser therapy in the treatment of chronic neck pain: a randomized double blinded placebo-control trial. Laser Med Sci 2016;31(4):687–94.

21. Basford JR. Low intensity laser therapy: still not an established clinical tool. Laser Surg Med 1995;16:331–42.

22. Barboza CA, Ginani F, Soares DM, et al. Low-level laser irradiation induces in vitro proliferation of mesenchymal stem cells. Einstein (Sao Paulo) 2014;12(1):75–81.

23. Min KH, Byun JH, Heo CY, et al. Effect of low- level laser therapy on human adipose-derived stem cells: in vitro and in vivo studies. Aesthetic Plast Surg 2015;39(5):778–82.

24. Iacopetti I, Perazzi A, Maniero V, et al. Effect of MLS laser therapy with different dose regimes for the treatment of experimentally induced tendinopathy in sheep: pilot study. Photomed Laser Surg 2015;33(3):154–63.

25. Peat FJ, Colbath AC, Bentsen LM, et al. In vitro effects of high-intensity laser photobiomodulation on equine bone marrow-derived mesenchymal stem cell viability and cytokine expression. Photomed Laser Surg 2018;36:83–91.

26. De Paiva Carvalho RL, Leal-Junior EC, Petrellis MC, et al. Effects of low-level laser therapy (LLLT) and diclofenac (topical and intramuscular) as single and combined therapy in experimental model of controlled muscle strain in rats. Photochem Photobiol 2013;89:508Y12.

27. Klopp RC, Niemer W, Schmidt W. Effects of various physical treatment methods on arteriolar vasomotion and microhemodynamic functional characteristics in case of deficient regulation of organ blood flow. Results of a placebo-controlled, double-blind study. J Compl Integr Med 2013;10:S39–41.

28. Klopp RC, Niemer W, Schulz J. Complementary-therapeutic stimulation of deficient autorhythmic arteriolar vasomotion by means of a biorhythmically physical stimulus on the microcirculation and the immune system in 50-year-old rehabilitation patients. J Compl Integr Med 2013;10:S29–37.

29. Gaynor JS, Hagberg S, Gurfein BT. Veterinary applications of electromagnetic field therapy. Res Vet Sci 2018;119:1–8.

30. Bogdan C. Nitric oxide and the immune response. Nat Immunol 2001;2:907–16.

31. Calabrese V, Mancuso C, Calvani M, et al. Nitric oxide in the central nervous system: neuroprotection versus neurotoxicity. Nat Rev Neurosci 2007;8:766–75.

32. Gyulai F, Raba K, Baranyai I, et al. BEMER therapy combined with physiotherapy in patients with musculoskeletal diseases: a randomised, controlled double blind follow-up pilot study. Evid base Compl Alternative Med 2015;1–8. https://doi.org/10.1155/2015/245742.

33. Thomas AW, Graham K, Prato FS, et al. A randomized, double-blind, placebo-controlled clinical trial using a low- frequency magnetic field in the treatment of musculoskeletal chronic pain. Pain Res Manag 2007;12(4):249–58.

34. Berna t SI. Effectiveness of pentoxifylline and of bio- electromagnetic therapy in lower limb obliterative arterial disease. Orv Hetil 2013;154(42):1674–9.

35. Piatkowski J, Kern S, Ziemssen TJ. Effect of BEMER magnetic field therapy on the level of fatigue in patients with multiple sclerosis: a randomized, double-blind controlled trial. J Alternative Compl Med 2009;15(5):507–11.

36. Piatkowski J, Haase R, Ziemssen TJ. Long-term effects of Bio-electromagnetic-energy regulation therapy on fatigue in patients with multiple sclerosis. Alternative Ther Health Med 2011;17(6):22–8.

37. Zidan N, Fenn J, Griffith E, et al. The effect of electromagnetic fields on postoperative pain and locomotor recovery in dogs with acute, severe thoracolumbar intervertebral disc extrusion: a randomized placebo-controlled, prospective clinical trial. J Neurotrauma 2018;35(15):1726–36.

38. Sullivan MO, Gordon-Evans WJ, Knap KE, et al. Randomized, controlled clinical trial evaluating the efficacy of pulsed signal therapy in dogs with osteoarthritis. Vet Surg 2013;42:250–4.

39. King MR, Seabaugh KA, Frisbie DD. Effects of a bio-electromagnetic energy regulation blanket on thoracolumbar epaxial muscle pain in horses. J Equine Vet Sci 2022;111:103867.

40. Callaghan MJ, McKie S, Richardson P, et al. Effects of patellar taping on brain activity during knee joint proprioception tests using functional magnetic resonance imaging. Phys Ther 2012;92(6):821–30.

41. King MR, Pavsek H, Ellis KL, et al. Effects of elastic therapeutic tape on thoracolumbar epaxial muscle pain in horses. J Equine Rehabilitation 2024;2:100007. ISSN 2949-9054.

42. Molle S. Kinesio taping fundamentals for the equine athlete. Vet Clin N Am Equine Pract 2016;32:103–13.

43. Miklovitz SL. Thermal agents in rehabilitation. 2nd edition. Philadelphia: FA Davis Co; 1996.

44. Hayes KW. Conductive heat. In: Hayes KW, editor. Manual for physical agents. East Norwalk, NJ: Appleton and Lange; 1993.

45. Beltrame R, Ronconi G, Ferrara PE, et al. Capacitive and resistive electric transfer therapy in rehabilitation: a systematic review. Int J Rehabil Res 2020;43(4):291–8.

46. Lopez-de-Celis C, Hidalgo-García C, Pérez-Bellmunt A, et al. Thermal and non-thermal effects off capacitive-resistive electric transfer application on the Achilles tendon and musculotendinous junction of the gastrocnemius muscle: a cadaveric study. BMC Musculoskelet Disord 2020;21(1):46.

47. Clijsen R, Leoni D, Schneebeli A, et al. Does the application of tecar therapy affect temperature and perfusion of skin and muscle microcirculation? a pilot feasibility study on healthy subjects. J Alternative Compl Med 2020;26(2):147–53.

48. Parkinson SD, Zanotto GM, Maldonado MD, et al. The effect of capacitive-resistive electrical therapy on neck pain and dysfunction in horses. J Equine Vet Sci 2022;117.

49. Tascioglu F, Kuzgun S, Armagan O, et al. Short-term effectiveness of ultrasound therapy in knee osteoarthritis. J Int Med Res 2010;38:1233–42.

50. Rutjes AW, Nuesch E, Sterchi R, et al. Therapeutic ultrasound for osteoarthritis of the knee or hip. Cochrane Database Syst Rev 2010;CD003132.

51. Montgomery L, Elliott SB, Adair HS. Muscle and tendon heating rates with therapeutic ultrasound in horses. Vet Surg 2013;42:243–9.

52. Nakano J, Yamabayashi C, Scott A, et al. The effect of heat applied with stretch to increase range of motion: a systematic review. Phys Ther Sport 2012;13(3):180–8.

53. Lewek MD, Rudolph KS, Snyder-Mackler L. Quadriceps femoris muscle weakness and activation failure in patients with symptomatic knee osteoarthritis. J Orthop Res 2004;22:110–5.

54. Elboim-Gabyzon M, Rozen N, Laufer Y. Does neuromuscular electrical stimulation enhance the effectiveness of an exercise programme in subjects with knee osteoarthritis? A randomized controlled trial. Clin Rehabil 2012;27:246–57.

55. Yow BG, Tennet DJ, Dowd TC, et al. Blood flow restriction training after achilles tendon rupture. J Foot Ankle Surg 2018;57:635–8.

56. Shimizu R, Hotta K, Yamamoto S, et al. Low-intensity resistance training with blood flow restriction improves vascular endothelial function and peripheral blood circulation in healthy elderly people. Eur J Appl Physiol 2016;116:749–57.

57. Tennent D, Hylden C, Johnson A, et al. Blood flow restriction training after knee arthroscopy: a randomized controlled pilot study. Clin J Sport Med 2017;27(3): 245–52.

58. Greve K, Domeij-Arverud E, Labruto F, et al. Metabolic activity in early tendon repair can be enhanced by intermittent pneumatic compression. Scand J Med Sci Sports 2012;22:e55–63.

59. Valerio DF, Berton R, Conceicao MS, et al. Early metabolic response after resistance exercise with blood flow restriction in well-trained men: a metabolomics approach. Appl Physiol Nutr Metabol 2018;43:240–6.

60. Tsukamoto S, Shibasaki A, Naka A, et al. Lactate promotes myoblast differentiation and myotube hypertrophy via a pathway involving myoD in vitro and enhances muscle regeneration in vivo. Int J Mol Sciences 2018;19:3649.

61. Yuan Y, Xu Y, Xu J, et al. Succinate promotes skeletal muscle protein synthesis via Erk1/2 signaling pathway. Mol Med Rep 2017;16:7361–6.

62. Kawada S. What phenomena do occur in blood flow-restricted muscle? Int. J. KAATSU Training Res 2005;1:37–44.

63. Johnson SA, Sikes KJ, Johnson JW, et al. Blood flow restriction training does not negatively alter the mechanical strength or histomorphology of uninjured equine superficial digital flexor tendons. Equine Vet J 2025;57(2):480–91.

64. Johnson SA, Frisbie DD, Griffenhagen GM, et al. Equine blood flow restriction training: safety validation 2023;55(5):872–83.

65. Tabor G, Williams J. Equine rehabilitation: a review of trunk and hind limb muscle activity and exercise selection. J Equine Vet Sci 2018;60:97–103.e3.

66. King MR. Rehabilitation. Vet Clin N Am Equine Pract 2022;38(3):557–68.

67. Lucas RG, Rodríguez-Hurtado I, Álvarez CT, et al. Effectiveness of neuromuscular electrical stimulation and dynamic mobilization exercises on equine multifidus muscle cross-sectional area. J Equine Vet Sci 2022;113:103934.

68. Stubbs NC, Kaiser LJ, Hauptman J, et al. Dynamic mobilisation exercises increase cross sectional area of musculus multifidus. Equine Vet J 2011;43(5): 522–9.

69. Pfau T, Simons V, Rombach N, et al. Effect of a 4-week elastic resistance band training regimen on back kinematics in horses trotting in-hand and on the lunge. Equive Vet J 2017;49:829–35.

70. Ursini T, Shaw K, Levine D, et al. Electromyography of the multifidus muscle in horses trotting during therapeutic exercises. Front Vet Sci 2022;9:844776.

71. Walker VA, Dyson SJ, Murray RC. Effect of a Pessoa training aid on temporal, linear and angular variables of the working trot. Vet J 2013;198:404–11.

72. Isbell DA, Schils SJ, Oakley SC, et al. Functional Electrical Stimulation (FES) and the effect on equine multifidi asymmetry. J Equine Vet Sci 2020;95:103255.

73. Carraro U, Kern H, Gava P, et al. Biology of muscle atrophy and of its recovery by FES in aging and mobility impairments: roots and by-products. Eur J Transl Myol 2015;25(4):221.
74. Ravara B, Gobbo V, Carraro U, et al. Functional electrical stimulation as a safe and effective treatment for equine epaxial muscle spasms: clinical evaluations and histochemical morphometry of mitochondria in muscle biopsies. Eur J Trans Myol 2015;25(2):4910.
75. Schils S, Carraro U, Turner T, et al. Functional electrical stimulation for equine muscle hypertonicity: histological changes in mitochondrial density and distribution. J Equine Vet Sci 2015;35(11–12):907–16.
76. Riemann B, Lephart S. The sensorimotor system, part 1: the physiologic basis of functional joint stability. J Athl Train 2002;37:71–9.
77. Lyytinen T, Liikavainio T, Bragge T, et al. Postural control and thigh muscle activity in men with knee osteoarthritis. J Electromyogr Kinesiol 2010;20(6):1066–74.
78. Sayenko DG, Masani K, Vette AH, et al. Effects of balance training with visual feedback during mechanically unperturbed standing on postural corrective responses. Gait Posture 2012;35(2):339–44.
79. Xie L, Wang J. Anticipatory and compensatory postural adjustments in response to loading perturbation of unknown magnitude. Exp Brain Res 2019;237(1): 173–80.
80. Rogind H, Lykkegaard JJ, Bliddal H, et al. Postural sway in normal subjects aged 20-70 years. Clin Physiol Funct Imag 2003;23:171–6.
81. Fisher AR, Bacon CJ, Mannion JV. The effect of cervical spine manipulation on postural sway in patients with nonspecific neck pain. J Manip Physiol Ther 2015;38(1):65–73.
82. Holme E, Magnusson SP, Becher K, et al. The effect of supervised rehabilitation on strength, postural sway, position sense and re-injury risk after acute ankle sprain. Scand J Med Sci Sports 1999;9:104–9.
83. Ellis KL, King MR. Relationship between postural stability and paraspinal muscle adaptation in lame horses undergoing rehabilitation. J Equine Vet Sci 2020;91: 103108.

Therapeutic Exercises for Rehabilitation of Muscle Injury

Melissa R. King, DVM, PhD*, Sandro Colla, DVM, MSc

KEYWORDS

- Muscle • Horse • Therapeutic • Exercises

KEY POINTS

- Muscle recovery is divided into 3 phases: inflammatory, regenerative, and remodeling.
- Early mobilization through controlled walking and isometric exercises supports healing by improving muscle strength and fiber alignment.
- Dynamic mobilization and core strengthening exercises stabilize postural muscles and improve neuromotor control.
- Proprioceptive balance exercises improve postural stability and proprioception, enhancing neuromotor control.
- Aquatic exercises are usually incorporated in the late regenerative to the remodeling phase.

INTRODUCTION

Muscle injuries are frequent and can affect all horses regardless of age or physical activity. A detailed understanding of the mechanisms and phases of muscle injury, including physical modalities and therapeutic exercises utilized during the rehabilitation process, is fundamental for a successful functional muscle recovery. The previous article covered the mechanisms of muscle injury, physical modalities, and injury prevention. This article will focus on therapeutic exercises to rehabilitate muscle injuries. The therapeutic exercises are divided into the 3 phases of muscle recovery: inflammatory, regenerative, and remodeling, but it is important to note that the exercises frequently overlap among the phases.

Department of Clinical Sciences, College of Veterinary Medicine and Biomedical Sciences, Colorado State University, Colorado State University Veterinary Teaching Hospital, Equine Orthopaedic Research Center, 2250 Gillette Drive, Fort Collins, CO 80523, USA
* Corresponding author.
E-mail address: Melissa.king@colostate.edu

Vet Clin Equine 41 (2025) 213–225
https://doi.org/10.1016/j.cveq.2024.11.011
0749-0739/25/Published by Elsevier Inc.

INFLAMMATORY PHASE THERAPEUTIC EXERCISES
Immobilization

Following injury, a short period of immobilization should be considered to avoid repetitive muscle contractions. The duration of relative immobility should be limited to a period of less than 5 days. This allows the newly formed granulation tissue connecting the traumatized myofibril ends to gain the required tensile strength to withstand the forces created by muscle contraction. For equine patients, minimizing activation or, more importantly, avoiding stretching of the injured muscle immediately after injury reduces the likelihood of excessive scar tissue formation and the risk for re-rupture at the injury site.[1] It is paramount that the period of immobility be limited to avoid the adverse effects of atrophy of healthy muscle fibers, excessive deposition of fibrotic tissue, and delayed strength gains associated with prolonged periods of immobilization.[2]

Isometric Exercises

Early mobilization of the injured muscle is strongly recommended and should be tailored to the horse's comfort level and the severity and extent of injury. Various rodent models of experimentally induced muscle injuries demonstrate that beginning active mobilization exercises after the short period of immobilization enhances the ingrowth of muscle fibers through the granulation tissue bed, decreases the amount of persistent fibrotic tissue, orchestrates alignment of the regenerating muscles fibers along the physiologic planes of loading, and assists in regaining the tensile strength of the injured muscle.[2] Early mobilization within 3 to 5 days should begin with controlled walking exercise and gradual increases in isometric training. Isometric exercises involve initiating a muscle contraction in which the length of muscle does not change, but the tension within the muscle increases. Isometric contractions in the early phases of rehabilitation are critical to regaining muscle strength and neuromotor control. Isometric exercises for the horse include wither pulls, lateral tail pulls, and caudal tail pulls.

- *Wither pulls:* With the horse standing square, stand on the left side and place both hands over the withers. Gently pull the withers toward yourself until the right fetlock extends slightly. Hold for 10 seconds, then gently release. Perform 5 times on the left and 5 times on the right. You should appreciate isometric contractions occurring within the forelimb stabilizing muscles and the thoracic sling muscles (**Fig. 1**).
- *Lateral tail pulls:* Have the horse standing square. Stand to the side of the horse at 90°, grasp the top of the tail with both hands and gently pull to encourage the horse to shift its weight onto that hindlimb and hold for 10 seconds. Note the contraction of the pelvic and stifle musculature. Perform 5 repetitions on each side (**Fig. 2**).
- *Caudal tail pulls*: Stand behind the hindquarters, ensuring you stay close to the horse to be in a safer position. Grab hold of the horse's tail, ensuring that you are holding the top of the tail (grasp bone, not just the hair). Gently apply traction on the tail at an angle along the line of the pelvis (approximately a 45° downward angle) by pulling backward, you should see the horse's weight shift back slightly. Hold for 10 seconds and then relax. Perform 5 repetitions. You should appreciate isometric contractions within the gluteal, bicep femoris, thoracolumbar epaxial, and pectoral muscles (**Fig. 3**).

Dynamic Mobilization Exercises

Rehabilitation programs should also incorporate core stability and trunk stabilization exercises beginning in the early phases of rehabilitation and progressing through

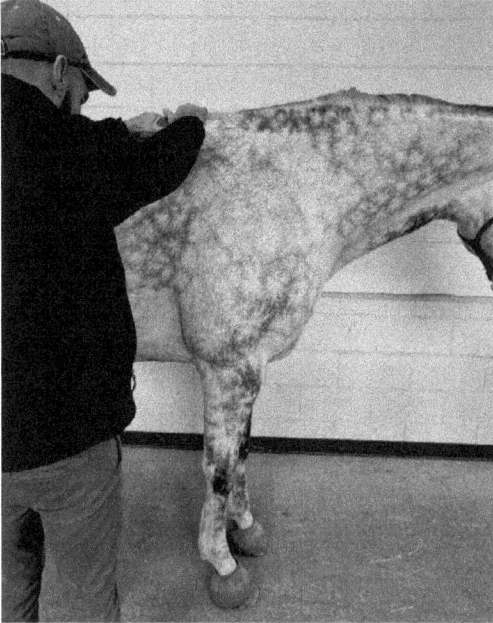

Fig. 1. Wither pull to the right.

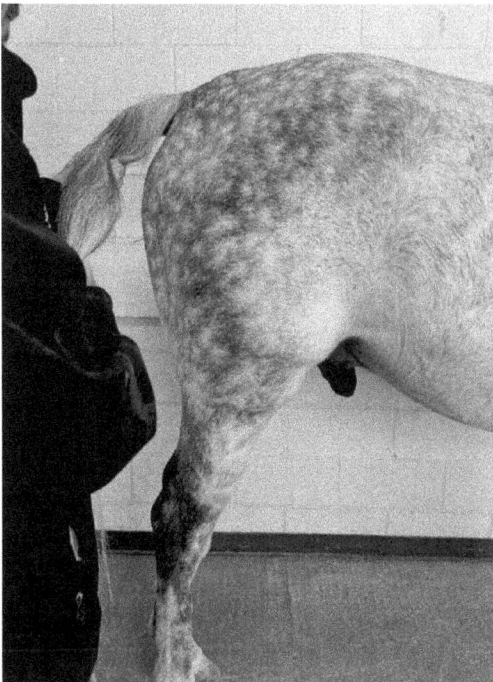

Fig. 2. Lateral tail pull to the right.

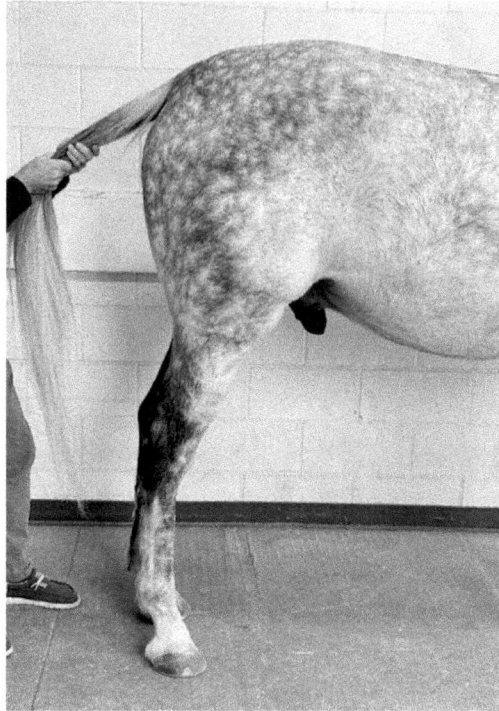

Fig. 3. Caudal tail pull.

the entire program. In a randomized prospective study on human athletes with hamstring muscle strains, those individuals that participated in protocols involving trunk stabilization exercises reduced their reinjury rate and had a quicker return-to-sport activity compared to protocols focusing only on stretching and strengthening of the injured hamstring muscle.[3] This demonstrates the need to develop a global whole body rehabilitation protocol and avoid placing all the emphasis on the injured muscle. In horses, core training exercises are intended to activate and strengthen not only the epaxial muscles but also the abdominal and sublumbar muscles that are critical for static and dynamic balance control. The primary focus in the early phases of any rehabilitation program is to restore motor control, improve stability, and regain muscle strength before targeting flexibility. Pursuant to the equine patient, several core strengthening exercises and their role in activating deep epaxial musculature to subsequently improve postural motor control and alter thoracolumbar kinematics have been investigated.[4,5] Institution of dynamic mobilization exercises over a 3 month time period has been shown to increase both size and symmetry of the multifidus muscle as assessed through longitudinal ultrasonographic evaluation. Dynamic spinal mobilization involves having the horse move in a controlled manner that involves rounding and/or bending the neck and back in a manner that recruits both the long mobilizing musculature and the deep stabilizing musculature to round or bend the neck and back. Performing a series of dynamic mobilization exercises with 5 repetitions of each exercise 3 times weekly for 6 weeks is sufficient to stimulate significant hypertrophy of the multifidus muscles. Performing more repetitions or with a higher frequency does not appear to provide greater hypertrophy.[5,6] Each target position (chin to chest, chin to carpi, chin to forelimb fetlocks, chin to girth, chin to hip, chin to tarsus, and neck extension; **Figs. 4** and **5**) should be conducted in a set of 5 holding for 10 seconds at each position, 3 times a week. The optimal time to perform dynamic mobilization exercises is immediately before exercise to preactivate the postural control muscles.

Core Strengthening Exercises

Core strengthening exercises are designed so that the axial and appendicular neuromuscular systems can respond appropriately to the numerous destabilizing forces that occur during functional movement, thereby reducing the chances of injury. These exercises are regarded as a progression from the dynamic mobilization exercises. The exercises are based on the horse's response to pressure applied over specific anatomic areas to induce muscular contractions that move the intervertebral joints in a manner that is regarded as being beneficial during locomotion or performance. As with dynamic mobilization exercises, the most effective time to use core strengthening exercises is immediately before exercise to preactivate the muscles that will round and stabilize the spine during athletic activity. Equine electromyographic studies have shown that the longissimus dorsi muscle is activated during stimulated extension or lateral bending of the thoracolumbar spine with activity being greater at T12 than at T16 or L3.[7] Core strengthening exercises combined with dynamic mobilization exercises conducted in horses following colic surgery improves the level of performance and results in an earlier return to training compared to a similar group of horses that had colic surgery but did not have core or dynamic mobilization exercises in the recovery period.[8]

Core strengthening exercises for the horse include

- *Induced thoracic spinal flexion*
  - Upward pressure is applied over the sternum on ventral midline between the pectoral muscles and moving slowly caudally while maintaining steady pressure (**Fig. 6**).
  - Horse responds by contracting the abdominal muscles and lifting through the cranial to midthoracic region.
  - This exercise increases strength in the abdominal musculature and improves thoracolumbar motion.
  - Conduct a set of 5 holding for 10 seconds, 3 to 4 times a week.
- *Lumbosacral-induced flexion*
  - Pressure is applied on dorsal midline above the tail head or bilaterally in the intermuscular groove between the biceps femoris and semitendinosus muscles (**Fig. 7**).
  - The lumbosacral joint and caudal lumbar intervertebral joints are flexed primarily by the sublumbar muscles, iliacus, and psoas minor.

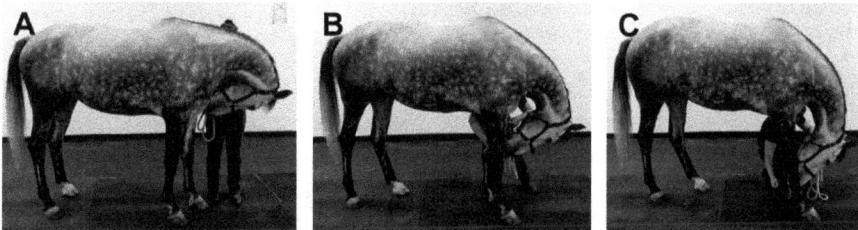

Fig. 4. Dynamic mobilization exercises. (*A*) Demonstrates chin to chest, (*B*) chin to carpi, and (*C*) chin between forelimb fetlocks.

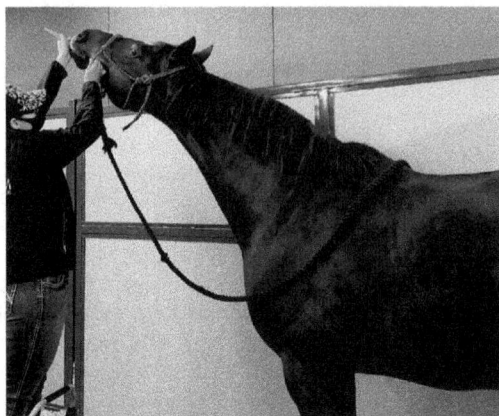

Fig. 5. Neck extension.

- ○ This exercise encourages lumbosacral flexion, and strengthens and activates the abdominal and sublumbar musculature to lift the lumbar region.
- ○ Useful in all horses, particularly those performing high-level dressage, jumping, reining, and cutting.
- ○ Conduct a set of 5 holding for 10 seconds, 3 to 4 times a week.
- • *Axial pelvic rotation*
  - ○ Pressure is applied across midline, 10 to 20 cm lateral from midline, and midway between the tuber coxae and tail head. The therapist applies pressure in a ventromedial direction (**Fig. 8**).
  - ○ For example, the therapist will stand on the left side and reach across the croup placing a hand 10 to 20 cm off midline and midway between the right tuber coxae and right side of the tail head.
  - ○ The horse responds by lifting the lumbar region and flexing the lumbosacral joint while simultaneously laterally bending toward the therapist.
  - ○ Conduct a set of 5 holding for 10 seconds, 3 to 4 times a week, bilaterally.
- • *Advanced thoracic spinal and lumbosacral flexion coupled exercise*
  - ○ This is an advanced coupled exercise that should be conducted once the horse has gained strength conducting the 2 exercises independently.
  - ○ It requires 2 people performing the 2 relevant exercises simultaneously.
  - ○ Conduct a set of 5 holding for 10 seconds, 3 to 4 times a week.

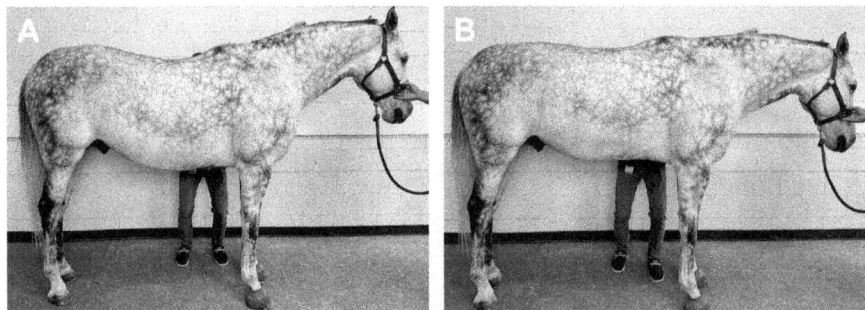

Fig. 6. Induced thoracic spinal flexion. The red line shows the difference before (*A*) and during (*B*) thoracic flexion.

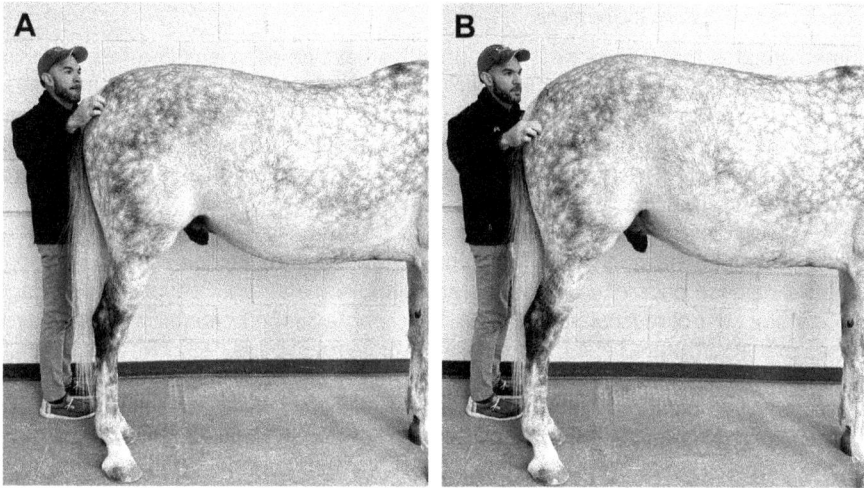

Fig. 7. Lumbosacral-induced flexion. This image demonstrates pressure being applied to the intermuscular groove between the semitendinosus and the biceps femoris muscles to lift the lumbar and lumbosacral regions. The *red line* demonstrates the change in contour of the caudal thoracic and lumbar region as the exercise induces lumbosacral flexion. The movements should occur smoothly and slowly, not in a fast, jerky manner. (*A*) Before and (*B*) during the lumbosacral flexion.

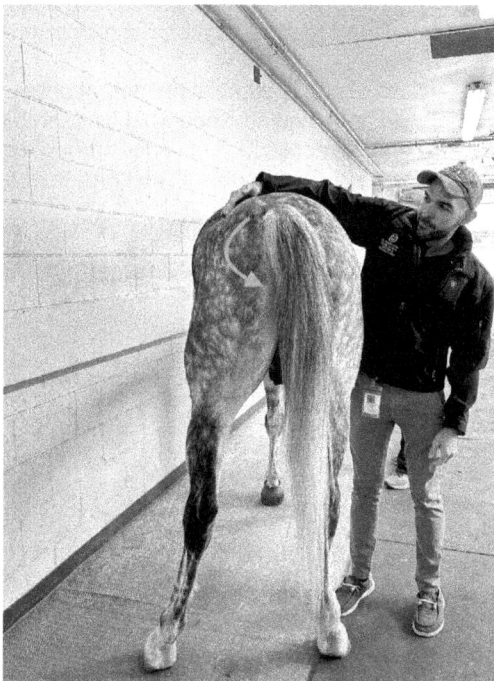

Fig. 8. Axial pelvic rotation to the left. The red line shows the apex of the sacrum deviated to the right and the green arrow shows the direction of the pelvic rotation.

Proprioceptive Balance Exercises

Human athletes that incorporate proprioceptive balance exercises into their rehabilitation programs are significantly less likely to suffer reinjury during a 12 month period following injury, compared to those individuals with similar injuries that did not emphasize core strength (7% reinjury rate in the balance training group vs 29% reinjury rate in the control group).[9] Strengthening and improving proprioception and balance control following injury remains a central focus of human physical therapy programs, and while standardized investigations have yet to focus on equine applications, there are several mechanisms through which neuromotor control can be recruited. Proprioceptive balance pads can be used to stimulate isometric contractions and engage the postural control musculature (**Fig. 9**). Following a 3 month rehabilitation program, horses that incorporated standing daily on balance foam pads demonstrated a significant strong correlation between multifidus muscle hypertrophy and functional improvements in postural stability.[10] This suggests that with improved postural stability, there is enhanced proprioception and neuromotor control critical to protecting the axial and appendicular skeleton. When incorporating proprioceptive balance pads, initially start with 1 to 3 minutes, once to twice daily, progressing to 5 minutes twice daily. Begin with firm pads and progress to less firm material. Initially place the targeted paired limbs on pads and progress to all 4 limbs on pads. Similar to the above modalities and exercises the utilization of proprioceptive balance pads should continue into the regenerative and remodeling phases of muscle injury utilizing a stepwise progressive approach.

REGENERATIVE PHASE THERAPEUTIC EXERCISES

Therapeutic exercises during this phase are designed to progressively improve proprioception, neuromotor control, and to gradually load and strengthen musculoskeletal tissues.

Physiotherapeutic exercises aimed at stimulating motor control, flexibility, and stability can be designed to build upon and advance what was established in the inflammatory phase of rehabilitation. The application of various proprioceptive techniques is frequently utilized to increase joint range of motion, re-establish appropriate

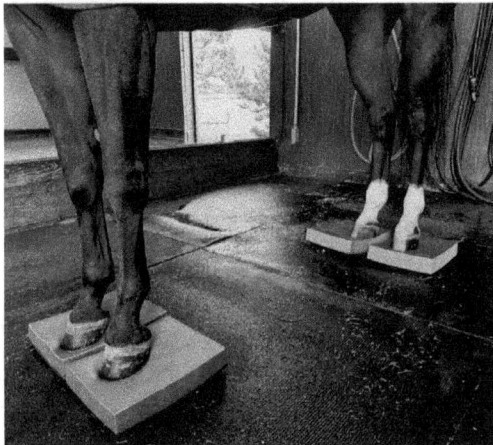

Fig. 9. A horse standing on proprioceptive balance pads in order to increase core stability. In this image, the horse is standing on firm (*green*) pads in front and softer (*purple*) pads behind to increase the level of difficulty of the exercise.

neuromuscular firing patterns, and improve the strength of targeted muscles that function to move and stabilize the joints.

Tactile Stimulators

The use of tactile stimulators applied around the hind limb pastern joints demonstrated a significantly higher hoof flight arc, with increased flexion of the fetlock, hock, and stifle joints.[11] Additional application of ankle weights (700 g) plus hind pastern tactile devices provided added increases in hip flexion and increased positive work performed by the hip, stifle, and tarsal musculature.[11] Long-term application of a hind limb bell boot (82 g) every 3 days for 6 weeks significantly improved superficial gluteal muscle imbalances detected via acoustic myography.[12] There is often habituation to the proprioceptive devices and limb weights, whereby they induce the greatest effects initially, followed by a rapid decrease in altered limb kinematics.[13] The use of these proprioceptive techniques supports the facilitation of enhanced afferent input to indirectly produce and modulate a targeted efferent response for the purpose of re-establishing motor control and improving joint range of motion. While further studies are needed to establish specific recommendations regarding use, initial biomechanic effects for targeted rehabilitation are encouraging.

Resistance Bands and Training Lines

Resistance band training is successfully used in human physical therapy programs to improve core strength and stability.[14,15] The use of resistance bands as a therapeutic technique for equine rehabilitation has been purported to provide a proprioceptive stimuli, whose sensory input drives a targeted motor output. Commonly referred to as a Theraband,[16] the 2 piece equine elastic band system is thought to stimulate core abdominal muscles with the abdominal band and engage hind limb musculature with the hindquarter band. Its use in horses at a trot was recently investigated and found to reduce mediolateral and rotational movement throughout the thoracolumbar region.[16] Optical motion capture analysis at the walk and trot during application of the hindquarter band demonstrates significant stabilization of the lumbar region, improving working posture and core stability.[17] Similarly, surface electromyography studies demonstrate increased rectus abdominus muscle activity at a trot in the presence of both abdominal and hindquarter resistance bands.[18] Further studies investigating long-term use and potential mechanistic pathways will help refine its use in the rehabilitation setting. Also pertinent to rehabilitation is the use of training lines. Pessoa training aids were demonstrated to increase both lumbosacral angles and thoracolumbar dorsoventral excursion when used in horses trotting on a lunge line.[19] While further studies are needed to establish specific recommendations regarding use, initial biomechanic effects for targeted rehabilitation are encouraging.

Ground Poles

Ground poles when arranged at various distances, heights, and configurations can encourage increases in range of motion, spinal flexibility, and core abdominal muscle activation. Walking over ground poles increases the activation of the rectus abdominus and longissimus dorsi muscles, while trotting over ground poles increases the activation of the thoracolumbar multifidi and rectus abdominus muscles.[18,20] The increases in active joint range of motion required for the horse to successfully complete the task subsequently activates and strengthens the corresponding musculature. Unlike the use of tactile devices, the effect of exercising over ground poles does not appear to diminish during an exercise session, as the number of repetitions and height of the poles will determine the intensity.

Dry Treadmills and Inclination Effects

Dry treadmills can be beneficial during this phase of rehabilitation due to the ability to control the speed, surface, direction (working in a straight line) and incorporation of an incline. A number of electromyographic studies have demonstrated that the use of inclines and changes in speed progressively recruit the muscles responsible for hind limb propulsion and back mobility.[21] However, it should also be noted that working on an incline increases the force distribution on the hind limbs and that increases in speed increase the ground reaction forces within each limb.[21] Therefore, careful consideration is important when developing rehabilitation protocols utilizing changes in treadmill speed and incline. Similarly to inclined treadmills, hill work and incorporating backing exercises into hill work can also be used to simultaneously improve muscular strength and challenge proprioceptive acuity.

Aquatic Modalities

Aquatic modalities are often used to optimize the treatment of sensory and motor disturbances associated with muscular injuries. Aquatic therapies, including underwater treadmills and swimming, have been reported in humans to improve muscle strength and timing, increase cardiovascular endurance, decrease limb edema, improve range of motion, decrease pain, and reduce mechanical stresses applied to the limb.[22–26] Humans with lower extremity injuries demonstrated a significant increase in limb-loading parameters, improved joint range of motion and a significant reduction in the severity of balance deficits following aquatic exercise.[22–26] Following a 3 month rehabilitation program, horses that had regimens incorporating underwater treadmill exercises significantly improved muscle strength, joint range of motion, neuromotor control, balance, and proprioception.[10]

Underwater treadmill exercise may provide a mechanism to control mechanical loading by decreasing axial loading on the limb depending on the depth of the water. The attenuation of distal limb forces generated by walking in water at increased depths must be balanced against the resistance of the water at higher water depths. The increase in water depth results in a higher coefficient of drag, which enhances muscle recruitment, activation, and strength. The prescription of underwater treadmill exercise must consider the stage of muscle healing and consider if the healing tissue is strong enough to undergo active contractions against resistance depending on the depth of water. The changes in water depth can produce both kinetic and kinematic effects that are directly applicable to the clinical management of musculoskeletal morbidities in horses.

REMODELING PHASE REHABILITATION

Frequently overlapping the regenerative phase, exercises during the remodeling phase aim to continue improving proprioception, range of motion, muscular strength, and cardiovascular fitness.

The diverse physical characteristics of aquatic exercise discussed earlier provide unique approaches to individualized rehabilitation for musculoskeletal issues in horses. Swim training programs have demonstrated an improvement in cardiovascular function, a reduction in locomotor disease, and an increase in the development of fast-twitch, high-oxidative muscle fibers, reflecting improved aerobic capacity.[27,28] Fine-wire electromyography has also been used to measure increases in muscle activation of the thoracic limb musculature during pool swimming exercise, compared to overground walking.[29]

Kinematic analysis of the pelvic limbs during equine swimming exercise demonstrated that horses spend more time ($\sim$60%) in protraction (limb flexion) compared to retraction (limb extension).[30,31] The horse adopts this difference in phase duration as a mechanism to increase thrust and decrease drag during swimming.[30,31] Consequently, along with the vertical orientation of the limbs the forces required to overcome the drag are primarily generated by the pelvic limbs. The stifle and tarsal joints undergo the greatest angular velocities throughout the swimming cycle with the largest difference appreciated during the retraction phase. Careful consideration should be applied to swimming protocols as exercising in water is profoundly different in terms of physiologic responses and changes in locomotion patterns compared to overground exercise.

CLINICS CARE POINTS

- Limit immobilization to less than 5 days after injury where possible, to prevent muscle atrophy and excessive scar tissue formation.
- Therapeutic exercises and modalities can be utilized in different phases of the rehabilitation program to aid recovery from and prevention of future muscle injuries.
- The progression of the therapeutic exercises should be adjusted based on the horse's functional reassessment.

DISCLOSURE

The authors have nothing to disclose.

REFERENCES

1. Järvinen TAH, Järvinen TLN, Kääriäinen M, et al. Muscle Injuries: optimising recovery. Best Pract Res Clin Rheumatol 2007;21(2):317–31.
2. Järvinen TAH, Järvinen TLN, Kääriäinen M, et al. Biology of muscle trauma. Am J Sports Med 2005;33:745–66.
3. Sherry MA, Best TM. A comparison of 2 rehabilitation programs in the treatment of acute hamstring strains. J Orthop Sports Phys Ther 2004;34:116–25.
4. Kavcic N, Grenier S, McGill SM. Determining the stabilizing role of individual torso muscles during rehabilitation exercises. Spine 2004;29(11):1254–65.
5. Clayton HM, Clayton HM, Lavagnino M, et al. Dynamic mobilisations in cervical flexion: effects on intervertebral angulations. Equine Vet J 2010;42:688–94.
6. Stubbs NC, Kaiser LJ, Hauptman J, et al. Dynamic mobilisation exercises increase cross sectional area of *musculus multifidus*. Equine Vet J 2011;43(5): 522–9.
7. Peham C, Frey A, Licka T, et al. Evaluation of the EMG activity of the long back muscle during induced back movements in stance. Equine Vet 2001;33:165–8.
8. Holcombe SJ, Shearer TR, Valberg SJ. The effect of core abdominal muscle rehabilitation exercises on return to training and performance in horses after colic surgery. J Equine Vet Sci 2019;75:14–8. ISSN 0737-0806.
9. Holme E, Magnusson SP, Becher K, et al. The effect of supervised rehabilitation on strength, postural sway, position sense and re-injury risk after acute ankle sprain. Scan J Med Sci Sports 1999;9:104–9.
10. Ellis KL, King MR. Relationship between postural stability and paraspinal muscle adaptation in lame horses undergoing rehabilitation. J Equine Vet Sci 2020;91: 103108.

11. Clayton HM, White AD, Kaiser LJ, et al. Hindlimb response to tactile stimulation of the pastern and coronet. Equine Vet J 2010;42:227–33.

12. Jensen AM, Ahmed W, Elbrond VS, et al. The efficacy of intermittent long-term bell boot application for the correction of muscle asymmetry in equine subjects. J Equine Vet Sci 2018;68:73–80.

13. Clayton HM, White AD, Kaiser LJ, et al. Short-term habituation of equine limb kinematics to tactile stimulation of the coronet. Vet Comp Orthop Traumatol 2008; 21:211–4.

14. Kell RT, Asmundson GJG. A comparison of two forms of periodized exercise rehabilitation programs in the management of chronic nonspecific low-back pain. J Strength Cond Res 2009;23:513–23.

15. Macedo LG, Maher CG, Latimer J, et al. Motor control exercise for persistent, nonspecific low back pain: a systematic review. Phys Ther 2009;89:9–25.

16. Pfau T, Simons V, Rombach N, et al. Effect of a 4-week elastic resistance band training regimen on back kinematics in horses trotting in-hand and on the lunge. Equine Vet J 2017;49:829–35.

17. Stenfeldt P, Ericson C, Jacobson I. The effect of an elastic resistance band around the hindquarters on equine dorsoventral back kinematics. Acta Vet Scand 2016;58(Suppl 2):A38.

18. Shaw K, Ursini T, Levine D, et al. The effect of ground poles and elastic resistance bands on longissimus dorsi and rectus abdominus muscle activity during equine walk and trot. J Equine Vet Sci 2021;107. https://doi.org/10.1016/j.jevs.2021. 103772.

19. Walker VA, Dyson SJ, Murray RC. Effect of a Pessoa training aid on temporal, linear and angular variables of the working trot. Vet J 2013;198:404–11.

20. Ursini T, Shaw K, Levine D, et al. Electromyography of the multifidus muscle in horses trotting during therapeutic exercises. Front Vet Sci 2022; 9:844776.

21. Tabor G, Williams J. Equine rehabilitation: a review of trunk and hind limb muscle activity and exercise selection. J Equine Vet Sci 2018;60:97–103.e3.

22. Prins J, Cutner D. Aquatic therapy in the rehabilitation of athletic injuries. Clin Sports Med 1999;18:447–61.

23. Miyoshi T, Shirota T, Yamamoto S-I, et al. Effect of the walking speed to the lower limb joint angular displacements, joint moments and ground reaction forces during walking in water. Disabil Rehabil 2004;26(12):724–32.

24. Messier S, Royer T, Craven T, et al. Long-term exercise and its effect on balance in older, osteoarthritic adults: results from the Fitness, Arthritis, and Seniors Trial (FAST). J Am Geriatr Soc 2000;48:131–8.

25. Kamioka H, Tsutanji K, Okuizumi H, et al. Effectiveness of aquatic exercise and balneotherapy: a summary of systematic reviews based on randomized controlled trials of water immersion therapies. J Epidemiol 2010; 20:2–12.

26. Moreira LD, Oliveira ML, Lirani-Galvão AP, et al. Physical exercise and osteoporosis: effects of different types of exercises on bone and physical function of postmenopausal women. Arquivos Brasileiros Endocrinol Metabol 2014;58(5): 514–22.

27. Misumi K, Sakamoto H, Shimizu R. Changes in skeletal muscle composition in response to swimming training in young horses. J Vet Med Sci 1995;57:959–61.

28. Misumi K, Sakamoto H, Shimizu R. The validity of swimming training for two-year-old Thoroughbreds. J Vet Med Sci 1994;56:217–22.

29. Tokuriki M, Ohtsuki R, Kai M, et al. EMG activity of the muscles of the neck and forelimbs during different forms of locomotion. Equine Vet J 1999;30:231–4.
30. Santosuosso E, Leguillette R, Vinardell T, et al. Kinematic analysis during straight line free swimming in horses: Part 2 - hindlimbs. Front Vet Sci 2022;8:761500.
31. Santosuosso E, Leguillette R, Vinardell T, et al. Kinematic analysis during straight line free swimming in horses: Part 1 - forelimbs. Front Vet Sci 2021;8:752375.

Moving?

Make sure your subscription moves with you!

To notify us of your new address, find your **Clinics Account Number** (located on your mailing label above your name), and contact customer service at:

Email: journalscustomerservice-usa@elsevier.com

800-654-2452 (subscribers in the U.S. & Canada)
314-447-8871 (subscribers outside of the U.S. & Canada)

Fax number: 314-447-8029

Elsevier Health Sciences Division
Subscription Customer Service
3251 Riverport Lane
Maryland Heights, MO 63043

*To ensure uninterrupted delivery of your subscription, please notify us at least 4 weeks in advance of move.

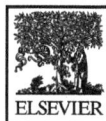

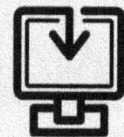

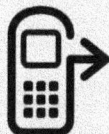

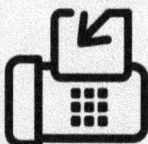

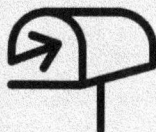

ELSEVIER

www.ingramcontent.com/pod-product-compliance
Lightning Source LLC
Chambersburg PA
CBHW050457190326
41458CB00005B/1322